MARKETING
FOR THE
DENTAL PRACTICE

CHARLES L. MILONE, D.D.S.
Associate Professor of Dental Ecology
School of Dentistry
University of North Carolina
Chapel Hill, North Carolina

W. CHARLES BLAIR, D.D.S.
Private Practice
Kings Mountain, North Carolina

JAMES E. LITTLEFIELD, PH.D.
Professor, School of Business Administration
University of North Carolina
Chapel Hill, North Carolina

1982
W. B. SAUNDERS COMPANY
Philadelphia   London   Toronto   Mexico City   Rio de Janeiro   Sydney   Tokyo

W. B. Saunders Company: West Washington Square
Philadelphia, PA   19105

1 St. Anne's Road
Eastbourne, East Sussex BN21 3UN, England

1 Goldthorne Avenue
Toronto, Ontario M8Z 5T9, Canada

Apartado 26370 — Cedro 512
Mexico 4, D.F., Mexico

Rua Coronel Cabrita, 8
Sao Cristovao Caixa Postal 21176
Rio de Janeiro, Brazil

9 Waltham Street
Artarmon, N.S.W. 2064, Australia

Ichibancho, Central Bldg., 22-1 Ichibancho
Chiyoda-ku, Tokyo 102, Japan

Library of Congress Cataloging in Publication Data

Milone, Charles L.

Marketing for the dental practice.

Includes index.

1. Dentistry — Practice.   2. Dental care — Marketing.
   I. Blair, W. Charles.   II. Littlefield, James E.
   III. Title.

RK58.M525   617.6′0068′8   81–40800

ISBN 0-7216-6391-5   AACR2

Editorial   J. Patrick Grace
coordination: Grace Associates

Photography: Ramona Hutton-Howe
             UNC School of Dentistry
             Learning Resources Center

Marketing for the Dental Practice   ISBN 0-7216-6391-5

Last digit is the print number: 9   8   7   6   5   4   3   2   1

In Memoriam
EDIE BLAIR
1941–1981

Foreword _____

This book is very timely. Appearing at a time of rapid and profound social and economic change, *Marketing for the Dental Practice* addresses the problems of developing and sustaining a successful dental practice.

The dental profession desperately needs to develop marketing skills based on the behavioral sciences and economics. Drawing on these fields, the authors' primary purpose in this book is to explain the application of marketing principles in the dental practice. The material the authors develop is soundly based in economics and the behavioral sciences, and does provide dentists with a direct, pragmatic approach to developing their practices.

To date, a limited number of dentists have benefited from the work of such organizations as the Pankey Institute, the Group at Cox, the Nexus Group, the Update Foundation, and the Napili Seminars. This book covers much of the basic information provided by such groups. Geniuses such as Dr. Robert Barkley have drawn from the creative developments in other fields and applied them to dental practice. Likewise, the authors draw heavily from other fields to bolster their application of sound theory to the problem of marketing dental services.

Rampant dental disease has stimulated advanced reparative techniques as well as preventive efforts. Advances in preventive dentistry have reduced the incidence of dental disease and will continue to do so. The reduction of dental disease has encouraged dentists to adopt a holistic approach to dental care. The new service perspective requires a new marketing approach. Although the authors make no claim to an ability to foretell the future, they do present principles and techniques that will be relevant to the future dental practice. The dentist who can apply the principles described in this book will surely thrive, not merely survive, in this rapidly changing environment.

As merchandising by such complex organizations as Sears becomes more comprehensive, so dentistry must present more options in dental care delivery. Although the authors do not predict the nature of such developments, they certainly lead one to believe that dentists must be prepared for change. Such preparation is the foundation for successful dental marketing.

I believe that *Marketing for the Dental Practice* is a seminal work and that it provides a basis on which we can all proceed in our marketing efforts. Certainly the authors expect and hope that this book will be helpful to dentistry at a time when lack of busyness is acknowledged as a primary problem. This is surely an exciting, not merely a frustrating, time. Marketing as presented by the authors can increase the excitement and reduce the frustration. I hope that it does that for each of you.

OMER K. REED, D.D.S.

Preface _____

Dentistry is not immune to the rapid changes that buffet American society. Recently, dental consumers have found themselves faced with a greater variety of choices in selecting dental services than ever before, primarily because of a relative increase in dental manpower. Also, inflation has taken more and more out of the typical American family's budget. This has spurred consumers to be even more careful in their choices. And this affects dentists. One key to economic survival for dental practitioners in an era of shortages, inflation, and cautious consumers will be an ability to market their services.

That is precisely what this book is about, and if you are like many dentists today, marketing is a word you have come to accept as a fact of life for the 80s and 90s.

In an era of scarcity, when dentists were few and the demands upon their time and talent were great, dentists easily "sold" all the services they could provide. Less desirable patients were even excluded from practices. The supply of patients was plentiful. Now, in an era of an abundant number of dentists, a marketing approach to attracting and keeping patients is imperative.

Some dentists have been understandably distressed over the growing need for marketing in the profession. Such dentists express concern that this practice will lead to a decline in ethics and in the quality of dental care. These critics, however, have not yet fully understood what marketing is about. They may, for instance, equate marketing with selling; but marketing is much *more* than selling. Properly conceived, marketing is the art of understanding the needs of consumers and satisfying, or meeting, those needs in such a way as to earn a profit.

Marketing is both ethical and profitable. This book will show you why — and how.

Most successful dentists already market their services, even if they don't see what they do as "marketing" per se. And even if they themselves may still be uncomfortable with terms such as "marketing," "promotion," and "advertising," at a minimum every dentist attempts to understand the needs of his patients — or to determine those needs. And every dentist addresses himself to meeting the patient needs he determines. Such an approach is the essence of marketing. Thus, what we are talking about here are ways to improve or refine marketing concepts or approaches that you, the practitioner, already use, and ways to expand upon those techniques.

Each dentist must, naturally, decide upon his own individual level of comfort in the marketing arena. For some, marketing will come more easily than for others; all, however, need to consciously participate in the arena — else they will find themselves with a minimal practice while colleagues thrive.

Today's successful dentist will accomplish the difficult task of blending astute business practices with professional caring. As an astute business person he will learn what people in his community want and need. He will provide considerate and desired care as a professional.

The competent marketer in dentistry will have a keen advantage in an era of an abundant supply of dentists. Especially will this be so because marketing in dentistry is relatively new, and most practitioners are not yet proficient at it. As we shall show, however, the most successful dentists were effective marketers even before marketing became so crucial.

This book will show you how principles of marketing, widely and successfully used for many years in business, can help the modern dentist gain and retain patients and boost his earnings—and also feel good about the new marketing techniques that he may employ. The dentist who is able to develop an effective marketing approach to his practice will not merely survive but will thrive in the evolving era of dental marketing. Why not be one of them?

Life is a marketplace in which we all attempt to identify and satisfy our needs. We hope this book satisfies a need or yours.

CLM
WCB
JEL

Acknowledgments _____

The authors are indebted to many friends and associates in dentistry and in marketing for their creative ideas, freely offered.

For the arduous task of typing countless drafts of the manuscript we are deeply grateful to Edie Blair, Lucille Brooks, Sharon Byrd, Thomas McIntyre, and Betty Pearson.

Finally, our families deserve great thanks for their support and understanding over the year or so that we were immersed in producing this book.

Contents _____

1

Why Marketing?

We are in a new era of dental practice. Gone is the old era of scarcity, of overburdened practices, of overwork, of turning away patients. Here is a time of challenge, when each dentist must stake out his practice with the sense and vision of a businessman starting a new enterprise. Dentists no longer have only the problem of producing all the services that consumers require. They now have the problem of finding the consumers to serve, and of keeping them satisfied and happy amid a plethora of burgeoning alternatives to traditional dentistry, such as cut-rate, no-frills dental clinics with aggressive advertising campaigns.

Over the last few years, for the first time in American dental history, many dentists have been caring for fewer patients than they would optimally like to treat. How has this come about? There are many reasons, and here are some (but probably not all) of them:

— relatively diminished demand for dental services (attributable, in part, to better preventive care and longer-lasting dental restorations)

— an increased number of young dentists being turned out by the schools

— leveling off of the U.S. population

— inflation and other economic factors pinching the family pocketbook

— government red tape

— the growing threat of malpractice suits and other legal problems, and the attendant rising cost of malpractice insurance

— increase of nondentist providers

— increase of dental practice operating costs

— inefficiency of the traditional solo dental practice

— increased risks in entrepreneurship (in general, but also as applied specifically to dentistry)

— an increase in the number of female and minority dentists

— political weakness of the dental profession

— changing demographics (e.g., the move to the sunbelt states, depleting some northern urban areas)

— changes in the way people perceive the need for dental services and changes in people's attitudes toward dentists

> . . . for the first time in American dental history, many dentists have been caring for fewer patients than they would optimally like to treat.

Economic Changes

Inflation has hurt all Americans. We can really wince over the inflation rate when we notice that a ten-year-old can recall when a thirty-five-cent candy bar cost only ten cents. Everywhere we look, we see that products and services are costing more. It has become apparent in recent years that we Americans have overindulged ourselves in material acquisition, driving cars that were gas guzzlers and building houses that now cost too much to heat. We have all been urged to get back to the essentials, trim the fat from our lifestyles, and become more efficient. This bitter medicine might be more acceptable if we could be sure it would be effective. Many economists agree that our economy has a rather high rate of inflation built into it, which will require changes in lifestyle and changes in government policy to bring under control.

It should be no surprise, then, to find those of us in the dental profession caught in the economic vise of the times. Inflation and graduated income tax schedules have cut into the purchasing power of most upper-middle-income earners, including dentists. This unpleasant fact of life has driven many dentists to consider marketing their services in order to achieve something more than a minimal degree of financial success. Unless dentists manage to obtain a larger share of the consumer dollar, they will not be able to enhance, or perhaps even maintain, their own standards of living.

One of the most salient constraints upon the dental practitioner has been the decreasing ratio of general population to dentists. Although the U.S. population *is* increasing, the rate of growth is less than had been projected when health planners were assessing the needs for increased manpower in the profession. Because of these projections, new dental schools were created. Government capitation programs encouraged larger and larger class sizes. Result: a marked increase in the number of dentists (and physicians as well) over and above the number that would have been correct had the projections been on target. To complicate matters further, many recent dental graduates have chosen to establish themselves in the more densely populated areas, avoiding the needier rural areas, and thus contributing to the maldistribution of dentists to patients.

Whether or not we are on the verge of an oversupply of dentists in our country is a point of debate. Clearly, though, we have engendered a higher ratio of dentists to population than anybody ever planned.

So long as dentists were in short supply relative to the expressed consumer demand, they could be readily absorbed into the U.S. economic system, regardless of where they settled and regardless of whether or not they consciously marketed their services. This kind of absorption into the system can no longer be taken for granted. The current oversupply of dentists, relative to consumer demand, mandates that individual dentists — at least those just getting their practices started — market their skills if they are to assure themselves of a viable economic situation. And with a decreased number of patients available to them, even older, established dentists are finding that they need to cultivate the consumer, increase the quality and variety of their services — and market their practices.

It should be no surprise . . . to find those of us in the dental profession caught in the economic vise of the times.

Clearly . . . we have engendered a higher ratio of dentists to population than anybody ever planned.

Government Regulations

Is our "free enterprise system" truly free? We all know that it is not. Rather it is tightly hedged in by government controls. In attempting to safeguard the rights of workers and of consumers, government has swamped businesses with laws, codes, standards, and forms in triplicate. Dentistry has not escaped this barrage. Employees must not be exposed to harmful radiation or other emitted substances. Overtime hours must be limited or compensated at time and a half. Employees may work only with approved, up-to-date equipment. Reports regarding radiation and analgesic safety must be forwarded to state and local agencies. Granted, these regulations are designed to ensure safe work places and even though they are acceptably effective, they nevertheless increase the cost of doing business. Then there are seemingly never ending taxes, retirement plans, and Social Security regulations. All these add to the cost in materials and personnel time for already overburdened small businesses, such as dental practices.

Besides these considerations, public disenchantment with the total health-care establishment has been growing. The escalation of costs in this sector has prompted consumers to think twice about how much they are really willing to pay for various levels of care. Within recent years there has been a mood for adopting legislation to put dentistry, as well as medicine, within a totally regulated framework. Costs for dental services have been subject to a lower rate of inflation than have costs for hospital services. However, the public frustration over escalating hospital costs may sweep dentistry into the net, too. Meanwhile, other major Western countries have been spending less for health care, proportionately, than has the United States. This fact boosts the stock of those pushing for total control. And what is the effect of controls on income? Controls will tend to mandate the continuance of a high level of dental service while placing a ceiling on fees; unfortunately, supplies and other costs, such as rent, utilities, salaries, and so on, may keep on rising. It is the dentist who will be caught in the squeeze.

Although dentistry may be tarred with the same brush used for hospitals, dentists ought to continue to control their costs and give their patients a good buy in health care. By doing this dentists will uphold the positive image the polls have shown that they enjoy. What's more, we may be able to convince the government that more controls or regulations for dentistry are excessive — even if other segments of the health-care establishment are being more tightly regulated. Such an accomplishment by dentists would indeed create a favorable marketing climate.

Public disenchantment with the total health-care establishment has been growing.

Legal Risk

During the late 1960s and throughout the 1970s and into the 1980s the esteem that professionals such as physicians, lawyers, and dentists once enjoyed has suffered erosion. One consequence of this has been that patients have become much more prone to sue for

malpractice than in the past. This unpleasant reality makes it mandatory for dentists to carry liability insurance with higher limits. More
and more lawsuits are being filed, and greater and greater judgments
are being awarded. Malpractice liability rates, then, are rising. Besides
paying more for his insurance, today's dentist also has been forced to
keep more complex records. He* spends more time on diagnostic
workups to cover himself in the event of a lawsuit. Again, these trends
make for a higher quality of care, but may be taken to the point of
excessive care, which is more costly.

Increase of Non-Dentist Providers

We are in the midst of an outgrowth of non-dentist providers of
dental services, including denturists and dental hygienists. Some of
the denturist market is new, but a significant portion has come from
established or growing dental practices. Compared to the independent denturist, the denture auxiliary who is under the supervision of
a dentist, as provided for in some states, is a favorable development.
This arrangement, if well managed, lends itself to increasing a
dentist's market. The bad news, though, is that developing a pool of
consumers sufficient to justify such an auxiliary is difficult for most
practitioners. Underutilization or poor management of this type of
auxiliary usually creates more economic problems for dentists than it
solves.

We are in the midst of an outgrowth of non-dentist providers of dental services.

Recent trends are for the development of independent practice
for dental hygienists. Independent hygienists with effective marketing techniques must definitely be counted as a threat to dentists'
traditional practices. A referral relationship between hygienists and
dentists, however, must be seen as a plus. Therefore, the independent
hygiene practice presents interesting opportunities for the dentist
who is competent in marketing.

Increase of Operating Costs

It costs more every day to run a dental practice. And the rate of
increase of operating costs continues to outpace the rate by which
dentists have been able to raise their fees. Inflation as measured by
the Consumer Price Index has risen more rapidly than have dental
fees. Overhead costs, thus, have kept going up faster than fee
increases have offset them. Supply costs and laboratory costs especially have increased faster than fees. Finally, almost needless to add,
fluctuating prices for precious metals have been a source of frustration for dentists.

Although personnel costs have hardly kept pace with the cost of
living, they have risen significantly. It's nice to know that, according to

---

*We realize that many dentists are female, and some auxiliaries are male. In this
book we strive to use language that recognizes these facts, but if the language becomes
awkward, we will refer to the dentist by the masculine pronoun "he" and to the
auxiliary by the feminine pronoun "she."

a recent ADA Survey of Dental Practice, dentists with the highest personnel costs enjoy the highest net incomes. Still, personnel costs present a problem. One aspect of the problem is the high turnover rate of dental assistants. This has been attributed, in part, to low salaries. A low salary schedule may create more hidden costs in lost production and training than a high salary schedule would. All extra personnel costs, whether out front or hidden, must be made up by additional receipts. Otherwise the dentist suffers a loss in his real income.

... depending upon the age of a practitioner, or even his geography or what dental school he attended, the resistance to marketing of a given dentist may still be high.

Other alternatives, however, in dentists' quest for economic security can, and should be, explored. These include working longer hours, delegating more duties to employees, and becoming effective marketers of dentistry. Without going into the first two options in an exhaustive fashion, let it be said that many dentists find the prospect of longer working hours unattractive. Such an increase in workload often is undertaken at a detriment to one's personal health and to a happy and stable family life. As for the second option, depending upon the state in which a dentist practices, he may find himself sharply restricted regarding the delegation of technical responsibilities to auxiliary personnel.

Lately within the dental profession, resistance to option three, marketing, has been abating, as it has within several other health-care professions. However, depending upon the age of a practitioner, or even his geography or what dental school he attended, the resistance to marketing of a given dentist may still be high. Nonetheless, it is in the area of marketing that the dental practitioner will find the widest possibilities for combating the economic pressures he has lately been under. The pressures have surely been exasperating and the idea of relieving them ought to increase a dentist's interest in the marketing alternative.

Increased Demand for Goods and Services

Since the close of World War II, American society has gone through a series of evolutions in taste and sophistication in its demands for goods and services. Each succeeding generation came to expect a higher "quality of life" than the previous generation had enjoyed. As marketers became more perceptive and creative, demands increased. Goods such as designer clothing and recreational equipment appealed to higher-level ego needs. Marketers of travel, vacation, and other recreational services grew to understand people's total needs and became adept at targeting their marketing approach to meet those needs. As a result, a significant share of the consumer dollar went to such "higher-level ego" services.

If dentists are to obtain a larger share of the market, they need first of all to understand the nature of their competition. That competition includes other goods and services for which marketers have fostered needs. An understanding of the full range of consumer needs and desires would help dentists to design their services to fit into that total range, not merely with dental requirements in mind. Service in accord with total needs is much more acceptable to consumers than a service that is presented as isolated from, or without regard to, the full spectrum of human needs. Fitting into the spectrum of needs in a conscious way should enable dentists to gain a larger share of the consumer dollar.

Leveling of Dental Insurance

Dental insurance has increased dramatically during the last decade. As of 1980, 70 million Americans were under dental insurance coverage (see Table 1–1).

The rate of increase of those buying coverage certainly will diminish, but the increase, in absolute numbers, will continue to be compelling. Dental insurance coverage is expected to stabilize at about 45 per cent of the population around 1990. Some highly industrialized areas (which are also unionized) may now be approaching saturation. Less unionized areas, such as the South, will likely experience significant growth in numbers insured. With the increase in dental insurance come measures, on the part of the carriers, to hold down claim outlays. Major plans that pay by a schedule rather than on a usual, customary, and routine basis are increasing. These trends in dental insurance call for greater attentiveness on the part of practitioners — and for a comprehensive marketing approach that takes dental insurance plans fully into account.

Sophisticated Marketing

. . . we in the dental profession need to realize that these other marketers are competing against us for consumer dollars.

Let us look, briefly, at concepts of marketing as applied to other products and services in American society. Despite some spottiness — an erratic rate of success or failure — the pattern in American marketing history has been one of increasing sophistication. This is to say, as marketers have become more and more proficient at their work, their chances of suffering failure have decreased markedly. Before introducing a new product, most U.S. companies conduct market research studies. With these studies they try to discover consumer needs and then develop products that meet those needs. The sales volume of any given product is likely to reflect the degree to which the product satisfies needs perceived by the marketing surveys. Whether advertising can actually create needs in the minds of consumers is still a subject of controversy. No one argues, however, that advertising is not an essential step in the calling of the consumers' attention to a new product in the mass marketplace.

TABLE 1–1. DENTAL INSURANCE COVERAGE*

Year	Number Covered
1970	4,000,000
1975	42,000,000
1980	70,000,000
1985	99,000,000 (projected)

*Source: Delta Dental Update, Summer-Fall, 1979.

The sheer abundance of goods and services in the American economy has made it incumbent upon producers to develop increasingly sophisticated marketing techniques. And, once again, we in the dental profession need to realize that these other marketers are competing against *us* for consumer dollars.

There's no denying, of course, that most dentists are in a competitive environment. Even in most small towns now, the average person has a choice of dentists. Such a choice, for small-town dwellers, once would have been a rarity. Although most people are more concerned about the dentist's competence than they are about his fees, they must consider fees. The high-fee dentist is likely to eliminate himself from consideration for many people. Consumerism has heightened interest in fees to the point where fees are a major element for more and more people in their selection of a dentist. The dentist whose fees are modest has a marketing advantage. If a particular dentist's treatment is substandard or if his fees are unreasonable, he can now expect little improvement in his income.

In the marketing of the general range of consumer goods and services, warranties (which guarantee replacement of work or redoing of service within a certain time frame if the customer finds the original work defective) have become quite common. This shows us that the real need, in consumers' minds, is not for the product itself, but for what the product will do. It is because of this trend that consumers are beginning to expect satisfaction from services rendered by health-care professionals, including dentists.

Dentists may perceive themselves as delivering a health service similar to that delivered by physicians. Most consumers, however, think of the products that dentists generate — dentures, crowns, fillings — rather than of the service. Although many dentists already in effect guarantee satisfaction even to the point of refunding full fee for a prosthetic appliance with which the patient is not pleased, most are very guarded so as to not imply warranty or guarantee. Perhaps the time has come for the dentist to be more definite in assuring patients of satisfaction. This assurance fits in with the trend of consumers' expectations and is likely to be financially advantageous to the competent dentist.

It has been said that the consumer movement is the result of the failure of marketing. If all goods and services were properly marketed — not foisted on the public but rather directed toward specific, well-identified needs — providers would quickly become aware of consumer problems and correct them. In other words, the providers would respond to complaints before the complaints reached the protest or product-boycott stage. Dentists, certainly, have always been advocates for their patients. And dentists have only infrequently been the target of any consumer anger. We need to note, though, that the majority of people are *not* regular dental patients, and hence they may be inclined to adopt a consumerist attitude toward the dental profession. Alvin Toffler, author of *The Third Wave,* predicts further popular disenchantment with professionals and a corresponding loss of prestige by professionals. Given this possibility, the dentist who wants thrive must become aware of consumerist trends. And he needs to head off unfavorable consequences for himself by instituting a sound marketing program.

Perhaps the time has come for the dentist to be more definite in assuring patients of satisfaction.

Attitude Toward Cost

The dentist ... needs to ask himself: ... "What would I want done if I were this patient — with his knowledge and his values, not mine?"

People tend to think that dentistry costs too much. They usually associate dentistry with over-all rising health-care costs — especially hospital costs. There has been a public movement toward demanding controls of dental-care costs in relation to the cost of other goods and services. On the other hand, while most consumers probably want acceptable quality at an affordable price, there still exists a minority of consumers who want the best that money can buy them. The dentist, therefore, needs to ask himself in regard to each patient: "What treatment is in the best interest of this patient, given his total needs?" Or one may decide what to offer on the basis of "What would I want done if I were this patient — with his knowledge and his values, not mine? If I were this patient, what could I afford that would do me the most good?"

When a person purchases an airline ticket, he has several options: first class, tourist, excursion, charter, and so on. All tickets get him to the same destination. Cost, service, and convenience vary. For some individuals who are offered *only* a first-class accommodation, the only real choice they may have is not to go at all. For some patients, the optimal treatment by professional standards may be economically out of reach. The practitioner, thus, needs to offer *more than one choice.* Deciding which choices to offer is part of marketing. Instead of offering different types of treatment, many dentists believe that they can serve their patients better by offering to provide treatment in phases. Thus, the financial limitations of the patient do not control the type of dentistry, but rather how long it takes to accomplish the treatment. Optimal treatment may take a number of years. Of course, people of very limited means may be unable to obtain optimal treatment regardless of the length of time.

Deciding which choices to offer is part of marketing.

Consumer Trends

Shopping trends are in great flux. In many areas, downtown shopping has gone the way of the horse and buggy. In other areas

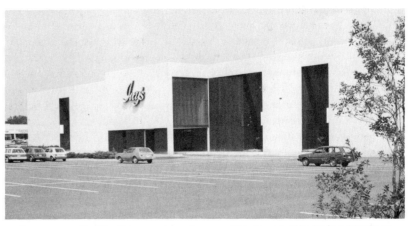

Shopping malls, like this one, have become the mecca of today's consumers.

efforts are underway for a renaissance of the downtown section. Neighborhood shopping centers and large regional malls have been drawing throngs, primarily because of easy accessibility and free parking. Besides having department and specialty stores, such centers and malls also offer food, movie theaters, and other entertainment locations.

No longer does almost everyone eat meals at the same regular times. Nor does everyone do shopping, banking, and other chores during normal daylight hours. The shopping centers and malls cater to people's changing shopping habits by remaining open at night. Toffler says that Americans are beginning to structure their time much differently and that further changes are likely. For example, a person who is able to buy groceries or get cash from a bank at midnight is likely to be interested in dental services offered in the evening. This is especially so since many two-worker families have difficulty finding time to obtain dental care. Many dentists, consequently, alert to this new need, have already extended their practices to some evening and weekend hours. We see this as a trend that is likely to accelerate.

Another important consumer trend through the 1960s and 1970s and into the 1980s has been the use of credit. We have been living in a credit society. In many instances, people bought goods or services based on the level of a monthly payment — not on the total cost. As interest rates for credit cards have soared, however, there has been some hesitation about indulging in credit. This is an area that the perceptive dentist-marketer needs to monitor carefully. In general, though, offering patients various payment alternatives is a good way to help build a practice.

Age Distribution and Population Mobility

Good marketing notes demographic changes. Many Americans were born during the postwar years of peak birthrates (which began to decline in the 1960s), and the percentage of people living past age 65 continues to increase. The needs of the senior citizen groups are receiving increasing attention from marketers of many goods and services. Dentists ought to pay attention, too. Then we have a large cohort of Americans now in their twenties who will require dental services of all kinds. As they enter their fourth, fifth, and sixth decades, they will need considerable care for periodontal disease and edentulism, partial and complete. Another factor: many mothers are bringing children in for dental examinations at younger ages than mothers did in former years.

The practicing dentist must look out and see the needs of the public as a whole in a way that the traditional dentist never had to bother to do. The traditional dentist, as we have noted, had more work than he could handle. He did not need to seek new patients actively — and he didn't. The successful practice of today depends on attracting many patients from a large cross section of the public. Dentists who are prepared to satisfy the needs of many diverse age and economic groups will enjoy a marketing advantage.

The successful practice of today depends on attracting many patients from a large cross section of the public.

Another shift of population has been geographic. The migration to the sunbelt to secure the "right" job and living environment has markedly boosted the population in much of the southern United States. (Dentists seem to have preceded this migratory pattern in an almost uncanny fashion, proving that there already is a fairly good innate sense of marketing among practitioners.) In general, today, whether moving to the sunbelt or not, people change residences more frequently than in past decades. As a result the once stable dental practice is kept in a state of flux. Every year, most practices lose a significant number of patients who must be replaced by newcomers.

Changes in Perception Toward Health/Preventive Services

Perceptions about health are changing. The holistic health movement, for example, is based on the idea that health relates to the whole person — not merely to body parts, such as the masticatory system. People who regard health in a holistic way are apt to be content only with dental service planned with a view to the whole person. Nutritional and exercise regimens and other preventive health practices are an integral part of life for holistic-health disciples. They are likely to appreciate such treatment modalities as biofeedback and acupuncture. The dentist who understands this kind of value system, or who, indeed, espouses such values himself, has an advantage with this group. He should be proficient in various treatment modalities associated with the holistic philosophy.

People also perceive differently today the relationship of health to the provision of health services. They notice, for instance, that despite an abundance of health services, there also is an abundance of endemic diseases, such as coronary artery disease for affluent upper-middle-class individuals who are heavy utilizers of health services. Such perceptions remind people that health services alone cannot

People who regard health in a holistic way are apt to be content only with dental service planned with a view to the whole person.

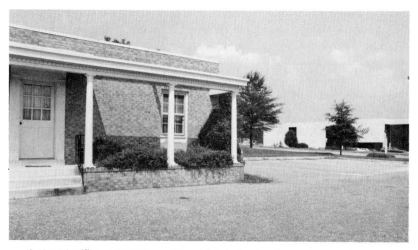

A dental office adjacent to the mall takes advantage of current consumer trends.

provide health. People are becoming aware that lifestyle habits, such as smoking or living in a polluted area, or lack of exercise, or stress from work or family appear to impact on health more than do health services. These prevention-minded people are aware that they can do much to foster their own good health through their lifestyle habits or choice of environment.

Such people are also likely to view dental services in somewhat the same way. They will be more inclined to take responsibility for their own dental health. They will thus have a less dependent relationship with the dentist than in times past. Consequently, they will be more likely to question his procedures and his restorative techniques. The dentist who understands the thinking of such health-conscious individuals can function in an interdependent role with them and can better serve their needs. At the same time, he must retain the capacity to function with people who prefer a dependent role — unless he wishes to limit his market appeal.

... the necessary level (of dental care) may be affordable to patients, whereas the optimal level may be excessively costly.

A stickier issue is the question of whether many people actually need or can afford the sophisticated level of dental services that many dentists are now trained to provide — and very much want to provide. What is *necessary* for dental health may be less than what is *optimal.* Moreover, the necessary level may be affordable to patients, whereas the optimal level may be excessively costly. Obviously, dentists and patients have varying perceptions here. Nobody wants a provision of services that would have to be called inadequate; however, some patients are suspicious that they are being sold more than they actually need. Some consumers apparently believe that dentists, if left to their own devices, will perform more complicated, and costly, procedures than necessary. Therefore, it is incumbent upon each dentist to ensure that each of his patients understands the dental problem sufficiently to come to agreement with the kind of treatment that is planned. Clearly, once a patient has the perception that he has been oversold, that he has bought a first-class ticket when an excursion ticket would have been enough, he may remove himself from the dentist's roster of patients.

The degree to which dentists have failed to justify their treatment plans to patients may account, in part, for the failure to convert people from nonusers to users of dental services. Approximately 50 percent of all adults visit a dentist for professional services during any twelve-month period. Estimates vary, but perhaps only 50 percent of these, or 25 percent of the total population, are on some kind of regular maintenance program. In other words, dentists do not provide regular care for 75 percent of the population. This large segment may be viewed as a tremendous untapped market. A retail marketing organization, such as Sears Roebuck, would look upon this large potential market as a golden opportunity. Because dentistry is only now evolving out of an era of an overabundance of work, or scarcity of dentists, professionals in the dental field may have a different view. However, dentists who are able to identify with the marketing approach and take the time and trouble to understand the needs of the nonusers should succeed admirably in filling their appointment books.

One aspect of prevention has been good for children's teeth but has, correspondingly, cut dental needs drastically: fluoridation. If, as has been said, the obligation of the profession is to reduce the need for its services, dentistry has succeeded remarkably well. Professional success, however, carries with it the penalty of making personal success harder to achieve. Certainly, children who drink fluoridated water still need dental treatment. But what they need is dental treatment of a sophisticated type, such as monitoring of and appropriate intervention in growth and development. Studies have shown that dental procedures are different in fluoridated areas, but that the volume of treatment is about the same as in nonfluoridated areas. Fluoridated areas, however, tend to be fairly sophisticated in their development, and are therefore also the kind of places that dentists like to live. Hence, there is usually an overabundance of dentists in fluoridated communities. These dentists, therefore, need to become more adept at marketing their services.

Inefficiency of Traditional Dentist

Since the development of the highspeed handpiece, the productivity of dentists has increased markedly. Even so, dentistry still is in a primitive stage when compared to much of industry. In other sectors, delegation of low-level tasks to persons with minimal training is an established principle. Applying this principle would greatly increase dental productivity. Yet, in "protecting the patient," the traditional dentist has been highly restrictive of what he would delegate. He has limited his auxiliary personnel to extra-oral tasks. This antiquated thinking has led to low output amid soaring costs. In jurisdictions where laws permit delegation of duties, dentists who can manage enough auxiliaries to perform all of the tasks they can possibly delegate produce several times the volume of dental services as dentists who do not delegate. (Needless to add, they also produce considerably higher incomes.)

> The volume of income that one dentist can generate is closely related to the efficiency with which he schedules his patients, completes his dental work, and administers his office.

Having more help and delegating more duties are not enough, in themselves, to increase income. The volume of income that one dentist can generate is closely related to the efficiency with which he schedules his patients, completes his dental work, and administers his office. These are areas that dental education touches upon lightly, perhaps because learning technical dentistry with little attention to management is very challenging for dental students. Efficient dentists have learned most of their efficiency in their own practices and through continuing education.

The notion of performing tasks with the most expertise in the least amount of time and with the least expense of motion, as applied within industry to increase profits, will work in modern dental practices, too. Waste of any kind — of time, of motion, of efficiency — will mean less income. The dentist who has firm control over these principles of industry will find he has developed an efficient practice.

Efficiency is a two-edged sword, however. Without it a dentist will limit his income; with it, he will find that he has to market his practice more effectively in order to use the capability he has developed.

Dentist as Entrepreneur

Private dental practice requires significant capital investment, as all recently graduated dentists have surely experienced. Once, such an investment was a very safe risk. Today, especially with aggravated interest rates, the entrepreneurial risk for dentists is higher. Once, the initial expense of office rental, equipment, and supplies was within easy reach; today, it is staggering. The entrepreneurial risk of our new era makes it mandatory that the dentist develop a conscious and well-delineated program to attract the clientele he needs for a quality, high-income practice.

> The dentist must develop a conscious and well-delineated program to attract the clientele he needs.

Female and Minority Dentists

The number of females and minority members who have become dentists recently has grown rapidly. This fact presents an interesting marketing situation both for them and for the majority white male dentist. Female dentists may appeal to a certain segment of the female population as feminist symbols, and to a certain segment of the male population as a "gentler touch" for dental services. The appeal of black, chicano, or other minority dentists to members of their respective minorities is obvious.

At first glance, it might appear that the presence of these new groups in the dental marketplace would tend to restrict the market-

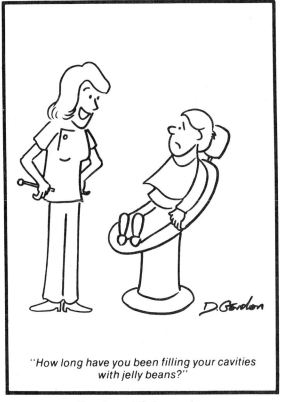

"How long have you been filling your cavities with jelly beans?"

Courtesy of *Cal* magazine.

ability of the traditional white male practitioner. On a deeper level, however, the new minorities in dentistry — females and nonwhite males — are not guaranteed any lasting advantage. They, too, will be faced, sooner or later, with all the other ramifications of today's consumer situation — preventive health consciousness, suspicion of being overcharged or overserved, concern for a total health-care approach, and so on. The color of skin or the sex of a female may be an initial calling card, but the total marketing approach, services offered, fee schedules, and personal compatibility with patients will come to overshadow all else. Each dentist must market his — or her — own services acceptably to his clientele, even though the initial contact with a patient may come about on the basis of being female or a member of the same minority group.

Political Weakness of Dental Profession

As a political force, the dental profession has never been noted for its strength. Dentists have been unaggressive, compared with some other health-care professionals, in competing for the spending of tax dollars for dentistry. The primary reason that traditional dentists avoided seeking a piece of the federal pie or cultivating political friends is that they had so little economic need of them. Their practices were full, patients were plentiful, and they were too busy to consider politics. This lack of interest or skill in advocating in political forums the need for dental health has resulted in weak public dental programs in most parts of the country. This inadequacy not only limits the potential income for dentists through these programs, but it also does little to improve the dental health of people of limited resources. This poor dental health translates into a community problem, which individual dentists may find themselves attempting to solve at their own expense and to the peril of their practices.

Non-dentist entrepreneurs who invest in dentistry . . . pose a threat to the control of the dental practice which is provided by ownership.

Here now is an even greater threat. Dentists may stand to lose the control of the dental practice which is provided by ownership. If outside investors decide that dental practice is a good investment, they are likely to exert pressure on legislators to permit non-dentist ownership. The dental profession may not be strong enough politically to prevent this from happening. Non-dentist entrepreneurs who invest in dentistry are likely to be much more proficient at marketing than are dentists. The entry into the dental marketplace of such investors places private dentists at a great disadvantage. Proper marketing by individual dentists is one way to counter this potential problem.

Attitudes of Dentist and Staff

Dentists may be their own worst enemies in the marketplace. Until very recently, the attitudes of most dentists have been rather anti-marketing. Dentists can no longer afford to look upon marketing as "unprofessional." A dentist needs to see to it, also, that his own staff is brought aboard his marketing team. His staff is a mirror of his own attitude. If he is anti-marketing, his staff will be anti-marketing. If he decides to be a marketer, his staff will join him in his new effort. And his staff may well market his service at least as effectively as he can himself.

Lest we convey the impression that we see marketing as only for the purpose of obtaining a higher income, may we add another thought. Marketing skills and the resulting success can be thought of in terms other than economic. If he is an effective marketer and competent dentist, the dentist can have more free time instead of more money, if he chooses. A dentist may choose to work fewer hours, work less hard, talk more with people, or use time however he likes. Work may be more fun if you control your work situation. Staff persons may find more fulfillment in a less hectic pace. The rewards may be intangible and spiritual as well as economic. Marketing proficiency gives the dentist these choices.

Finally, we hope that you, the dentist, will understand marketing better through reading this book. We hope that as you read, you will come to view marketing as *professional* — in that it is a way of serving more people more effectively.

Work may be more fun if you control your work situation.

REFERENCES

Ginzberg, E.: An economist's view of dentistry in the 80s. Dental Economics, January, 1981, pp. 77–78.
King, A. E.: A survival guide for independent dentists. The Nexus Group, Inc., Cave Creek, AZ, 1979.
Toffler, A.: The Third Wave. New York, Bantam Publishers, 1981.

2

The Dental Marketplace

Dr. James Nesbitt has just returned from the annual midwinter meeting in Chicago where he heard a program on *Marketing For The Dental Practice.* His feelings are very mixed. He always thought of marketing as something tricky that a seller had to do to get a buyer to buy. The advertising that even some of his friends have begun to do is offensive to him. It all seems so unprofessional — maybe even unethical. Yet what the speaker said made a lot of sense. Maybe he had not understood what marketing was. Maybe he should look into it more. In this chapter we are addressing some of these concerns.

HISTORICAL REVIEW

A dentist exchanges his skills in detecting and repairing maladies or malformations of teeth or gum tissue for something of value — usually money. In this he participates in the general phenomenon we call "the marketplace." The marketplace has an old and honorable history in human society. It would be worthwhile here to take a brief look at how this phenomenon has evolved in the Western world, and understand the dentist's place in this realm. The eras of development of the marketplace are: scarcity, production, selling, and marketing.

The eras of development of the marketplace are: scarcity, production, selling, and marketing.

Scarcity Era

The scarcity era was characterized by a shortage of goods and services. Early in this period, people lived just above a survival level. Most people were self-sufficient, producing all of the absolute necessities for themselves with little excess. At a certain point, specialization began to emerge, and people started to produce what they could do best. Exchange became necessary. So places were set aside for exchange (barter mostly), and these came to be called "markets." They were usually within a day's round trip for all citizens. Money — gold and silver pieces — soon found a role as a medium of exchange.

Prior to the Industrial Revolution a system developed in which certain people began to distribute goods produced by others. They bought the output so that the producers no longer had to bring their goods to market and sell them. Instead the distributors, the first retailers, bought a variety of products from producers in their workplaces and sold them to the consumers in the marketplaces. This more efficient system of distributing goods enabled consumers to purchase most of what they needed in one place. This explains the evolution of the general store, such as flourished in frontier America.

The industrial revolution concentrated the means of production in a factory. The factories were able to produce many more goods than were required in the community. Consequently, there developed transportation systems that could move large quantities of goods over long distances.

Production Era

These developments brought about the production era. During this period consumers readily bought all the goods the factories could produce. The problem for the producers was to increase the efficiency of production, so that they could keep up with consumer demand. Eventually, efficiency increased in most well-known product lines to a point at which producers *could* readily produce more than consumers wanted to buy.

The marketer starts with the consumers' needs. He then figures out how he can help to satisfy those needs.

Selling Era

As a result, producers began to develop sales departments to push their products. This was the selling era. Now the problem was how to sell all the goods the factories could manufacture. We are speaking now of the early twentieth century. Just as production had caught up with demand, so selling eventually seemed to reach a point beyond which further efforts produced little or no further results. Selling had reached the limits of its potency as a solution to the problem of moving goods.

Marketing Era

Clever managers reasoned at this point that they ought to find out what consumers really wanted and needed, and then put *those* goods on the market. This was marketing. No longer was it enough to produce efficiently and sell products. It became the vogue to develop an "outside-in" approach: study the needs of consumers and develop products to satisfy those needs. The marketer starts with the consumers' needs. He then figures out how he can help to satisfy those needs. Whereas the seller is concerned with his need to sell whatever he already has, the marketer is concerned with the needs of the consumer and how he can satisfy them. If selling is getting rid of what you have, marketing is having what you can get rid of (what people want)!

Marketing may be defined as "the management of exchanges for the benefit of the consumer at a profit to the producer." First, the producer needs to develop a product that will benefit a consumer, and second, he needs to make a profit on it. Henry Ford is a case in point. Ford saw that the American people needed and would buy automobiles at $500 each. So he set himself the task of developing the means of production to turn out cars that could be sold at that price, and then he got the word out and sold millions of cars. Thus, Henry Ford can be thought of as not only a production genius but as a marketing genius as well. He certainly undertook to concern himself with benefiting the consumer, and he made a substantial profit in the process. (Incidentally, he also paid the highest wages for his time, creating higher purchasing power among the group of consumers who were his own workers.)

> Marketing may be defined as "the management of exchanges for the benefit of the consumer at a profit to the producer."

IMPLICATIONS FOR DENTISTRY

Dentistry has not yet entered completely into the marketing era. In some sense — and especially in certain geographic areas — the scarcity era may yet prevail. If we can borrow an image from an earlier era of business, in which it was said that customers "were cleaning off the shelves," in some areas of America today, consumers of dental services are still "cleaning off the shelves." That is to say, they are keeping their local dentist working at full capacity. This is a characteristic of the production era.

Indeed dental practice management has for some time emphasized efficiency of production — utilization of auxiliaries and technol-

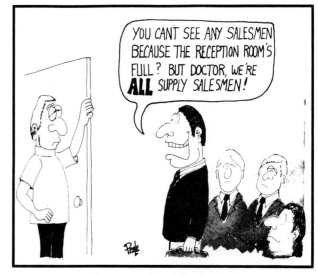

Courtesy of Dr. Mike Peele.

ogy, which enables dentists to be many times as productive as they once were. As in industry, efficiency of production is necessary in order to produce goods and services at a reasonable cost. As we have said, emphasis on production leads to an availability of goods or services that exceeds the ready demand of the consumer. So it would seem that in relationship to industry, dentistry has been in a production era, at least in areas where dentists are in short supply. In geographic areas where the supply of dentists is adequate for the demand, certainly in most urban areas, dentistry is at the threshold of the selling era. The introduction and increase in dental advertising would seem to be evidence for this.

If we are to learn from history, a good lesson would seem to be that we should attempt to leap over the selling era and enter directly into the marketing era. Look again at the automobile industry, and you can see the danger of "selling." The American automobile producers, until recently, seemed most interested in selling what they could produce readily and efficiently, rather than in producing what they came to realize Americans needed and wanted. They lingered in the selling era too long, and at a great cost to their profitability.

> If we are to learn from history, a good lesson would seem to be that we should attempt to leap over the selling era and enter directly into the marketing era.

If we can learn from the mistakes of others rather than making those same mistakes, we ought not to continue to produce what WE want to and then try to sell it. The greatest hazard in advertising is that it appears to enable us to continue selling what we are already producing. If our service fails to meet the perceived and real needs of consumers, advertising will soon become ineffective just as selling became ineffective. This one-way communication is very limited.

MARKETING IN DENTISTRY

Rather, we ought to try to figure out what people want and need and attempt to satisfy those wants and those needs. This is not to say that we should compromise principles of treatment because people don't want the treatment we propose. It does say that we need to know how our patients' circumstances, health, and personality bear on dental treatment. In this way we can offer treatment that best meets their individual needs. Also, we need to understand the people and their circumstances in the communities where we practice. We must be aware of personal and community characteristics. To succeed we must satisfy the needs that arise out of those particular characteristics.

If a dentist practices in a community where a large proportion of the people are employed in factories, he must consider their particular needs. If the worker loses pay to come to the dental office, he is unlikely to come unless he is in pain. Certainly, if a dentist expects to treat workers in this group, he must provide some hours when a worker can come in without losing pay. Likewise, if workers have an insurance plan for dental care, the dentist should understand the plan and assist them in getting the most benefit from the plan. What are all the circumstances bearing on dental treatment in your community? To serve your community effectively — and to build your practice — you will need to learn what they are.

Dental Office Encounter

Figure 2–1 indicates the approach of most consumers to the dental practice. Although the technology is the province of the dentist, the "process factors" are shared and are important to the patient. Although the responsibility may be shared to some extent, the dentist must be responsible for criteria that have biological implications. The dentist who best satisfies his patient's total needs will relate to him in such a way that treatment can be discussed openly and freely. The patient will have the opportunity, and in fact will be encouraged, to enter into the process, so he can better ensure that the treatment is acceptable to him in every way. The dentist, in a sense, is actually a consultant to the patient in the decision-making process rather than the one deciding for the patient. This works best when the patient and the dentist are capable of an interdependent relationship. In fact, if either is incapable of such a relationship, the model that views the patient as decider and the dentist as consultant will collapse.

Dentists traditionally have tended to assume the decision-making function. The authoritarian dentist is likely to be quite comfortable in this role. He will attract patients who are looking for someone else to make their decisions. Some patients may require this dependent role with the dentist making decisions, which they accept or reject. The effective marketing dentist will figure out what kind of role the patient wants to play (i.e., what the patient's needs are) and make it possible for the patient to play that role. The dentist must be aware of his patients' needs and must be responsive to them. As he succeeds in assessing needs and in responding to them, he will succeed in marketing his services to patients.

In spite of modern preventive techniques, there is still a vast amount of dental disease in America. The priority placed on having this disease treated varies among the population. It is difficult to accurately predict who will choose full dental treatment and who will opt for emergency procedures only, but it is probably a safe generalization to say that people who have dental insurance or social welfare at their disposal will be more likely to follow through with complete treatment, and that the more educated patient will want treatment from the standpoint of overall health and personal appearance. Of course, there are always exceptions, and many times the acceptance of

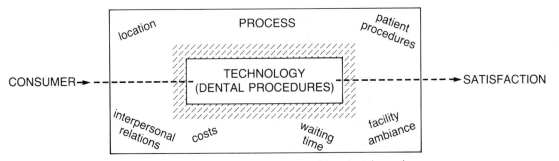

Figure 2–1. Consumer encounter with a dental practice.

treatment by certain patients will exceed or fall short of the dentist's expectation.

In any event, the actual need for services outweighs the current demand, which places the dentist in a financial and sometimes ethical dilemma. If the traditional dentist has been averse to the idea of marketing his services, the modern dentist has begun to realize that he must consider doing so out of necessity in order to bring the demand for his services in line with the need of people within his immediate marketplace.

Variables in Increasing Dental Demand

How can the dentist go about this? There are many avenues to explore. The dentist should look at the spectrum of clinical services he offers. Does he restrict his market to certain types of procedures, or does he include a full range of services that will appeal to and fill the needs of the most people? If he refuses to take denture patients or does not particularly like root canal treatment, he may be limiting his income. While it is true that mental acceptance of a task is important, just how much of a financial loss through limiting his market is the dentist willing to accept in order to do only those procedures he enjoys?

As the dentist succeeds in assessing his patients' needs and responding to them, he will succeed in marketing his services.

Another important factor in attracting more patients is the spectrum of financial services offered by the dentist. If he insists on cash only from patients not covered by insurance and extends no credit, he severely limits the size of his patient load. If he would consider time payments, discounts for cash, and other payment alternatives, he could probably increase his market share by a significant margin.

Does he accept third party payments (insurance)? Since a great many industries now offer dental insurance as a benefit, larger numbers of individuals are seeking dental services. The dentist should investigate whether or not to accept assignment from the insurance company or require cash from the patient. If he does accept assignment, he should explore methods of collecting additional fees not paid by insurance. Charging a fee for filing insurance forms can be a negative factor in attracting new patients.

Capitation funding for dental care is increasing rather dramatically. Some dentists contract with industries to treat their employees for a given flat fee. These capitation programs can be a boost to a practice because even though some employees will require extensive work that far exceeds the rate paid per person, others will not even take advantage of the benefit. In some areas, the HMO (Health Maintenance Organization) is catching on. Dentists who participate are usually paid a given amount per person per year. When the patients require treatment, it is done at no additional charge.

Some dentists prefer not to treat patients who participate in programs such as Medicaid, Headstart, Veterans Administration benefits, and School Health Funds. Whether their reluctance stems from the extra paperwork, problems with broken appointments, or other factors, there are many patients of this type who could enhance the financial state of most practices.

The range of technical dental treatment that is offered can also be extremely important. If a patient can choose from viable alternatives at different fees, his acceptance of some type of treatment will be a greater possibility.

This discussion on variables points to the marketing fact that the more varied the services offered, the more types of patients accepted into the practice, and the more varied the financial arrangements and treatment alternatives, the greater the impact a given dental practice will have on the public. Even if the dentist is satisfied with the level of his workload and income, he should structure his strategy to ensure that he maintains these levels over the years. The practitioner who has not reached his desired level ought to consider setting goals to increase his market share of patients and therefore his profit margin.

CONSTITUENCIES

There are several groups of people with whom the dentist must relate in some way in his marketing program (managing exchanges). Surely the most obvious group is patients, or as some prefer to call them, clients. Another group is the dental team or staff. The team is involved in day-to-day care of patients and must be thoroughly briefed in marketing. Other less obvious constituents are to be found in the community, such as other members of the dental professions, professionals, businesspersons, and the general public.

Dentists

Colleagues may be quite helpful in one's marketing program. Established dentists can be helpful to each other and better meet community needs by open cooperation. Consulting a colleague with permission and active involvement of the patient fosters cooperation among dentists, which is apparent to patients. Such concern for patients impresses both patients and fellow dentists.

Consulting a colleague with permission and active involvement of the patient fosters cooperation among dentists.

Wherever dentists are in short supply, most established dentists refer patients to beginning dentists. In areas where there are enough dentists, that is, not a surplus of patients, fewer dentists refer patients to new dentists. Even in these latter areas, the dentist needing new patients should call on established dentists and ask for suggestions on how to attract patients. The collegial relationship is often strong enough that the established dentist will assist the beginning dentist. The assistance may not necessarily be by referring patients but by helping the new dentist to understand better the community and its needs. With this understanding, the dentist can succeed with many patients where before he might have failed.

The successful established dentist knows that if all dentists are satisfying patients' needs, there is a more favorable dental climate in the community. Such a climate enables all dentists to relate more successfully to their patients than they otherwise could. General dental awareness (dental

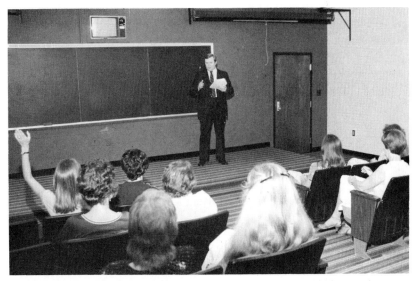

A practicing dentist speaking to an assembly of dental auxiliaries — who are a potential source for referrals.

IQ) is higher in such a community. Community dentists set the tone for dental health by how they affect attitudes as well as by their technical dental skills.

Dental Auxiliaries

Dental auxiliaries are part of the dental community and are to be considered in the dentist's marketing program. Your willingness to speak at programs for auxiliary organizations and your personal acquaintance with individual auxiliaries will help you to learn more about community characteristics. Auxiliaries (particularly reception-ists) who know you will refer overflow patients from their offices to you. They may also refer their friends or even come to you as patients, especially if they work for specialists. More will be said later about your own auxiliaries.

Physicians

Contacts with other health professionals will also foster market-ing within the community. Relating to a pediatrician obviously will benefit the dentist who wants to care for children. Since mothers make most of the health-care decisions for the family, it is easy to see the advantage of knowing the obstetrician and the family practitioner. Thus, a dentist can cultivate relationships according to whichever segments of the population he most seeks to appeal.

The dentist should share with local physicians any information or knowledge that will assist them to: (1) refer patients for dental care, and (2) manage medical treatment with consideration for dental problems. Staining of teeth from antibiotic medication is an example of such information. At times various kinds of information, in printed

The dentist should share with local physicians any informa-tion or knowledge that will as-sist them to: (1) refer patients for dental care, and (2) man-age medical treatment with consideration for dental prob-lems.

form, should be shared with referring physicians. The physician who is aware of your expertise in areas such as myofascial pain or dental care for the medically compromised is more likely to refer such patients to you. The well-informed physician will be able to recognize dental disease at least in moderately advanced stages. Certainly physicians see a great many patients who are not under regular dental care; the marketing dentist can gain access to such patients through his medical colleagues.

Non-Physician Health Professionals

Health-care colleagues may be a source of referrals.

Non-physicians — nurses, nutritionists, dieticians, laboratory technologists — within the medical profession should be viewed similarly to dental auxiliaries. All professionals in the health community may be able to refer a friend to a dentist. The dentist who is marketing successfully will know a great many health-care colleagues. And this broad acquaintance will inevitably bring him many referrals.

Pharmacists deserve special attention. They function almost in the role of primary care. They receive numerous questions about health problems. The retail pharmacist is in a position to refer a great many people to a dentist.

Dental Technicians

Community dental laboratory technicians also deserve mention. Laboratory technicians who live in the community may be a rich source of referrals. Their knowledge of the dentist's technical excellence gives them a special credibility among their friends and acquaintances. The dentist who sends excellent preparations, impressions, and records to the laboratory is likely to be noticed. Such notice may result in the referral of fastidious patients.

Dental Suppliers

Valuable assistance can also be obtained from dental suppliers. Especially helpful is suppliers' knowledge of the community for a dentist who is selecting a location. After locating, one can still learn from suppliers about the needs of the community and how to satisfy them. Suppliers can talk about what already goes on in the dental community; such information is invaluable for planning purposes.

Other Professions

Non-health-care professionals — teachers, lawyers, and so forth — should receive attention in one's marketing program. Certainly other entrepreneur professionals understand some of the problems of simultaneously practicing a profession and conducting a business. Marketing problems for attorneys, for instance, are very similar to those of dentists. Successful attorneys may be especially helpful to a beginning dentist and may be solicited for ideas. During the selection of an attorney for legal services, the dentist should attempt to interview several. This may be done in a relaxed manner over lunch, when it is possible to inquire about means of marketing. Much valuable information can be obtained in this way—especially about the needs of the community.

A prime referral source for the general dentist, pedodontist, or orthodontist is the school teacher. If he is willing to spend a little time out of the office, the dentist will be readily welcomed into classrooms to give programs on dental health.

Community businesspeople may be very valuable in a dentist's marketing program.

Businesspersons

Community businesspeople are a widespread constituency that can be very valuable in a dentist's marketing program. You can meet many of them through community organizations, such as the Chamber of Commerce and service clubs. The dentist entering a community should call on them at their places of business and inquire as to how they might suggest that he could best satisfy community needs. Committee work — beyond mere membership — in a community organization is advisable. Service club members may have less opportunity to refer patients than people in the health professions. However, the service club facilitates making a great many contacts, which very probably will result in patient referrals. Members of service clubs usually understand the problems of promoting a business and are likely to be helpful.

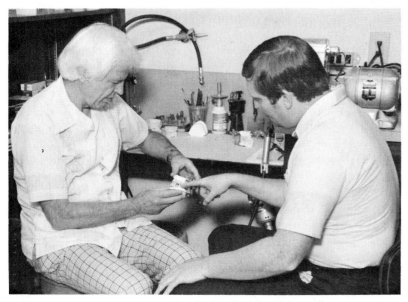

Colleagues gain much by sharing the latest information.

General Public

Finally, there is the general public. It is from this group that the majority of patients come. It may be considered the target group of the marketing program. A dentist beginning practice in the community has innumerable opportunities to interact with the public. Religious groups, Scout troops, and parent-teacher groups, among many others, provide such opportunities. As social networks develop from those groups and others, the dentist will find himself gaining a place in the community. If he is energetic and outgoing, opportunities are almost unlimited. In fact, he may have to limit such relationships to maintain his practice and his family responsibilities. As he is able to become of real value in community life and if he manages his practice well, his business and professional success is almost assured. The dentist who is a productive citizen is likely to be successful as a dentist.

DYNAMICS OF THE MARKETPLACE

By definition, the marketplace is dynamic — a place where changes occur constantly. Changes include the number of people in the market, demographics, characteristics of these people, numbers of dentists, numbers of non-dentist providers, and the money available for dental care.

Numbers of People

The population of communities changes constantly. One in five families moves every year. Some remain in the same community; others move away. On this basis alone, the annual turnover in any dental practice could be approximately 20 percent. The stability of communities varies. In a community where industry transfers executives frequently the turnover rate may exceed 20 percent. In more stable communities it may be less. The dentist should be aware of the degree of stability of his community. If turnover is high, marketing needs to be more effective if the practice is to thrive. Where turnover is high, the established dentist needs to market aggressively. The new dentist has more opportunity where turnover is high.

A growing community, like the high-turnover communities, presents a favorable opportunity to the new dentist and a problem to the established dentist who is an ineffective marketer. The effective marketer will be getting his share of new patients in the growing community. A shrinking population is a problem for both, but it is more severe for the new dentist. Again, the dentist should be aware of the change in population (increase or decrease) and manage his marketing program accordingly.

Demographic Characteristics

Birth rates and mortality rates are a part of demographics. Improved health and increased life expectancy are lowering mortality and increasing the numbers of the aged. Health problems of the aged are receiving more and more attention. There is considerable concern among the dental profession that dental problems for older people have not been dealt with adequately. Research is not conclusive as to the needs of this group. It seems safe to assume that the dental needs are likely to be prosthetic, periodontic, and complex restorative. Also, personal needs are likely to include consideration for limited economic resources, for problems of mobility, for complex health problems, for more personal attention, and for more time for dental treatment. Many elderly people have much free time and don't like to be rushed. Actually the dentist may be able to accomplish his procedures quickly and delegate someone else to spend additional time with the patient. In states that permit delegation of many intraoral tasks, this can occur naturally. The patient may view the dental visit primarily as a social occasion. Certainly the dentist who understands the needs of the aged and formulates a program to satisfy those needs has a considerable marketing advantage with this growing percentage of the population.

Certainly the dentist who understands the needs of the aged and formulates a program to satisfy those needs has a considerable marketing advantage with this growing percentage of the population.

At the same time the over-65 group is becoming a larger percentage of our population, children are becoming a smaller percentage. The number of births peaked in 1960 and declined rather steadily until the early 1970s when it again began to increase. If the persons born in peak birth years have the expected number of children, numbers of births will again increase during the 1980s. If, as happened in the 1930s, a period of economic distress, the birthrate for the 1980s declines, absolute numbers are likely to increase very little if at all.

Treatment Needs

Generally speaking, for the foreseeable future the market for dental treatment for children, principally orthodontics and pedodontics, will be limited. As the median age of the people increases, more complex restorative treatment, periodontics, and prosthodontics are likely to be needed. If the 1980s are increasingly economically stressful, as some predict, dental health may deteriorate because of neglect. The combination of an aging population and increasing dental disease is likely to create a need for significantly more dental treatment of the complex variety. *The general dentist who is competent to treat complex dental problems will enjoy a distinct marketing advantage.*

Numbers of Dentists

Not only is the number of dentists increasing, but the proportion of dentists per capita is also increasing. The federal policy of increasing dental manpower has been based on the large unmet need for dental treatment. A small surplus of dentists is now projected for 1990 based on a demand model developed by federal health manpower planners. This projection assumes that dental care will not be provided by National Health Insurance.

TABLE 2–1. PROJECTED NUMBER OF DENTAL GRADUATES, TOTAL STOCK OF DENTISTS, AND DENTIST POPULATION RATIO, 1980–1995*

Year	Number of New Graduates	Total Stock of Dentists	Dentists Per 100,000 Population
1980	5150	141,272	63.6
1981	5320	144,258	64.6
1982	5400	147,313	65.1
1983	5400	150,353	65.8
1984	5400	153,340	66.5
1985	5400	156,336	67.1
1986	5400	159,306	67.8
1987	5400	162,259	68.4
1988	5400	165,200	69.0
1989	5400	168,110	69.6
1990	5400	170,978	70.2
1991	5400	173,835	70.8
1992	5400	176,660	71.4
1993	5400	179,448	72.0
1994	5400	182,198	72.6
1995	5400	184,901	73.2

*Source: Department of Health, Education, and Welfare, DHEW (HRA) 79–6, Sept., 1979. Forecast of Employment in the Dental Sector.

Table 2–1 shows these projections through 1995. Possibly the number of new graduates may decrease by reduction of class size and by the phasing out of some dental schools. Otherwise, *if population projections are accurate, the ratio of dentists to population would increase approximately 15 percent from 1980 to 1995.* Demand is such a complex factor that it is virtually impossible to predict with any degree of assurance whether the demand will require this increased supply of dentists.

There are vast numbers of insured persons who are not demanding dental care. Marketing efforts should be directed to this group.

Traditionally approximately 25 percent of the people have received regular dental care. With the increased supply of dentists, marketing efforts must be directed to the majority not receiving comprehensive dental care. Dental insurance is bringing into dental offices people who previously did not utilize dental services. Still, there are vast numbers of insured persons who are not demanding dental care. Marketing efforts should be directed to this group. Also, other groups not previously attracted to dental offices should be targeted. The individual dentist who studies the nonutilizers in his community, and develops a program to satisfy their needs, will be able to thrive even in the face of an increased supply of dentists.

Numbers of Non-Dentist Providers

If, as Alvin Toffler says in *The Third Wave,* there is a trend toward less respect for the professional, there is likely to be an increase in nonprofessional providers of dental care. The trend toward midwifery and physician's assistants in medicine may indicate what can be expected for dentistry. In fact, the provision of prosthetic replacements by denturists in certain states may be the beginning of such a trend. Previously, all dental care, whether by the hygienist or the expanded function dental auxiliary, or even the prosthetic auxiliary, has been in dentists' offices under the supervision of dentists. Dental hygienists are beginning to exert pressure in the political arena to enable them to practice independently. Given the societal inclinations of less awe for the professional and an interest in broadening consumer choice, the trend toward more non-dentist providers seems clear.

More non-dentist providers need not dismay dentists. This additional constituency should be viewed as exactly that — another group to be included in one's marketing program. The additional points of entry into the dental care system surely improve access; improved access is likely to increase demand. The elasticity of demand seems not to be well understood by many dentists. The dentist who understands that improved access increases demand need not worry about the competition provided by the non-dentist.

Rather, the competent marketing dentist will consider non-dentist providers a constituency in his marketing program. As with all constituencies, he will attempt to understand their needs and how he can assist them to do a better job. He will be available to speak to their groups in the interest of better dental health. Individual relationships should be cultivated in a helpful mode. Many of these non-dentist providers will refer patients. If hygienists gain true independence, they will see many patients who need the care of a dentist. The independent hygienist will surely refer these patients to the dentist who is helpful. Even the denturist who has such a relationship with a dentist competent in prosthodontics will refer more difficult patients to the dentist. Non-dentist providers may well create *more* business for dentists than they take from them. At a minimum, the dentist who is an effective marketer with this constituency will derive business from it.

Money Available for Dental Care

Federal planners project an increase in real income for dentists. This might seem overly optimistic in view of the increased number of dentists and some of the more gloomy economic forecasts. In fact, it may turn out to be more optimistic than realistic. Dentists should be prepared for whatever comes and not depend on the increased income that is projected. Given the dynamics of the economy, much of which is under governmental control and much of which is not, dentists ought to keep abreast of economic trends and plan their marketing programs accordingly.

> Given the dynamics of the economy . . . dentists ought to keep abreast of economic trends and plan their marketing programs accordingly.

The dental marketplace is also affected by government health clinics, which offer services directly to the public at little or no cost. When a potential patient can choose from a number of dental facilities that offer a wide range of services and costs, the private practitioner has to be aware of his own strong points as a competitor in the market place, so he can develop and capitalize on them. Selected large industries have begun dental and health clinics in areas where they have large numbers of employees. The workers have the option of going to these clinics at company cost or paying at least the insurance copayments to go to a private dentist.

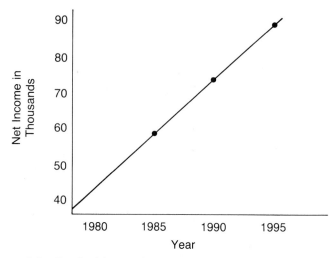

Figure 2–2. Dentists' income in constant dollars. (From DHEW (HRA) 79–6, Sept., 1979: Forecast of Employment in the Dental Sector.)

Not only is patient volume shrinking (patients available to the dentist on fee for service basis), but the health-care dollar is also decreasing. While the money available for dental services will actually rise for a few years owing to increases in insurance benefits, this money will continue to decrease in value because of inflation. This means that consumers will have less buying power in general, and dental care will be placed lower on a list of priorities. The trend will then be toward less costly dentistry. Money for dental care through social programs may decrease because of pressure for other expenditures of the governmental budgets.

Opinions vary as to whether dentists should give more or less credit in periods of economic slump. Those who argue for less credit maintain that the dentist is likely to collect less money at the time when he needs it most. They maintain that he simply cannot afford such losses. Others argue that credit is necessary at such times in order to maintain a level of production essential to the health of the practice. A practice geared for a given level of production cannot easily reduce it. Such reduction might require less staff. To dismiss staff in slow times and increase later is costly. According to this argument, short-term borrowing of money is preferred over reduction of expenses required by tight credit.

We believe that the dentist intent on meeting the needs of the community will continue to do that even during economic slumps. Obviously, costly elective dental treatment should be deferred for people in dire economic straits. But the essential needs should be cared for regardless of the financial arrangements. However, whatever financial arrangements people commit themselves to in the face of economic problems should be honored. Even though more credit may be extended, collection efforts should be rigorous. Payment schedules should be lenient but collection policies firm. Treat seasonal economic differences, such as in resort or farming communities, in the same way.

Payment schedules should be lenient but collection policies firm.

The effective marketer's first concern must be to meet community needs and then to manage his practice in such a way as to satisfy his own financial needs. Concern for community is his obligation as a professional, and efficient management is his obligation to himself as well as to the community.

PLANNING

Figure 2–3 (developed by marketing consultant Jurgen Haver) illustrates the marketing process and environment. The triangle represents the process of planning, which we are about to discuss, and execution and control, which we will be discussing throughout the book. The focus of the process represented by the inner circle is the consumer or patient/client. Planning, execution, and control concern product, promotion, place, price, and organization people. These processes occur in an uncontrolled environment of factors: economic,

Planning, execution, and control concern product, promotion, place, price, and organization people.

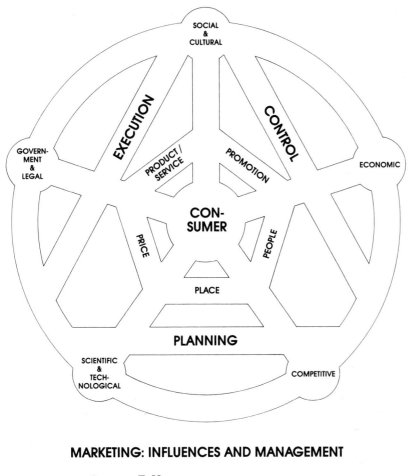

MARKETING: INFLUENCES AND MANAGEMENT

Jurgen F. Haver Marketing/Communications

Bingen Road · R. D. #5 · Bethlehem, PA 18015

Figure 2–3.

Developing a marketing strategy involves . . . (1) selecting a target market . . . and (2) developing a marketing mix. . . .

scientific and technological, social and cultural, competitive, political and legal. These we will refer to throughout the book. Also, later we will discuss promotion, place, price, and organization people. Let us now direct our attention to product or service (for a profession).

The purpose of a marketing program is to maintain one's share of the market, if it is satisfactory, or, if not, to increase one's share. Developing a marketing strategy involves two distinct but interrelated steps. These are: (1) selecting a target market, that is, groups of people to whom to appeal, and (2) developing a marketing mix, that is, elements of dental service designed to satisfy the needs of the target groups.

Selecting Target Market

We have made and will continue to make suggestions as to how you can broaden your market appeal, that is, attract a diversity of people to your office. This we as a dental profession must do. As a diverse group of people ourselves, we can appeal to all. But, as individuals we cannot be all things to all people, and must concentrate on certain groups with whom we can relate to our mutual benefit. For this purpose, we select a target market.

Segmentation of the market is the first step in selecting the target group. Division of the general population into subgroups can be done by demographic variables such as age and socioeconomic factors. Although clinical specialties, except for pedodontics, are focused on particular kinds of dental conditions or diseases, the treatment tends to be of certain age groups. Thus, prosthodontists usually treat elderly people; oral surgeons and orthodontists, young people; and periodontists and endodontists, middle-aged people. Fees for specialty care tend to limit services to persons with upper middle incomes or persons with third party funding. Lower socioeconomic groups have tended to eliminate from their priorities all but the most essential dental service, such as the relief of pain and infection. In this way many people have eliminated themselves from the market for dental care.

The time has come for the dentists to seek out the most interested non-users.

In the evolving dental market, the dentist will find it much to his advantage to bring back into the market as many of these nonutilizers as possible. In the past, nonutilizers have opted out of the dental care system. Dentists have paid little attention to them because they could stay busy treating people who were interested. Now, dentists in many communities can no longer stay busy solely with people who come to them. The time has come for the dentists to seek out the most interested of the nonusers. Both dentists and people may be better off because of this change in busyness. Dentists can now practice at a less hectic pace, and more people will receive much needed dental treatment.

Some industries have tended to segment the market according to their product lines, rather than according to the characteristics and needs of the segments. A modern example of this marketing failure is the American automobile industry, which has until recently segmented the market according to the size of the car. An apparent assumption was that small cars did not require the same quality as large cars. Acceptance of the small, high quality foreign car has proved the fallacy of segmentation by product line. Indeed many Americans have bought small, expensive, high quality foreign cars, rather than the small, cheap, low quality American cars. Segmentation should be by groups whose needs *are* similar, rather than by groups who *appear* similar in their selection of products or services.

Segmentation by specialty is analogous to segmentation by product line and may place the specialist at a marketing disadvantage vis-a-vis the general dentist. The general dentist has the flexibility to segment the population according to needs, to study those needs, to determine whether he can satisfy them, and based on that determination, to select a group or groups for special attention.

In the dental market, segmentation may be obvious by some criteria but certainly less obvious by others. Edentulous people all need prosthetic replacements but vary considerably in what the service must include to satisfy their needs. Some are very fastidious and require the highest level of skill to satisfy their needs for esthetics, phonetics, and mastication. If they are wealthy, their only problem is to find a very skillful prosthodontist whose fee covers a highly sophisticated service. Others may be much less demanding and more concerned with cost. These people are more inclined to patronize the high-volume denture practice. It is up to the dentist to decide what segment(s) he can best satisfy and tailor his service to that segment or those segments.

> Segmentation should be by groups whose needs *are* similar.

Segmentation may be done in a reasonably scientific manner by using demographic traits. Data are readily available for many of these, such as age, sex, occupation, and education. Other, more qualitative traits represent needs for such things as status, privacy, economy, variety, and security.

However, we need not consider limitless possibilities. They must be limited in order to be manageable. The Stanford Research Institute, in a study of values and lifestyles, came up with a reasonable segmentation method and it can be applied in the dental market.

The need-driven group, composed of approximately 19 million adults, is described as follows: average family income $5,500; racial composition — one-third black; average education — nine years; age — one-third under 30 and 39 percent over 50; sex — 63 percent female. The forecast is for no change in number. Forced by low income to buy to satisfy basic needs, they are worried about survival and security and have little interest in cultural matters.

The belongers, 58 million adults, are described as follows: median family income $13,000; racial composition — blacks underrepresented; occupations — hard hat and ' clerical; age — average over 50; sex — two-thirds female. The forecast is for very mild growth. Income level does permit some discretionary purchases, most of which are for the purpose of fitting in or conforming. They tend to be puritanical, formal, matriarchal, reliable, and dependable.

Achievers are 37 million adults described as follows: income — 40 percent have family incomes over $25,000; race — 97 percent white; occupations — professional and managerial; age — average about

42; education — 60 percent have attended college; sex — most male of the groups. Very mild growth is forecast. These people are driving and driven, successful, able to buy the best, and willing to work hard for it.

Inner-directed, 26 million adults, are described as follows: income — average family income $20,000; race — about 90 percent white; occupations — professional and technical; age — average 32; education — highest of all groups; sex — evenly divided. Rapid growth is forecast. The most liberal and permissive of the groups, they strongly favor nontraditional political and moral views. More concerned with social than with personal needs, they buy to meet inner and expressive needs, which are very diverse and thus difficult to characterize.

How does the dentist approach these groups? As has been said many times, by understanding and satisfying their needs. If one is to serve the *need-driven* group, price is a dominant factor along with the ability to plan for the most basic kinds of treatment. Government-funded care is available to many of this group. If the *belongers* are concerned that a certain level of dental care is necessary to belong, they will attempt to purchase it. Fortunately many of them have dental insurance. If *achievers* are convinced that dental care is necessary for success, they have the means and will purchase it. Dental insurance is available to many of them, as it is to the inner-directed also. The motivation of the *inner-directed* is less clear, and they are perhaps the most challenging group. An individual (in this group) who values dental service will purchase it, but may be quite demanding as to its quality and perhaps as to its price.

Another system of segmentation is by social class, as shown in Table 2–2. The upper and middle classes include about 85 percent of the population and comprise most of the paying dental patients. The lower class, which is unemployed or employed in very menial jobs, can only obtain dentistry as part of a social benefit, or hardly at all.

Identification of people in these classes is easier than identification according to segmentation by the Stanford Research Institute. Answers to questions about (1) occupation and title, (2) education and age, and (3) neighborhood and mobility will usually be sufficient for classification.

We should be careful in applying these classifications and remember that no system of segmentation is perfect. A significant number of people do not fit into any particular group relative to

TABLE 2–2. SEGMENTATION OF THE U.S. POPULATION BY SOCIAL CLASS

Upper	15%
Middle	70%
Lower	15%

Source: Richard P. Coleman: The Significance of Social Stratification in Selling. Classics in Consumer Behavior. Lewis E. Boone, editor. Tulsa, Oklahoma, P.P.C. Books, 1977.

buying habits. Nevertheless, segmentation is helpful in making rough determinations as to the behavior expected from various groups. We believe that you should consider much of the behavior in groups to be similar, but that individuals are unique. Although promotion is to groups, the final decision to purchase a service is made by an individual.

Marketing Mix

After one has selected the target groups, one must then develop a marketing mix that appeals to that group. The marketing mix used in the commercial world consists of: product, price, promotion, and location. These have been translated for health to CAPS as described by McStravic in *Marketing Health Care.*

> C = consideration (price)
> A = access (place)
> P = promotion (promotion)
> S = service (product)

For our purposes, product will be considered service. The dentist may wish to refer to price as fee.

Given the target group and the parameters for the marketing mix, we can construct a grid, which is what marketers in industry do. The grid for segmentation by Stanford Research Institute is shown in Figure 2–4. As stated earlier the grid could be made much more complex by segmentation into more population groups and by further breaking down the marketing mix. The checks within the grid indicate what each group primarily seeks; the absence of a check within a square does *not* indicate total absence of interest.

The grid construction is based on certain assumptions. We assumed the segmentation method developed by Stanford Research Institute and arbitrarily selected the features of the marketing mix. You may choose to segment your market differently and to select a

A significant number of people do not fit into any particular group relative to buying habits.

	Crisis Oriented	Future Focused	Relief of Pain	Esthetics	Function	Comfort	Economy	Convenient Location	Artistic Decor of Office	Sophistication of Staff	Prestigious Location
Need Driven	X		X			X	X	X			
Belongers	X			X		X	X		X		
Achievers		X		X	X	X			X	X	X
Inner Directed		X				X	X			X	

Figure 2–4. Market grid for dentistry.

different marketing mix. Figure 2–4 is meant to suggest a practical segmentation and mix, but many other possibilities exist.

Another approach to the marketing mix is based on the segmentation by social class shown in Table 2–2. A problem in using this approach is that these groups may appear to have similar needs, but their needs vary just as the needs of purchasers of small automobiles do. People within these groups do not necessarily share values, and values tend to determine needs more than does social class.

Segmentation according to values as done by the Stanford Research Institute works best in a heterogeneous urban community where any of these groups is likely to be large enough to justify targeting. In small communities, segmentation by social class is easier. The mix of classes will vary in specific communities. As you plan your marketing mix, you may choose other elements to describe your practice, as well as other groupings more characteristic of your community. You need to segment the market and develop your marketing mix for your specific community.

Because treatment is provided to individuals not groups, the dentist must always assess individual needs and offer treatment to meet them.

Another caution regards the professional aspects of the marketing mix. We are not suggesting that a marketing mix less than professional is acceptable. Every patient should be treated in a caring considerate manner, but the different groups have different concerns in the service they seek. Certainly every group is concerned about relief of pain when hurting, but the *need-directed* group is most likely to require pain relief. Individuals may have needs more characteristic of another group than of their own. Because treatment is provided to individuals and not groups, the dentist must always assess individual needs and offer treatment to meet them.

Most of the comments about marketing mix referred to the service with some comments about price and place. More needs to be said now about price and later about place and promotion.

Pricing or setting fees can be done in various ways. The marketing rule of setting price in light of expected customer reaction may be as good as any. Classic ways of setting prices are according to cost or demand or competition. Defining competition for the dentist is difficult. The same nominal service, such as a two-surface amalgam, by another dentist may be far from equivalent, so that the fee charged by the other dentist may have little bearing on what your own fee should be. Many of us in dentistry take pride in establishing fair fees by cost of the service. Although this method appears fairest to us, it may not appear fair to the patient. They hardly want to pay for inefficiency which might account for a high fee. Nor do they enjoy paying out of meager earnings to support what they consider an outlandish lifestyle on the part of a dentist.

This brings us to "demand" as a means of pricing. Demand takes into account the reaction of the patient. This was what Henry Ford considered in determining the price of the Model T Ford. If we can determine that there is a significant market for our services in our communities at a given price level, we can, as Henry did, plan our methods of production so as to pay costs and derive a satisfactory profit. This may seem very commercial, but this general approach is necessary for successful marketing. Consumer needs include consideration for a fair price. The consumer cannot be expected to continue to pay a price that he considers exorbitant. However, he will pay a fair fee for a professional service that meets his needs rather than a lower price for a service that does not meet his needs. Services, carefully planned according to needs, will return a very adequate income to the professional provider.

SUMMARY

History shows that marketing is a natural result of progress in the marketplace. Dentistry is lagging in the development of a scientific marketing approach, but has an opportunity to make a quantum leap from the production era to the marketing era. Ethics demands marketing in its finest and most complete sense. The dentist should try to understand the characteristics and needs of his community. Once he understands the needs of various segments he can decide which group he can best serve. He should study that group or groups in depth and present his services in a form, at a price, and at a location most satisfactory to the target groups, and promote so as to make his potential patients aware of his service. By serving as needed in his community, he can manage exchanges at a profit. This is successful marketing.

Dentistry . . . has an opportunity to make a quantum leap from the production era to the marketing era.

REFERENCES

Coleman, R. P.: The Significance of Social Stratification in Selling. Classics in Consumer Behavior. Lewis E. Boone, editor. Tulsa, OK, P.P.C. Books, 1977.
Cooper, P. D.: Health Care Marketing. Germantown, MD, Aspen, 1979.
Heaton, H.: Economic History of Europe. New York, Harper and Brothers, 1948.
Journal of Marketing/Management for Professions, August, 1980, p. 5.
Levitt, T.: Marketing myopia. Harvard Business Review, July–August, 1960, pp. 45–56.
McCarthy, E. J.: Basic Marketing. Homewood, IL, Richard D. Irwin, Inc., 1971.
McCarthy, E. J.: Essentials of Marketing. Homewood, IL, Richard D. Irwin, Inc., 1979.
McStravic, R. E.: Marketing Health Care. Germantown, MD; Aspen, 1977.

3

The Ethics of Marketing

Dr. George Benton is disturbed about what is going on in dentistry and in his own practice. Several colleagues are under attack for their vigorous marketing activities. The ADA Principles of Ethics and Code of Professional Conduct appears to permit the activities in question, but many dentists feel that the tactics demean dentistry. George feels caught in a dilemma. Engaging in marketing as he understands it is distasteful to him personally. However, his practice is developing slowly. What is ethical? What is professional? What can he do to promote himself — without hurting others?

MEDICAL ETHICS

Medical ethics have varied greatly in different periods. The Hippocratic Oath emphasized one's obligation to colleagues and suggested how one should behave in the presence of patients. Love of humanity was an express concern of Galen's in the second century A.D. In 1240 Emperor Frederick II set high ideals in his law to regulate the practice of medicine. Thomas Percival of Manchester, England, in drawing up a code for his son about to enter medicine in the late 1700s, stressed good moral conduct of practitioners and patients, and disdained trickery. The original AMA Code (1846) was based in large part on Percival. At that time physicians were worried about homeopathic practitioners. Later concerns regarded fees, divulging information, membership, and service to humanity. As a result of German atrocities during World War II, the Nuremburg Code in 1946 dealt extensively with experimentation. Principles of Medical Ethics (1980), shown here, is the last of a half dozen major changes. The 1980 Code stresses obligations to patients and community and lessens attention to relationships with colleagues. Changes in the written principles of medical ethics have always reflected

> Changes in the written principles of medical ethics have always reflected contemporary societal ethics and the concerns of the profession at a given time.

contemporary societal ethics and the concerns of the profession at a given time.

ISSUES IN DENTAL ETHICS

Dental ethics have evolved in a fashion similar to medical ethics. It has been within the last twenty years that the most significant ethical changes have occurred, corresponding to a period of great changes in society as a whole. The ethical changes also relate directly to the production of an overabundance of dentists and increasing difficulty

---

PRINCIPLES OF MEDICAL ETHICS

PREAMBLE: The medical profession has long subscribed to a body of ethical statements developed primarily for the benefit of the patient. As a member of this profession, a physician must recognize responsibility not only to patients, but also to society, to other health professionals, and to self. The following Principles adopted by the American Medical Association are not laws, but standards of conduct which define the essentials of honorable behavior for the physician.

I. A physician shall be dedicated to providing competent medical service with compassion and respect for human dignity.

II. A physician shall deal honestly with patients and colleagues, and strive to expose those physicians deficient in character or competence, or who engage in fraud or deception.

III. A physician shall respect the law and also recognize a responsibility to seek changes in those requirements which are contrary to the best interests of the patient.

IV. A physician shall respect the rights of patients, of colleagues, and of other health professionals, and shall safeguard patient confidences within the constraints of the law.

V. A physician shall continue to study, apply and advance scientific knowledge, make relevant information available to patients, colleagues, and the public, obtain consultation, and use the talents of other health professionals when indicated.

VI. A physician shall, in the provision of appropriate patient care, except in emergencies, be free to choose whom to serve, with whom to associate, and the environment in which to provide medical services.

VII. A physician shall recognize a responsibility to participate in activities contributing to an improved community.

(Adopted by the HOUSE OF DELEGATES, American Medical Association on July 22, 1980, Chicago, Illinois.) Courtesy of the American Medical Association.

in building prosperous practices. In this section of the chapter, we shall look closely at changes in ethics as stated in the ADA code, quoting key passages at length. The overall tenor of the changes, as can be clearly seen, has been to allow dentists much greater freedom in marketing their services.

Presentation to the Public

The overall tenor of the changes . . . has been to allow dentists much greater freedom in marketing their services.

Restrictions as to how dentists may present or publicize themselves have gradually been lifted.

Cards, Letterheads, and Announcements (Section 13, 1962) stated: *A dentist may properly utilize professional cards, announcement cards, recall notices to patients of record and letterheads when the style and text are consistent with the dignity of the profession and with the custom of other dentists in the community.*

Announcement cards may be sent when there is a change in location or an alteration in the character of practice, but only to other dentists, to members of other health professions and to patients of record. This provision remained the same through 1978 when it was footnoted that *component and constituent dental societies be urged to refrain from initiating disciplinary proceedings for alleged violations of Sections 13, 14, 15, 16, 19, 20 and 21 of the Principles of Ethics until appropriate modifications can be considered by the 1979 House of Delegates.*

The 1980 Principles had no such provision. All restrictions on style of cards and to whom they might properly be sent had therefore been withdrawn.

Use of Professional Titles and Degrees (Section 15, 1962): *A dentist may use the titles or degrees, Doctor, Dentist, D.D.S., or D.M.D., in connection with his name on cards, letterheads, office door signs and announcements. A dentist who has been certified by a specialty board for one of the specialties approved by the American Dental Association may use the title "diplomate" in connection with his specialty on his cards, letterheads and announcements if such usage is consistent with the custom of dentists of the community. A dentist may not use his title or degree in connection with the promotion of any drug, agent, instrument or appliance.*

The use of eponyms in connection with drugs, agents, instruments or appliances is generally to be discouraged. This remained in effect until 1978, when it was footnoted as was Section 13. There was no such provision in 1980.

Directories (Section 19, 1962): *A dentist may permit the listing of his name in a directory provided that all dentists in similar circumstances have access to a similar listing and provided that such listing is consistent in style and text with the custom of the dentists in the community.* As did sections 13 and 15, this remained in effect until 1978 with the same footnote. It was absent from the 1980 Code.

Office Door Lettering and Signs (Section 14, 1962): *A dentist may properly utilize office door lettering and signs provided that their style and text are consistent with the dignity of the profession and with the custom of other dentists in the community.*

Use of the Terms "Clinic" and "Group Practice" (Section 16, 1962), also footnoted in 1978 and absent in 1980, strongly recommended against the use of the term "clinic" for private practice and suggested the term "group practice" when consistent "with existing statutes and the custom of the dentists in the community."

Name of the Practice (Section 20, 1972) essentially reworded Section 16 (1962) and was retained until 1978. It was reworded in 1980 to read: *The use of a trade name or an assumed name that is false or misleading in any material respect is unethical.*

Health Education of the Public (Section 20, 1962) stated: *A dentist may properly participate in a program of health education of the public involving such media as the press, radio, television and lecture, provided that such programs are in keeping with the dignity of the profession and the custom of the dental profession of the community.* This was also retained until 1978. It was eliminated from the 1980 Principles.

Contract Practice (Section 17, 1962): *A dentist may enter into an agreement with individuals and organizations to provide dental health care provided that the agreement does not permit or compel practices which are in violation of these Principles of Ethics.* This, too, remained unchanged until 1980, when it was dropped.

Advertising (Section 12, 1962): *Advertising reflects adversely on the dentist who employs it and lowers the public esteem of the dental profession. The dentist has the obligation of advancing his reputation for fidelity, judgment and skill solely through his professional services to his patients and to society. The use of advertising in any form to solicit patients is inconsistent with this obligation.* There were many advisory opinions interpreting this principle. Section 12, 1978, stated: *A dentist may advertise the availability of his services and the fees that he charges for routine procedures. No dentist shall advertise, in any form of communication, in a false, misleading, deceptive or fraudulent manner.* Advertising in Section 5A, 1980, was addressed in these words: *Although any dentist may advertise, no dentist shall advertise or solicit patients in any form of communication in a manner that is false or misleading in any material respect.*

> It is . . . easy to understand how many dentists . . . experience feelings toward dental advertising ranging from anguish to suspicion to uneasiness.

The foregoing change certainly is radical. Once advertising was not only described as something that reflected poorly on the individual dentist and on the profession as a whole but also was forbidden to dentists. Now advertising is allowed, the only provision being conformity to the law. It is therefore easy to understand how many dentists, especially those whose careers began well before the code changed, experience feelings toward dental advertising ranging from anguish to suspicion to uneasiness.

Announcement of specialization and limitation of practice as described in Section 5C, 1980, represents extensive change since 1962. At that time it was only possible to announce a "Practice limited to . . ." one specialty, and the word "Specialist . . . should be discouraged." The 1976 Principles permitted dentists to list themselves for all specialties for which they were qualified. Objection to the word "specialist" was dropped in 1980. Also, the 1980 Principles permit general dentists to announce the availability of services so long as they avoid any communications that express or imply "specialization."

The changes we have highlighted in the preceding paragraphs have enabled dentists to present themselves more directly to the public and to their colleagues as individuals. The Principles historically have discouraged individuality or any unique identification by a dentist. The 1980 Principles permit dentists to establish their own images with the public rather than restricting them to a rather indefinite image as a member of the group known as the dental profession. Such identification is considered essential to advertising for an individual business organization regardless of whether the business is providing a product or a service. Some even go so far as to say that the professional is obligated to today's public to characterize unique services (in advertising, if any) to help people make choices.

Relationships with Colleagues

Actually, no section of the ADA Code currently addresses itself directly to collegial relationships. An underlying theme of sections that relate to the dentists' presentation of themselves, however, is consideration for colleagues.

Justifiable Criticism and Expert Testimony

Section 1G, 1980, states: *Dentists shall be obliged to report to the appropriate reviewing agency instances of gross and/or continual faulty treatment by other dentists. If there is evidence of such treatment, the patient should be informed. Dentists shall be obliged to refrain from commenting disparagingly without justification about the services of other dentists. Dentists may provide expert testimony when that testimony is essential to a just and fair disposition of a judicial or administrative action.* This statement acknowledges concern for the interests of the patient, whereas prior to 1974 the primary concern seemed to be for the professional colleague, as expressed by this sentence: *The dentist has the obligation of not referring disparagingly to the services of another dentist in the presence of a patient.*

Service to the Public

Service to the Public and Quality of Care is addressed by Principle — Section 1 of the 1980 ADA Principles of Ethics and Code of Professional Conduct: *The dentist's primary obligation of service to the public shall include the delivery of quality care, competently and timely, within the bounds of the clinical circumstances presented by the patient. Quality of care shall be a primary consideration of the dental practitioner.*

Consultation (Section 7, 1962) states: *The dentist has the obligation of seeking consultation whenever the welfare of the patient will be safeguarded or advanced by having recourse to those who have special skills, knowledge and experience. A consultant will hold the details of a consultation in confidence and will not undertake treatment without the consent of the attending practitioner.* The 1978 and 1980 Principles specify the additional obligation of the consultant to *"return the patient . . . to the referring dentist"* and *"when there is no referring dentist . . . to inform patients when there is a need for further dental care."* The obligation of the specialist to the patient, which was ignored originally, is clarified. The current principle, by specifying the obligations of the consultant to the patient, expresses a concern for patients first articulated in 1978.

Use of Auxiliary Personnel (1F, 1980) says: *Dentists shall be obliged to protect the health of their patient by only assigning to qualified auxiliaries those duties which can be legally delegated. Dentists shall be further obliged to prescribe and supervise the work of all auxiliary personnel working under their direction and control.* Previous principles expressed a different orientation by the words *"not delegating . . . any service which requires the professional competence of a dentist."* Thus, what once was prohibited has become allowable, with dentists receiving approval for delegation of tasks they once had to perform strictly alone, so long as they supervise carefully.

Emergency Service (1D, 1980) provides: *Dentists shall be obliged to make reasonable arrangements for the emergency care of their patients of record. Dentists shall be obliged when consulted in an emergency by patients not of record to make reasonable arrangements for emergency care. If treatment is provided, the dentist, upon completion of such treatment, is obliged to return the patient to his or her regular dentist unless the patient expressly reveals a different preference.* Not until 1980 did the first statement appear which makes clear dentists' obligations to their own patients needing emergency services.

Patient Selection (1A, 1980) states: *While dentists, in serving the public, may exercise reasonable discretion in selecting patients for their practices, dentists shall not refuse to accept patients into their practice or deny dental service to patients because of the patient's race, creed, color, sex or national origin.* The reference to *"race, creed, color, sex or national origin"* first appeared in 1972.

Patient Records (1B, 1980): *Dentists are obliged to safeguard the confidentiality of patient records. Dentists shall maintain patient records in a manner consistent with the protection of the welfare of the patient. Upon request of a patient or another dental practitioner, dentists shall provide any information that will be beneficial for the future treatment of that patient.* This appeared for the first time in 1980.

Changes in dental ethics over the last twenty years have reached the point at which dentists may feel full approval for their efforts to expand their practices by advertising and by numerous other promotional techniques.

Professional Announcement Principle — Section 5 (1980) states: *In order to properly serve the public, dentists should represent themselves in a manner that contributes to the esteem of the profession. Dentists should not misrepresent their training and competence in any way that would be false or misleading in any material respect.* The provision about what contributes *"to the esteem of the profession"* is subject to interpretation.

Guidelines on advertising are as follows: *Advertising, solicitation of patients or business, or other promotional activities by dentists or dental care delivery organizations shall not be considered unethical or improper, except for those promotional activities which are false or misleading in any material respect. Notwithstanding any ADA* Principles of Ethics and Code of Professional Conduct *or other standards of dentist conduct which may be differently worded, this shall be the sole standard for determining the ethical propriety of such promotional activities. Any provision of an ADA constituent or component society's code of ethics or other standard of dentist conduct*

> What once was prohibited has become allowable, with dentists receiving approval for delegation of tasks they once had to perform strictly alone, so long as they supervise carefully.

relating to dentists' or dental care delivery organizations' advertising, solicitation, or other promotional activities which is worded differently from the above standard shall be deemed to be in conflict with the ADA Principles of Ethics and Code of Professional Conduct.

Only false and misleading advertising is unethical. Such advertising, of course, is also illegal.

State laws about advertising and promotion vary. Some are more restrictive than the current code. The trend is similar to that of the ADA Code so that eventually whatever is permitted by the code is likely to be permitted in each state. You may choose to challenge the law in order to accelerate change in your state. However, unless you want to challenge the law, you should carefully abide by your state law.

ETHICS AND PROFESSIONAL CONDUCT

The Development of Ethics

Professional ethics for health-care practitioners have long been subject to controversy. In interpretations of the Hippocratic Oath, for example, confusion developed between notions of what was acceptable professional conduct and notions about obligations of candor toward patients. Although "benefit of the sick" was an avowed aim of the oath, Pythagoreans tended to emphasize professionals' conduct in the view of their colleagues, and certain points of etiquette in the presence of patients.

Current principles of ethics in both medicine and dentistry put more emphasis on obligations to patients and to society than they do on obligations to colleagues.

In decades past the collegial relationship tended to take precedence over the relationship to patients. This precedence can be traced back to Hippocrates' day. Then, the young Greek physicians were indebted to their teachers for sharing knowledge that enabled the junior physicians to learn and practice medicine. Because of this sharing, a bond was struck between the young practitioners and their teachers, and others who had taken the oath.

Now, the current principles of ethics in both medicine and dentistry put more emphasis on obligations to patients and to society than they do on obligations to colleagues. Nevertheless, a sense of covenant with colleagues remains potent. It may be hard for some dentists to accept fully our present code and relinquish the emphasis on collegial relationships.

In fact the 1980 ADA Principles of Ethics and Code of Professional Conduct dispels much of the confusion regarding ethics and professionalism. The five principles of ethics address: (1) Service to the Public and Quality of Care; (2) Education; (3) Government of a Profession; (4) Research and Development; and (5) Professional Announcement. Under each of these principles except for 2 and 3 are stated the Code of Professional Conduct by subheadings. These items under the codes replace many of the sections formerly stated as principles. Although the current principles deal with professional issues, the basic concern is quality service to society as expressed in such phrases as "service to the public," "promoting the health of the public," and "properly serve the public."

Ethical Issues

Biomedical ethics is evolving with a great deal of input from philosophers, sociologists, political scientists, and theologians. Ethical issues in medicine potentially may have tremendous impact on all our lives. Threat to life is not to be taken lightly. Consequently many of our best thinkers have devoted themselves to questions of biomedical ethics.

What can we learn from these creative minds that will help us with the ethics of marketing? Let us look at some of the basic principles. According to Beauchamp and Childress these are: (1) autonomy, (2) nonmaleficence, (3) beneficence, and (4) justice.

Nonmaleficence was expressed in the Hippocratic Oath in terms of doing no harm. Ethical marketing must conform to this principle. Advertising or other promotion that is false or misleading is ruled out on this basis. Activity that detracts from the esteem of the profession is not permissible. Clearly, a marketing program that misleads patients or creates public suspicion of other dentists is wrong.

Beneficence is "the duty to help others further their important and legitimate interests when we can do so with minimal risks to ourselves." The foundation of marketing is the understanding of needs (interests) and the provision of a service to satisfy those needs in a manner acceptable to consumers. Doing good (beneficence) includes the removal of harmful conditions beyond the noninfliction of harm (nonmaleficence). If marketing does good for patients by informing them of a service in their interest, *it must be seen as beneficent.* Good can also be done for colleagues by marketing efforts that heighten dental awareness. Beneficent activities enhance the long-term effectiveness of marketing. We recommend that you do good (be beneficent) in your program.

Justice, as a principle, can be elusive. Some moral philosophers consider "fairness" the equivalent of "justice." Others say that justice prevails when people receive what they deserve. Thus, in regard to advertising, some say that it is only "fair" or "just" that the public be able to learn about dentists and their services through the media, the way they learn about other services and products. The courts so held and rendered it impossible to prohibit dentists from advertising. This ruling may trouble many of us who have practiced dentistry in different days, yet it is difficult to argue against the "fairness" of allowing dentists to tell the public about their services.

A case can surely be made, however, against those marketers of dental service who are inclined toward unethical and unprofessional advertising. They indeed threaten fairness, or justice, to all dentists. We should invoke the Principles and Codes to discourage questionable conduct. Outright illegal activity, of course, should be called to the attention of civil authorities.

"Autonomy is a form of personal liberty of action where the individual determines his or her own course of action in accordance with a plan chosen by himself or herself." Freedom of choice is everyone's right. In order to choose freely, one must obtain or be provided necessary information, which for the dental patient includes understanding of the problem, alternative solutions or treatments,

Clearly, a marketing program that misleads patients or creates public suspicion of other dentists is wrong.

A noncoercive climate ought to prevail in the office, so that patients can choose freely and can expect complete support from the dental team.

and consequences or expectations of the alternatives. A noncoercive climate ought to prevail in the office, so that patients can choose freely and can expect complete support from the dental team.

We will elaborate on this in Chapter 12, but for the moment let us explain a bit further. Patients should be autonomous in the dental office regarding the way they choose to deal with their dental problems. We are obliged to provide information to people and to market effectively, and we must support them in their decisions. We may, however, find ourselves in a bind if their decisions are harmful to themselves. If we are firmly convinced that the decision is harmful, we will probably find it necessary to provide more information. In no case must we promote treatment that we believe to be harmful. But we have no right to impose our values on patients to the extent that we will not allow them to believe that anything less than ideal treatment is adequate.

To be ethical, promotion also must provide *accurate*, though not complete, information to the public. The information should be accurate in spirit as well as literally so that the ordinary person is likely to understand the message. Again, subjective interpretation is necessary and differences of opinion will exist. With some difficulty the dental profession should be able to resolve these differences. Indeed, if we are to measure up as a profession capable of governing ourselves, we have no choice.

Not that facilitating autonomy for our patients is always easy or simple. Both dentists and their patients have for years interacted in communication patterns that have bordered on the paternalistic — and sometimes even the authoritarian. Dentists have been used to saying things such as "Now, Art, you're going to need some pretty deep endo work, followed by a couple of gold crowns and probably one gold inlay. When can we schedule that?" Or, "Mrs. Greenfield, your little Marcie is a prime candidate for braces. I'm afraid her teeth will just never be right without them." Or — the more authoritarian model: "Paul, come back next Tuesday and we'll get started on that bridgework. There's just no way around it; you need to have it done." Not only have dentists become accustomed to saying such things, patients have grown used to hearing them — and accepting them with few or no questions.

As Warner and Segal have observed, from the time of Hippocrates physicians have been caring for patients as they (the physicians) see fit. The healing arts have endorsed "doing what is best for a patient by a particular conception of 'what is best.'" We in dentistry have very naturally been treating our patients in a similar manner. If we believe that people, given sufficient information, can assume responsibility for their own problems, we must then avoid the overt paternalism that has characterized much of our practice. Covert paternalism is very difficult to avoid. In communicating with our patients about their treatment options, we are likely to provide information in such a manner that they will choose what we think is best. How can we let people go over the precipice with their dental health when we have the means to preserve their health?

Our dental philosophers such as Pankey, Barkley, Reed, and King tell us that we cannot preserve our patients' dental health.

Promotion information should be accurate in spirit as well as literally.

Individuals must preserve, conserve, and cultivate their own health; yet, surely, we can advise them. Indeed, we are ethically bound to do so, but we cannot ethically *decide for them* if we observe the ethical principle of autonomy.

The current Principles and Codes permit a high degree of autonomy to the dentist. The Association no longer relates to individual dentists in a paternalistic manner. Dentists enjoy a great deal of freedom in the way they relate to their colleagues and to their patients. Yet the interests of patients and of colleagues are sufficiently protected. Indeed, our Principles and Codes are quite soundly based in the general principles of biomedical ethics espoused by Beauchamp and Childress.

The Necessity of Ethics and Professional Conduct

The interests of patients and of society are the basis of dental ethics. Fortunately our current principles enable us to pay attention to our patients' interests without harming our colleagues' interests. However, many of us find it difficult "to report to the appropriate reviewing agency instances of gross and/or continual faulty treatment by other dentists" and to so inform the patient. We also have some difficulty with the line "any dentist may advertise." None of us is likely to argue that we should not police ourselves, difficult though it may be. All of us must face up to the fact that our code of professional conduct permits behavior that was formerly proscribed. Governmental agencies have maintained and won their point that such conduct opens up the profession and makes it more responsive to people's needs. Although many dentists are opposed to advertising, we must now acknowledge the right of any dentist to advertise so long as it is not "in a manner that is false or misleading." Other provisions of the code regarding patient records, emergency service, consultation, and referral enhance the benefit to patients. These provisions are evidence of concern for patients, surely an ethical foundation for professional practice.

Now that we no longer can ethically protect a colleague and fail to look out for the interests of patients, we run the risk of paying less attention to the welfare of colleagues than that consideration deserves. Concern for self and lack of concern for others, as expressed by the "me generation," detracts from the quality of collegial relationships. Traditional values, most of which are worthy of survival, appear beleaguered. Professional groups, because of their conservative attitudes toward change, may well be able to preserve and observe these values better than society generally. We believe that these values of concern for colleagues' welfare should continue among dentists. In no way, for instance, should a dentist's marketing program detract from another dentist's reputation.

However, the attempts to control marketing programs, especially advertising, may be quite arbitrary. Such attempts have occurred in certain geographic areas and have restricted rather severely the image that a dentist could project in his advertising. Discomfort with the idea of advertising, which is very understandable, may have

Although many dentists are opposed to advertising, we must now acknowledge the right of any dentist to advertise so long as it is not "in a manner that is false or misleading."

prompted these attempts. Nevertheless, the ADA Code clarifies this issue; it is only false or misleading advertising that is unethical. The Code uses these words: *Any provision of an ADA constituent or component society's code of ethics or other standard of dentist's conduct relating to dentists' or dental care delivery organizations' advertising, solicitation, or other promotional activities which is worded differently from the above standard shall be deemed to be in conflict with the ADA Principles of Ethics and Code of Professional Conduct.*

The question of what constitutes false or misleading advertising can only be answered definitely in the courts. Civil court action to define what started out to be a professional issue may be distasteful to most of us. Others would argue that the people have a protectable interest in this definition and deserve an open forum for its formulation. None of us could justifiably argue that our own professional concerns ought to take precedence over the concerns of the people at large.

We believe that ethical codes are necessary to protect the people and the profession. In this newly expressed concern for the people exemplified in the 1980 code, we are faced with the problems of implementation. Interpretation by individual dentists, and constituent and component societies is necessary. Variations in interpretation are likely and will probably create some differences among dentists. Out of this conflict ought to come a resolution of the differences that will benefit the people and also be acceptable to dentists.

MARKETING, ETHICS, AND PROFESSIONAL CONDUCT

What can George Benton do to promote himself or market his services without hurting his colleagues and without violating the Code of Professional Conduct? What reward is reasonable for him to expect for his efforts as a dentist? What can marketing do for him? For his patients? Let us see.

The Good Life

The "pursuit of happiness" is justified by one's concern for others' happiness. We may not, however, claim this pursuit for ourselves while we deny it to others.

Mortimer J. Adler describes the good life as: freedom of choice, freedom from coercion, and time for leisure or creativity. Individuals are entitled to the good life so long as they discharge their obligation of facilitating the good life for others. The "pursuit of happiness" is justified by one's concern for others' happiness. We may not, however, claim this pursuit for ourselves while we deny it to others.

Dentists' *freedom of choice* is enhanced by the new ethics and their consequent codes of conduct. The various delivery systems provide opportunities for dentists to practice in many different kinds of settings. From the restrictive code that declared closed panels unethical, we have come to the point where dentists are encouraged to behave in a *"manner that contributes to the esteem of the profession"* and are only forbidden to behave in a manner that is *"false or misleading."* Office door lettering and signs, cards, letterheads and announcements, and contract practice are no longer mentioned in the new code. More salaried positions are available than formerly. The number of dentists in group practice or cost-sharing arrangements is increasing. With more dentists accepting salaried positions, there are more opportunities in independent or small group practices for those with the necessary ability in management and marketing. Although risks have increased, the freedom of choice has been multiplied.

Coercion is not characteristic of the current principles and codes. Most requirements of the code, some more than others, are based on our obligations to patients. Thus they are no more coercive than our laws regarding individual rights. Surely we all believe that our neighbors' rights do not coerce our behavior unreasonably. In fact we are reassured that our own rights are not to be violated by others. As individuals we need to respect others' rights; as dentists we need to respect our patients' rights.

Time for leisure or creativity implies the ability to afford an appropriate use of such time. If we as dentists by our efforts enable others to enjoy the good life, we are entitled to appropriate compensation. Obviously we are obligated to relate to our patients in such a way as to honor their freedom of choice, as not to coerce them, and as not to interfere with their time for leisure or creativity. To enable them to exercise their freedom of choice, we have to provide them with information on which to base a choice in a noncoercive atmosphere. If we are not to interfere with their time for leisure or creativity, we must set fees that are reasonable enough not to deprive them of the ability to afford appropriate use of their leisure time.

> We must make treatment available that our patients can afford.

Not only must we set fees that do not deprive patients of such liberties, but we must make treatment available that they can afford. Of course, some rearrangement of their priorities may be necessary, but paying dental fees should not throw their lives into turmoil. Fortunately dental insurance has enabled many dentists to provide very adequate treatment without penalizing patients financially.

As professionals we surely believe that our services are useful to everybody. The 75 percent of the people who utilize us poorly could enjoy an improved quality of life from good dental care. Ethics and professionalism require our concern for everyone. Of course, our offices have always been open, and we provide care to everyone who seeks it. The time has come for us to reach out more to those who have not made the effort to get dental care. If we believe in the system of private practice (the most efficient in the world) we need to try to make it work for everyone. Our efforts will certainly improve our own professional lives and our economic status.

A logical extension from our private offices is to the public sector of dentistry. Local health departments provide care for people who cannot obtain care in private offices because of lack of personal resources or lack of third party funding. If by Adler's terms, we dentists are entitled to the good life, we must concern ourselves with dental service for people who cannot afford our services. Consequently we will take an interest in the public sector. We will make an effort to see that care is provided in such a way as to meet the needs of all people. As described by Graff (see References), care should be available which is:

1. accessible and convenient

2. of satisfactory quality
3. efficacious
4. provided in an environment acceptable to recipients.

Additionally, this care should provide freedom of choice — that is, freedom from coercion, and should not compromise leisure time. The attitude of a community toward its dentists will be favorable if the dentists show concern for the needs of the community, including its less fortunate members. We can expect people to value our services as we make them available to everyone.

The attitude of a community toward its dentists will be favorable if the dentists show concern for the needs of the community, including its less fortunate members.

Professional Conduct

Professional conduct presents a sticky problem for most of us in planning our marketing strategy. Health professionals have been more sensitive to what colleagues think than have other professionals. As Sperry has observed, lawyers and professors attack each other, theologians spar with each other, but not so the doctors. He goes on to point out that an outsider is struck by how much attention the code of ethics (prior to 1980) gives to relationships with colleagues. We dentists will surely continue to be sensitive to what our fellow dentists think about our marketing efforts.

But . . . times *have* changed. Formerly the dentist was expected to advance "his reputation . . . *solely* through his professional services to his patients and to society." The predominant ethic for accountants was that practice growth resulted from reputation and quality. Certainly, high quality professional service by both dentists and accountants is required, but it is no longer sufficient for the recent graduate attempting to build a practice in a community where patients and clients can already obtain appointments without delay.

To survive and preferably to thrive in most geographic areas, marketing is essential. When the old ethic of growth based solely on professional services was codified in our Principles, marketing as we are describing it was not essential. However, as we observe throughout this book, the most successful dentists have *always* been successful marketers. But in times past, effective marketing did not need to be as aggressive as it does now. Although most dentists who were effective marketers under the old ethic continue to do well, many find their patient volume decreasing, especially in crowded urban areas. Thus they find their marketing of services needs to become more pronounced. Yet marketing that is *too* aggressive may be hazardous to the profession's health. Advertising that verges on being misleading can create problems for the advertiser, for other dentists, and for patients. Clearly this is not desirable. As we have pointed out, dentists *do* have the right to advertise the uniqueness of their services. If people are misled by such advertising, the advertiser is behaving unethically. The autonomy of each individual is limited at the point at which it interferes with autonomy of another dentist or consumer. Sensitivity to the interests of others should ensure that we do no harm. Dentists, new in practice, find themselves in a buyers' market. If they merely open their doors and wait for patients to seek them out, as dentists could do successfully in the past, they may find little demand. Most new dentists discover early in practice that they must promote themselves.

"Practice promotion" has been an acceptable term and activity with most dentists for some time now. "Marketing" is a new term in dentistry and may offend some dentists. Actually we believe that "marketing" is a more accurate and less self-serving term than "promotion." If you are more comfortable with promotion, fine. We hope that you are, or will become, comfortable with marketing, according to the new ethic as defined in the 1980 Principles and Codes. We believe that it is in your interest and in that of your patients for you to market your service in your community in accord with the new ADA Principles of Ethics and Code of Professional Conduct, with a view to the public interest and with great sensitivity to the interests of your colleagues.

REFERENCES

Adler, F.: An Ethical Philosophy of Life. New York, Regina Press, 1975.

Adler, M. J.: The Time of Our Lives: The Ethics of Common Sense. New York, Holt, Rinehart & Winston, 1970.

Beauchamp, T. L., Childress, J. F.: Principles of Biomedical Ethics. New York, Oxford University Press, 1979.

Graff, L.: On patient satisfaction, marketing research, and other useful things. Hospitals 53(2):59–62, 1979.

Mahon, J. J.: The Marketing of Professional Accounting Services. New York, Wiley, 1978.

May, W. F.: Code and covenant or philanthropy and contract. Hastings Center Report 5:29–38, 1975.

Reiser, S. J., Dyck, A. J. (eds.): Ethics in Medicine. Boston, MIT Press, 1977.

Sperry, W. L.: The Ethical Basis of Medical Practice. New York, Paul B. Hoeber, Inc. (Med Book Dept of Harper & Brothers), 1956.

Warner, R., Segal, H.: Ethical Issues of Informed Consent in Dentistry, Chicago, Quintessence Publishing Company, 1980.

4

Changing Your Self-Image

Hal Longstreet wasn't sure he could take any more change. It seemed as though he had been changing all his life. Now, after seventeen years as a successful pedodontist, his patient load was slowly dwindling—to the point where he was going to have to take on patients other than children. He had, of course, on occasion treated adults, but now he was going to have to make a concerted effort to attract adults to his practice. In other words, Hal was going to have to change his way of practicing. "But," Hal wondered, "can I still change after all these years?"

REASONS FOR CHANGE

A dentist today can be compared to a musician who was reared on the Big Band sound but now, given changes in taste, attitude, and buying habits among the public, has to learn to play new tunes. He is still using the same instruments — that is, his office space, his dental equipment, his training, his staff. However, the way in which everything is orchestrated now must match up to the reality of an economy in which marketing dental care is not a frill, but a necessity.

Sometimes it is hard and even painful for a musician to learn to make new sounds with his familiar old instruments. The new sounds jar against his ear. He has been playing the old tunes for so long, and he is so comfortable with them, that it feels terribly risky and possibly also awkward to try something new. The new sounds appear to have such a tenuous relationship to the old ones; everything seems "turned around," "changed." And, although everything isn't, *some* things are.

A fair percentage of today's public thinks of dentistry as something of a "luxury" — except when pain occurs. This part of the public has to be wooed into the office if all dentists now practicing or coming into the profession in the 1980s and 1990s are to earn a

Many senior citizens have gone decades without dental care. Yet it will take a special sort of appeal to convince them of the merits of restoration.

livelihood. Many senior citizens have gone decades without dental care. Yet it will take a special sort of appeal to convince them of the merits of restoration.

The trouble is, dentists are still being trained primarily as technicians, very little as businesspersons or marketers. And the nontechnical skills are nowadays as important for the economic well-being of dentists as are the technical ones.

For many dentists today possibly the hardest thing to deal with is that in dental school no one mentioned to them that marketing was becoming increasingly important. So much time was spent on the biology of oral tissues, on identifying and treating caries, on prosthodontics, and on endodontics that hardly anybody spoke about the problems of attracting and holding on to patients. Patient availability, upon which an individual dentist's very livelihood depends, was virtually ignored. In fairness to the schools, it must be said that this area was not emphasized simply because the change to a marketing economy in dentistry has been so recent. Any school curriculum is molded over years, decades even, of trying out and proving certain subjects; it takes time for new coursework to be developed and become woven into the routine. (This is as true of history or economics as it is of dentistry.)

What today's dentist needs, in order to make a transition to becoming a marketer in addition to being a good dentist, is a certain degree of open-mindedness. As Ben Franklin remarked, "Be not the first by whom the new is tried, nor yet the last to lay the old aside." At this point, you certainly will not be the first by whom a new thing is tried if you absorb the information in this book and then proceed to apply as much of it as you think practical to your own situation. A small but progressive minority of dentists has been engaged in active marketing of their practices for at least five years now. Others are beginning to venture out with various marketing techniques, from restyling their offices, to altering their payment plans, to starting a newsletter.

If you adopt a posture of open-mindedness, you have a lot to gain and not much to lose — although it may, at first, *feel* as though you are losing a lot. What can you gain? You can, above all else, gain patients and consequently income. You can gain a more prominent status in the community in which you practice. You can, too, acquire a new sense of self-confidence, which comes to any successful businessman. As we have shown, in the scarcity era, and even later, in the selling era, dentists did not need to gain confidence as businessmen. Their problem was learning how to manage all the business that simply tumbled in the door. Today, however, a successful dentist is likely to be as adept at marketing as is the owner of a thriving restaurant or movie theater.

What you have to lose is a certain notion or concept that you may have long cherished about what it means to be a dentist. In considering the profession, in all probability your least worry was where to find patients. It may well be that one reason you chose to embark upon dentistry as a career was the sense of security that the idea of being a dentist conveyed to you. It may have seemed about as secure as the idea of being a physician. In actuality, a small percentage of den-

Possibly the hardest thing to deal with for many dentists today is that no one mentioned to them in dental school the fact that marketing was becoming increasingly important.

tists — perhaps 20 per cent or so — are said to enjoy thinking of themselves as physicians of the mouth and relate themselves, in their own self-images, with physicians. Obviously, oral surgeons would tend toward this self-image, but it is not an uncommon image among other dental practitioners as well. Physicians, even more than dentists, are having a difficult time these days coming to terms with fitting themselves into the role of marketer. Struggling with a shortage of patients was not part of the professional image they envisioned for themselves.

Dealing With Ego

The key to coming to terms with a change in your image of yourself as a professional lies in that old adage of Socrates, "Know thyself." It would be wrong, and harmful, to attempt to gloss over the pain and the depth of feeling involved in this sort of an image change. Your ego may well be "on the line." So may your need for security (which may have been high among your priorities when you chose to enter dentistry). What is more, your family is counting on you to project a successful image, to be a better-than-average provider, and perhaps even to be a community leader or prominent figure. These expectations are hard to reconcile with a dearth of patients and a backlog of loan payments and other bills. Therefore, it is first of all important for you to take stock of just what your notions of yourself as a dentist have been, how they were formed, and what they mean to you — and to those "significant others" in your life, such as your spouse and children, your parents, your in-laws, your close friends, and peers. So, admit the depth of your feelings, and get in touch with them. (For this purpose, it may be helpful to engage in some counseling with a psychologist or perhaps take part in a group counseling process.)

The next step in dealing with your ego is to attempt to rethink some of the old stereotypes of a dentist, to challenge them, and to see if some new images of a dentist cannot emerge from the process. Just because a dentist now has to make an effort to attract patients does not mean, for instance, that he is any less a professional than his counterpart of past years. Remember too, that dentists indeed have been marketing all along, in various ways. They have, no less than many other individuals in business practice, tried to spruce up their offices with plants, pictures, and warm carpeting. They have hired staff with pleasing personalities who would help increase the number of patients. And they have striven to become more visible members of their local communities through club work and other associations. And above all, they have tried to treat patients as they would members of their own families. Without anyone telling them about the marketing skills described in this book, these dentists have nonetheless adopted many of our points in building their practice. In a word, they have shown themselves to be "natural marketers."

Not everyone is a natural. Most of us have to be taught how to market. And there's nothing wrong with admitting that we may have to learn and consciously begin to apply what to someone else–even someone else in our own profession — is second nature.

Attempt to rethink some of the old stereotypes of a dentist, to challenge them, and to see if some new images of a dentist can emerge from the process.

Most of us have to be taught how to market. We may have to learn and consciously begin to apply what to someone else — even someone else in our own profession — is second nature.

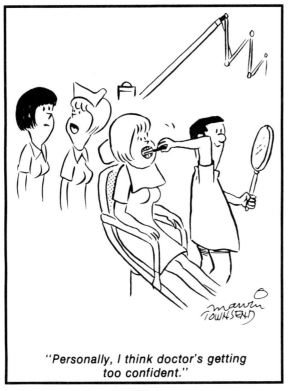

"Personally, I think doctor's getting too confident."

Courtesy of *Cal* magazine.

Barriers to Change

Deciding to make a change and effecting the change are two different things. Not that one is harder than the other. For various individuals, deciding may be harder; for others, effecting may be harder. The important thing to understand is that they are two separate processes, though not unrelated.

The fact that you purchased this book and that you have read this far suggests that you are 80 percent of the way toward deciding to make a change. It does not indicate that you have yet begun to make that change.

Typically, parents who enroll in a Parent Effectiveness Training course are having trouble coping with their children, and often have decided that some change in their (the parents') behavior may facilitate the parenting process. They enroll for the course, pay the registration fee, purchase the required books, and appear on time to attend the classes. Their actions indicate some readiness to make a change. What happens in the classes, however? Experienced PET instructors 'heave long "sighs" and tell of massive resistance on the part of many of the registrants. The parents listen to the teacher describe the new parenting techniques, take notes, and even go home determined to apply them. But some never do; they balk. Others fidget with their children and apply the techniques half-heartedly. They then return to class prepared to resist even more. A minority of PET registrants, it appears, actually make a breakthrough in their parenting habits and apply the new techniques.

A leader of "self-awareness" psychological workshops recounts stories of similar behavior on the part of people who fly to his center from great distances to raise their consciousness and achieve a breakthrough to their "real selves." They expend large sums of money and a significant block of time, then dig their heels in and refuse to drop their defenses and their rigid acquired behavior and let their "inner selves" come forth.

Effecting changes of attitudes — when old feelings and notions are deeply ingrained — can be extremely painful. When the pain begins to assert itself, the temptation is to draw back, to revoke the decision to change. That is why many people who decide to make ego changes, or image changes, fail to put the changes into practice. The changes remain merely mental notes — "things to do — someday."

Visiting another dentist can be very helpful. Pick out some friend or colleague who has made or is making some of the changes you are considering. Invite him to lunch or go to see him; tell him what you're considering; and ask about his experience. You may get some very good ideas that will make your change easier.

It is important to keep in mind that effecting the change of ego, or of image, once you have made a firm decision to do so, probably will "feel funny." It may even hurt, psychologically speaking. It is supposed to. That is to say, the "funny feelings" or even the "hurt" are natural reactions of your inner self to deep ego change. Let yourself feel funny, or hurt, and go forward with the changes you have decided upon. Gradually, the new ways will no longer cause you to feel strange or hurt; by and by, the techniques you begin to apply will become commonplace or normal. You will then be "catching up" with those colleagues who happen to be "natural marketers."

IMPLEMENTING CHANGE

Try to estimate to just what degree some technique or other would feel "strange." Don't push yourself beyond certain limits.

The changes that you may want to implement will have to be ones that you are convinced will affect your professional and personal situation for the better within a short time. These will vary from dentist to dentist. In subsequent chapters of this book, we will be discussing a wide range of marketing techniques, from the provision of insurance assignment and other financial incentives for patients and employees, to advertising in various media, to such interpersonal communications as newsletters and birthday greeting cards, and many others. Which of these techniques you decide to try, and in what order, will have to be your decision. Only you can tell how "funny" or how "painful" a change may feel. We would advise, however, that you pay careful attention to your feelings, right in the pit of your stomach, as you read. Try to estimate to just what degree some technique or other would feel "strange." Don't push yourself beyond certain limits. There is no point in trying, as a first step, what appears to you to be the most uncomfortable or outlandish technique. You will find that the psychological pain probably will be more than you can bear, and you may decide that you have had your fill of marketing. Choose the techniques that seem logical and that would stand a good chance of producing some fairly immediate results. There is nothing in the world like a positive result, such as a measurable increase in business, to confirm the change process for an individual.

A high degree of self-reliance, as described by John Cowan, is required. Research shows that most Americans are not high in this quality. Less courage and daring are required to be one of the crowd. Conformity is easier for most people in our culture, but not very rewarding. If you are to bring about change in yourself, you cannot be one of the herd. You must resolve to take responsibility and seek the necessary assistance to carry out your purpose. It takes tenacity.

Pay attention to the changes in attitude on the part of your staff. They too may have psychological barriers to the idea of being part of a marketing program. It is likely, however, that their degree of resistance to marketing will not be as strong as your own. As they see you, the dentist, begin to effect changes in your image of yourself, they will logically follow suit.

Of course watch your patients' reactions. The health-care professions have not kept strictly to themselves their notion that professionalism is separate from marketing. Inevitably, their ideas of professionalism have been communicated to the general public. Thus, some resistance to marketing may crop up among the public with whom you yourself deal. Your first advertisement in a local weekly newspaper, for example — should you venture in that direction — may evoke a skeptical comment or two from patients and peers. Again, however, resistance to dental marketing is not nearly so embedded in the public mind as it has been in the minds of dentists themselves. Therefore, if you are sensitive to good taste in all that you attempt, any public resistance that you perceive at the outset will gradually melt away.

> Some resistance to marketing may crop up among the public with whom you yourself deal. But if you are sensitive to good taste in all that you attempt, any public resistance that you perceive at the outset will gradually melt away.

Coping With Change

Hal Longstreet had decided to change. Instead of restricting his practice to people under the age of 16, he was going to open himself up for the full range. In other words, he would change from pedodontics to general practice. And he was going to have to do some unusual things to make the conversion.

He hesitated before calling a meeting of his staff — his receptionist-secretary-bookkeeper, Sally; his hygienist, Debbie; and his assistant, Paulette. Yet what was the choice? Sally knew the figures. It was not unlikely that she had dropped at least a hint or two to Debbie and Paulette during their frequent TGIFs together. The practice was in the doldrums and bills were backing up; credit was being stretched farther and farther by the suppliers and banks, but there would be limits — soon.

Hal was surprised when the three young women responded enthusiastically to the news of a change. "It's past due!" was their general reaction. "Let's do it! Lead the way!"

Fortunately, Hal lived in a metropolitan area in which the services of a marketing professional with some expertise in advising health-care professionals were available. The consultant, Peter Jamisson, advised Hal to send tastefully printed notes home with his juvenile patients, announcing the change to general practice but stressing that he would always remain devoted to treating youngsters. The next step would come later on, the consultant advised. One thing at a time.

When the adults began to come, first in a trickle, later in a steadier flow, Hal Longstreet, again upon Peter Jamisson's advice, made a point of asking each one whether he or she would feel more comfortable if the office were redecorated out of the children motif (a circus in full swing, with clowns, elephants, and tight-rope walkers painted on the walls). A few said a weak "maybe," but others said more emphatic "no's." Adults, like children, love a circus, the informal survey showed. Nonetheless, Hal redecorated one operatory into pleasingly traditional "adult" tones — a celestial blue — that yet held some attraction for his traditional pedodontic patients. He left the lobby, the halls and the other treatment room in the circus motif. And he offered free coffee along with the *The Wall Street Journal*, *Time*, *Harper's*, *Saturday Review*, and *Mademoiselle*.

That done, Peter Jamisson suggested some modest advertising. In the beginning, just announcements in the daily and weekly newspapers of the community stating: "Hal Longstreet is pleased to announce that he is now accepting adults as well as children in his practice of dentistry. A caring atmosphere at a minimum of pain to the mouth and the checkbook." Hal kept his ads in the paper for ten days. More adults came to the office.

Spacing Changes

Change usually proves to be a paper tiger: it is much scarier when you are thinking about it than when you go through it.

Hal Longstreet had more changes to make, but he had gotten under way. And, he found, considering his increased revenue and the

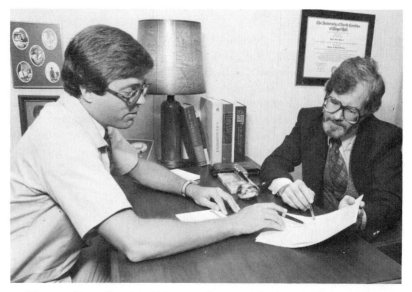

When making changes, it is sometimes worth the expense to engage a consultant for advice and feedback.

morale boost to himself and his staff, the pain to his ego and his checkbook had been kept to a minimum.

Change usually proves to be a paper tiger: it is much scarier when you are thinking about it than when you go through it. We are, in essence, flexible beings; we have within ourselves the resources to do things differently than we have done them before. We have the capacity to seize upon new ideas, to change, and to grow.

Once we have incorporated a new idea into our personal philosophy, we will never be the same. It is as if we have shed a skin and put on another — one that suits our situation.

It is, however, important to recognize that changes must be spaced, so that we can attempt and accomplish one thing before taking on the next. Too much change attempted in too short a period of time will doom us to failure, and leave us more anxious and depressed and behind than when we started.

There can be no hard and fast guidelines for "how much is too much." This will be a very individual matter. How can you know your limits? Pay attention to what you are feeling in the pit of your stomach. That is where you are fighting all your battles with your paper tigers, not up in your head (where you *think* you are fighting the battles but which is really just a decoy). Bluntly put, your "gut feelings" will tell you how much you can safely risk during each new attempt at change.

As the old chestnut goes, however, "Nothing succeeds like success." Hence, each time you change something about yourself, your staff or your office, or about your modes of promoting your practice, and that something "works," you enlarge your reservoir of courage for the next change that you want to make.

> However . . . too much change attempted in too short a period of time will doom us to failure, and leave us more anxious and depressed and behind than when we started.

MONITORING CHANGE

How can you keep track of the results of the changes you make? Here are a few thoughts (although we are sure you will come up with more methods on your own):

— Interview your staff *before* you inaugurate the changes. Ask them how they feel about the practice, about their specific jobs, about the attitudes of the patients, about prospects for the future. Record their comments in a notebook or else on a tape recording. Then interview the staff again several months after the changes have taken effect. Note the differences.

— Use the same technique for long-term patients, those who have been "with you" for years and who would be most sensitive to changes in the practice.

— Record and then graph the patient volume per day and the income per week before the change — and six months after the change.

— Interview *yourself,* before and after. Simply make up a list of questions the way you would for interviewing a staff member, then sit yourself down with a tape recorder and answer them. It may help to have a staff member ask you questions and be present while you record your answers. That way you will be talking to a person, not just to a machine.

Your accountant can suggest other ways of monitoring changes, according to their cost-effectiveness. If you find you are spending more money to produce the changes than the changes are bringing in as revenue, you will know you have gone too far (although some changes, by their nature, will be slow to deliver on results but still will prove worthwhile in the long term). Also you may find that some changes bring about positive results other than financial (such as a smoother operation or a happier staff), so that they are worthwhile for other reasons.

Last but scarcely least, don't forget to get feedback from your own family. They will notice the changes in *you*. Informally (unless you are the kind of person who could make your own kids fill out a questionnaire on how they perceive their Dad or Mom), some four to six months after the changes have gone into effect, check with your spouse and your children on how they think *you* have changed. Do you grouse less? Worry less? Are you a cheerier, more upbeat person? Easier to live with? Are you home more? And so on.

Evaluating the Effects of Change

When all is said and done, of course, what you are really after is the dollars and cents of the changes you have put into operation. In many cases one "change item" will have a one-time cost, such as Hal Longstreet's sending home notes with his pedodontic patients to try to recruit their adult family members, but an ongoing effect. The note was like dropping a pebble into a pond. The ripples, however, continue to grow and expand far beyond the spot where the pebble splashed in. The children's parents may mention the change to their neighbors, friends, or relatives, for example. Whatever adults come to Hal's practice and are pleased with the dental service they receive will likewise spread the word to their friends. And so forth.

In other cases the cost will be ongoing. This would be true, for instance, if you published a monthly newsletter for your patients. In such a case you would want to measure the cost of the newsletter against the increase in dollar volume to your practice over a period of months. At one point, you might want to ask your patients, as they leave after a visit, to fill out a short card on the newsletter to see if they are finding it helpful or a bother. Naturally, you cannot come straight out and ask a client, "Does receiving this newsletter remind you of your need to visit my office regularly?" But you could say something like: "Does the newsletter help you remember to take the best care of your teeth that you possibly can?"

Often it will be difficult to measure the exact effects of changes that you install.

Often, we must admit, it will be difficult to measure the exact effects of changes that you install. Who is to say whether your patient volume has increased because of: (a) your newspaper advertising, (b) your newsletter, or (c) your addition of new services to your practice. The likelihood is that all three changes had some effect on bolstering your volume.

One way to tell is to introduce changes one at a time, with an interval of several months between each significant change. Then keep a careful record of business increase within each period. If you try three changes, one at a time, and they all work, then go ahead and try the three together. If you find that only one has really made a difference, keep that one, drop the other two, and find something else that you can test out. As this book unfolds, you will find more suggested possibilities than any one dentist would ever be able to install in one practice.

Corrective Action

Sometimes a particular change will not work well not because the whole idea, say, a newsletter, was wrong, but because *some aspect* of the project is off base. It is all too easy to assume that if we make a change and we don't get the results we are seeking, we should just drop the idea. In many cases this may be precipitous. New ideas, systems, programs, and equipment often require fine tuning. The newsletter that doesn't seem to be bringing in any new clients or increasing the business of old clients may be judged by its readers as too jazzy — or too dull. If a dentist with no special training in graphic art and journalism attempts to produce his own newsletter, to cut corners on expenses, the result may be an unprofessional product that serves the practice poorly. Therefore, the corrective action may not be to drop the newsletter, but to upgrade it, recruiting an experienced journalist or public relations person to produce it as a sideline project.

Similarly with personnel. Perhaps you have decided to add a nutrition specialist to your practice, on a half-time basis. After two months, however, few of your clients are taking advantage of the nutrition counseling service, leaving you with a half-time salary to pay and few proceeds to help meet the added payroll expense. Well, have *you* and the other staff promoted the nutritional service energetically to the patients? Or . . . is the person you brought in fully qualified? Is he or she deficient in the delicate matter of personal rapport with clients? Is the nutritionist too "hard-sell" or too "soft-sell"? Could you perhaps support the nutritionist by making available to your patients booklets stressing the importance of proper diet for a healthy life-style?

In some exceptional cases you may have to terminate the person that you brought on board to help you effect a new program. Needless to say, this is extremely painful for both parties. Consequently, it is often best to negotiate a trial period with someone such as a nutrition specialist. Simply explain that this is a service that few dentists have ever offered, that you look upon yourself as somewhat revolutionary and that there is just the possibility that the experiment may fail. If it does, you hope that the "trial" staffer can be understanding and realize that your decision not to make the "trial" a permanent position does not necessarily reflect badly on his or her abilities. It may be that the public "isn't ready for this yet." Or some such similar explanation. In this way, if termination becomes imperative, both you and the nutritionist are braced for it and the matter does not need to be so personal.

It is important, in all these matters, that change be effected — and corrected — with adequate planning, with ample briefing of staff,

It is often best to negotiate a trial period with someone such as a nutrition specialist.

and in a reasonably measured fashion (not helter-skelter, one thing after another with no breathing room in between). It is equally important that all changes be communicated to your clientele in such a way as to guide them through the change process and to invite their candid reactions.

AFTERWORD

Manager Versus Leader?

As an "afterword" to this chapter, may we submit for your perusal some provocative comments by Avrom E. King that appeared in his newsletter, *NEXUS,* of April 17, 1978. King distinguishes between traits of managers and traits of leaders and insists that, on many levels, they are opposites. Some of us may find King's definitions of "leadership" too restrictive or his critique of "managerial skills" too severe, but we can all profit from mulling them over. This is especially so since King also believes that while the industrial model has favored managerial skills, those skills are now "maladaptive" in the postindustrial age currently emerging.

The following are the distinctions King makes:

— The emphasis of the manager is to be *effective,* not *affective.*

— Thus, managers *impersonally* relate to their tasks; motivation is in the *systems* of accomplishment.

— As part of the rationality of management, risk is rationally appraised.

— Work is seen by managers as an enabling process, and it is advanced by appropriate use of timing, persuasion, negotiation, rewards, and punishments.

— Managers are adept at shifting conflicts of interests and values in order to achieve a satisfactory balance that will facilitate a solution.

— For all of these reasons, managers tend to rationally *limit* available choices.

— Managers have a need to use an arm's length collaboration with others, sharing both risks and solace, especially with managers of comparable authority.

— Managers relate to people in terms of the role or function the people *then* occupy.

— Managers are more concerned with "how to" (technique and procedure) than "why."

— Ceremonial observances are important to managers.

— Managers believe that the passage of time generally will improve the tactics and strategies of management. (This relates to the manager's confidence in rational negotiation and compromise. *Managers focus on the process for decision-making rather than the decision itself.*)

— Managers tend to be people for whom life has been a straight-forward and relatively peaceful progression.

— Managers perceive themselves as being conservators and regulators of an existing order, and they identify with that order.

When compared with managers, leaders manifest important qualitative differences.

— Leaders depend more on intuition than rationality in making foundational decisions. Leaders relate intuitively to others — regardless of their work role, function, or social status.

— Thus, leaders are more passionate and so they are more comfortable in proceeding forward on desire, not need.

— Leaders are essentially *a*ffective personalities. Their *e*ffectiveness is a function of the validity of their intuitive processes.

— Leaders relate *personally* to task achievement, not in the impersonal modes of the manager.

— Leaders accept — even seek out — high-risk situations.

— Leaders perceive work as a break-through process. Highly energized spurts are separated by fallow periods.

— Leaders polarize those around them. They are loved or hated. Leaders utilize charisma rather than the negotiating skills of managers.

— Leaders are exceedingly impatient. The passage of time is looked upon as an irretrievable loss and antagonistic to progress.

— The process of leadership expands available choices.

— Leaders tend to respond to internal cues. They work effectively with others, but they do not need the emotional support or approval of others.

— Leaders are intolerant of ceremonial observances.

— Leaders have a pathological need to know "why" and a low level of concern for "how to." They are inclined to assume that knowledge of "why" automatically endows the knower with "how to."

— Leaders display relatively discontinuous, often erratic, personal histories.

— Leaders often work within a group, but they do not belong to it. They identify with individuals within the group but not the organization *per se*. They believe that with appropriate individuals, the organization can be reassembled.

—Leaders see themselves as being separate from the established order. (This is different than saying that leaders are hostile to it; hostility would imply that they care. In fact, leaders do not care about the established order. It is, for them, irrelevant.)

REFERENCES

Cowan J.: The Self Reliant Manager. New York, Amacom, 1977.

Gordon T.: Leadership Effectiveness Training. Scranton, PA, Harper & Row, Publisher, 1978.

Levoy R. P.: The Successful Professional Practice. Englewood Cliffs, NJ, Prentice-Hall, Inc., 1970.

5

Planning and Setting Realistic Goals

Dr. Jan Sutherland was puzzled. She had carefully instructed her appointments clerk in how to schedule her patients. She had tried her best to keep on schedule and had even given up her lunch period in order not to get behind. Further, she had sat down at the beginning of the year to determine her goals for the year. Yet, she always seemed to be behind in her work and never had time for herself or her family. In her darkest moments, she felt sometimes that she was missing half her life! "How could I be such a good goal setter and planner," Jan asked herself, "and yet not see the benefits of such work?"

Do you notice any parallels between what has happened to Jan Sutherland and what happens in your life? If so, this chapter should help you. We will discuss the importance of goals, how to set goals, and how to achieve goals once they are set. Among the many reasons for the failure of organizations, one of the most important is "failing to define goals" (Dormer). We hope the information that follows will help keep your organization, your dental practice, from failing to achieve its utmost.

WHY SET GOALS?

When we set goals, and only when we set goals, can we know how we are progressing on the road to success.

It has frequently been documented (*Nexus*) that the type of person who goes into dentistry normally is not a leader, or even a manager. How, then, can such a person be expected to do more than run a simple dental office (a solo dentist operating with one or two auxiliaries)? A larger, multifunction office operating with one or more dentists and several, even many, auxiliaries is quite beyond most present-day dentists. A complex operation, involving several dentists, necessary auxiliaries, complex systems (including data processing) is out of the question for all but the most talented managers. A partial answer is *goal setting* — an operation wherein each individual, including the dentist or dentists, knows what his or her job is, what level of performance is required, and what specifically must be accomplished in a given time period. In short, when we set goals, and only when we set goals, can we know how we are progressing on the road to success.

Teethtalk recently listed some key questions to help us indicate how important it is to set goals. The following are adapted from the list:

— How old are you, the dentist, going to be ten years from now?

— How old is your spouse going to be?

— How old are your children going to be?

— What will your financial responsibilities be in ten years?

— How much will tuition and other college expenses be?

— How much time would you like to be spending at the dental chair ten years from now?

— How many mortgages established now will you still be paying on?

— How old is your prime dental assistant going to be?

— What will be the rental payment for your office in ten years?

You will very likely be able to think of other challenging questions to justify goal setting.

WHAT ARE GOALS?

Goals can be conceptualized as *desired future states of affairs*. That is, what you want things to be like, in different areas of your life, in the future: tomorrow, next week, next year, or many years in the future. For our purposes, goals and objectives will be considered as synonymous terms. In order to achieve a goal, to bring about a desired future state of affairs, it is necessary for us to direct our efforts toward those ends. All of this requires making *changes* in the way we operate.

> To achieve a goal requires making *changes* in the way we operate.

If we are unable or unwilling to make changes in the way we live and operate our practices, we will not be able to achieve the goals we set. In fact, goal-setting under the constraint of no changes is self-defeating and a waste of time and effort. So, the first step in goal setting is to resolve to make whatever changes seem necessary in our lives and practices. This resolution should be considered carefully, for without a true resolve, nothing will happen. Nothing, that is, except that our level of frustration will go up! An excellent source for further information about goals and goal setting is the book *Motivation and Work Behavior* by R. M. Steers and L. W. Porter.

WHAT GOALS DO

Goals guide and direct behavior. They serve to focus our attention and to guide us in our everyday patterns. Although this simple explanation is appropriate and sufficient for most situations, goals do have other uses. They serve as a standard upon which we can judge the correctness of our actions at any given time. Further, they help us justify to ourselves and others the time and other resources we expend on specific activities.

TYPES OF GOALS

Three types of goals may be identified. First, there are *organizational* goals. In the case of the dentist, these are goals of the practice as a whole. These goals are known to and accepted by members of the organization, your partners, if any, you, and your employees. If stated correctly, this type of goal will affect employee effort by giving individuals at least a general idea of what performance is expected of each of them. These organizational goals will help give identification and an increased feeling of self-worth to all people associated with the dental practice.

The second type of goal we can identify is a *work-related goal* for individuals within the organization: dental assistants, receptionists, and the dentists themselves. These are *task goals*, specific objectives assigned to each individual. The broader organizational goals described above are necessary for the organization as a whole. Specific task goals, however, must be enumerated in order for each employee or person to know the extent of his or her responsibilities.

Specific task goals must be enumerated in order for each employee or person to know the extent of his or her responsibilities.

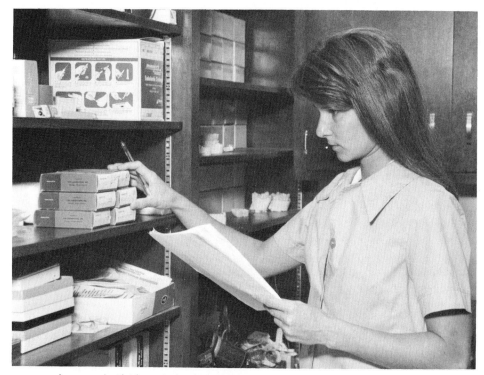

A young dentist inventories her storeroom, maintaining her efficiency goals.

A third type of goal is distinct from the others in that it is *personal*. One way to view personal goals is that they are personal aspirations. For example, Jan Sutherland may aspire to raise her practice income from $45,000 annually to $60,000. Or, she may aspire to arrange a three-week vacation instead of her normal one or two weeks, taken whenever she can get away and sometimes not at all.

At this juncture a number of points can be made. First, the task of setting goals depends upon the perspective one uses: the organization, the working individual, or the personal individual. Many problems in the past have come about because of a confusion of these perspectives. If the correct perspective is not recognized and used, conflicting and self-defeating goals can result.

Second, goal setting can be viewed as a type of negotiation. Dental practice employees negotiate with the dentist or dentists to determine their goals. Each employee must be helped in reconciling personal and task goals, and, in turn, organizational goals. By the same reasoning, the owner of a dental practice must view his own task goals and the organizational goals against his personal goals.

MANAGEMENT BY OBJECTIVES

One way to resolve potential goal setting problems is by using the familiar concept of management by objectives (MBO). In MBO, a person sets his or her own goal in collaboration with the supervisor. In dental practice terms, for example, the appointments clerk may set a goal of answering the telephone on the first ring. Presumably, this goal will be encouraged by you, the dentist, and you will do all you can to help her accomplish it. You and your employees may also set a goal of maintaining certain patients in the practice, say 95 percent. This is a common objective or goal, and all of you will coordinate your efforts toward accomplishing it. If done well, MBO can help employees at all levels of the organization to recognize the ways in which their particular jobs contribute to the larger organizational purposes.

Management by objectives does not imply, nor does it normally bring about, a situation wherein people try to set goals that are too low or too easy to achieve. It simply means that people have a hand in determining their destinies, in determining what they are accountable for. In fact, many people involved in setting objectives for themselves will set higher, more difficult goals for themselves than would someone else. So, ask your employees what they think they can accomplish. Let them have a major hand in setting goals for themselves. They will work harder to achieve goals they have helped set than they will to achieve goals set for them by someone else.

Another concept should be introduced here: employee involvement in job enrichment. This includes asking employees to suggest ways to make their jobs better, thereby making the office run better. Research has shown that involving employees in job enrichment and job design adds to employee job satisfaction. Using our appointments clerk example again, ask your clerk to suggest ways that patients can be reminded tactfully to keep appointments. Ask her to consider new

> Management by objectives simply means that people have a hand in determining their destinies and what they are accountable for.

ways to keep records — new ways to help the office operate more effectively and efficiently. You might be surprised by her suggestions! The lesson here? Involve employees in how the practice should operate. They will be more productive and happier in their work.

MODEL BUILDING

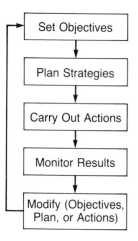

The goal-setting process has been called "model building" by *Teethtalk*. In their terms, model building consists of the steps in the accompanying diagram:

Perhaps the most difficult part of the model, at least initially, is setting the objectives. *Teethtalk* has an interesting suggestion about setting objectives. Many times, the *plans* and *actions* necessary for the short term seem too ambitious, even impossible to achieve, especially for your coworkers. If you believe that your plan and your action are unreal, then move your objective down the time line. Time can be a friend rather than an enemy in this regard, and the point of view of yourself, your staff, and your team (the total practice) can be more similar if the time moves the objective farther away. When things are closer to us as we visualize them, our viewpoints are more clouded with personal and emotional negatives. It is much easier to believe that something can be achieved if it's further away, timewise. In viewing an object that is close to us, a group of people will have very divergent points of view; if the object that we are observing is some distance away, our points of view are very similar because our vantage point in relationship to the object is quite similar. Time affects our view of "unachievable objectives" in this way, so if there is confusion and disagreement about any given objective, move it down the time line and it will become less objectionable. In other words, if someone associated with the practice believes that your goal of doubling the practice income is too ambitious, be sure to specify that you are referring to five years later. Doubling the practice income next year may indeed be too ambitious; doubling it in five years is far easier to imagine and accept as a goal.

It is much easier to believe that something can be achieved if it's further away, timewise.

WHAT KINDS OF GOALS SHOULD I SET?

At this point, you may be saying, "O.K., I agree that I need to set goals and to learn how to accomplish the ones that I set. But how do I know which goals to set?" This process is highly personal. Only you can do it. To some extent, your goals will depend upon your philosophy of practice. However, we can and do list and describe below some of the types of goals that successful dentists have set for themselves. Among these are:

 — Standards of care in the practice
 — Practice and personal income levels
 — Practice expense levels
 — Service to the community
 — Level of service fees

— Personal time off for the dentist
— Level of patient dental knowledge
— Level of community dental knowledge
— Size and extent of the dentist's community network

We will discuss some of these in detail below. You will probably have others to add to your list.

Standards of Care in the Practice

It is very difficult to define "undertreatment," or for that matter, "overtreatment." Obviously, standards of care vary by geographical area as well as by each professional's estimation. However difficult it is, each of us must determine at least the minimum level of quality of care we are willing to provide, plus a margin for error.

Clearly, however, we cannot provide perfection, even if we could define it. Perhaps a suitable quality of care standard for many of us is the following:

Discuss the quality of care question with the patient and speak frankly with him or her about the different alternatives. Make it clear that different amounts of time and different materials will produce different outcomes— all above the minimum level of acceptable quality. Let the patient help you decide what quality level he or she desires and wants to pay for.

The goal here is to set the quality of care based upon the wishes of the patient, certainly tempered by what the dentist would like to do and knows he must do. This goal is not based *only* on the type of dentistry the dentist would like to practice. Quality of care as a goal may need to give way to the larger goal of satisfying patients' total needs. This need not be viewed as a compromise, as we are wont to do, but as the optimum treatment for the individual patient in his or her unique circumstances.

> The goal is to set the quality of care based upon the wishes of the patient, certainly tempered by what the dentist would like to do and knows he must do.

Practice and Personal Income Levels

The economic goal, as with all others we will discuss here, cannot be set in isolation. All other goals will be affected by the level at which we set any one goal. If a $100,000 income is desired, then perhaps a $250,000 practice is required, which in turn determines the number of auxiliaries we must hire, and to an extent, the number of hours we must work. Also, this goal determines the amount of service we must perform for our patients, which in turn requires effective marketing. We *must*, however, set a number for the income we wish to have. How else will we be able to plan the rest of our practice and life?

Practice Expense Levels

How do we know when the expenses of operating the practice are too low or too high? We can do this only by setting a goal based on observing other practices, and by our own experience, and then periodically monitoring our progress. So far we have set goals for standards of care and for practice and personal income. These will, to a great extent, determine the levels of practice expenses. However, there are expense items that we can control directly. We must watch for material wastes; we must monitor water temperatures — many practices have water temperatures set higher than necessary for sanitation; we should even watch such items as office supplies. These items, taken a few at a time, can add up over the year. We should, of course, set a good example for the rest of the office by not taking office supplies or other materials for use at home.

It is critical to keep track of practice expenses and operational changes when necessary — not to just let the expenses *happen*. Many dentists find that salaries, materials, rent, and other identifiable expenses are a more or less uniform percentage of practice income over a period of time. Find out what your practice usually averages for each expense and make sure your bookkeeping system allows you to track your expenses. Also, spend some time on a regular basis thinking through how you can cut specific expenses. When can some procedure be dispensed with altogether? Can something be done as well or better, and at a lower cost, by an outside specialist?

A word of caution is in order here: be certain to consider not only expense but net practice income as well. Any expense that helps to increase net income (fees minus expenses) should be dropped only cautiously. Cutting an expense when net income falls more than the expense is obvious folly.

> Any expense that helps to increase net income (fees less expenses), should be dropped only cautiously. Cutting an expense when net income falls more than the expense is obvious folly.

Service to the Community

For many of us, it may seem strange at first to set a goal for service to the community. Doesn't such service "just happen?" Isn't such service a function of what we are called upon to perform? If we don't set a goal for it, that is exactly what happens; we let others determine where and how much we serve. Also, without control we perform service to the community in a cyclical fashion. For a while we spend little or no time in community involvement, then we seem to do little else. In community service we are either overworked or under-worked.

The secret to this apparent dilemma is to plan for such service in advance and to set goals for each type of service. For example, Jan Sutherland has set as a goal active membership in one service club and in the Lake Forest Owners' Association. She politely declines invitations to join other organizations and plans to spend one evening a week with the service club and two evenings a month with the Owners' Association.

Further, she sets aside one day a month for service to area schools. On some of these days, she gives slide shows and lectures on dental hygiene; on others, she joins colleagues in providing dental exams at the schools. She and her colleagues have purchased a portable examination chair, and it is taken to the schools when the exams are performed. These school services are done without recompense or other rewards. She has received patients on occasion as a result of this work, however.

Service Fees

As with some of the other goals, the level at which we price our services will be determined largely by the quality of care we and our patients choose, and by the type of clientele to which we cater. In addition, the fees will be strongly influenced by the prevailing dental fees in the community. In any event, it will be necessary to set a goal for the fee level and to monitor it periodically. As with all of the other goals, we are simply urging you to maintain control, not to just let the service fee level happen!

Personal Time Off

Many of us do not plan for personal leisure. We have time off whenever we are not busy with work, so of course, many of us do not get the leisure time that we need for our physical and mental health. Therefore, if we are to come close to an appropriate amount of time off, we must plan for it, set a goal, and monitor our progress.

Jan Sutherland has set aside every Sunday to be with her family. She has set aside every other Saturday to spend on herself, either in physical activity or on professional development activities. On the alternate Saturdays she sees patients from 9 a.m. until 2 p.m. She plans no less than two weeks vacation each year, and after the office vacation schedule is set, does not alter her plans. Although this may be similar to the approach many of us use, the difference is that we do not carry out our plans. We set too loose a goal and are too easily drawn away from the goal we have set.

> If we are to come close to an appropriate amount of time off, we must set a goal and monitor our progress.

Patient Dental Knowledge

It is clear to most dentists that the general public's level of knowledge about dentistry and dental hygiene is rather low. None of us can have much impact, at least in the short run, on the knowledge of the general public, but we *can* influence our patients. In order to know if we are having an influence on our patients, and in order to set a goal, it is necessary for us to measure the level of knowledge about dentistry and about dental hygiene when patients start in our practice and periodically thereafter. One way to do this is have one of your auxiliaries administer a short set of questions of your choosing when a patient first comes to you for treatment and from time to time thereafter. The question should be designed to tell you how much the patient knows about dentistry and about oral hygiene. Included in this list may be questions about how often the patient visits a dentist, how often he or she brushes, what type of brush is used, how often dental floss is used, and the like.

Community Dental Knowledge

Again, although we won't have much impact on the world's or even the country's or state's level of knowledge about dentistry or dental hygiene, we *can* have an impact on our community's level of awareness. Perhaps a good way to test this level and to set a goal to improve it is in your work with local schools. As you give lectures and slide presentations, as you perform dental exams in the schools, you can administer the same questionnaire you use in your practice. After you determine just how much the students know or don't know, you can better set goals for improving their level of knowledge over time.

Size and Extent of the Dentist's Community Network

By community network, we mean the number and extent of relationships we develop with the various constituencies discussed in an earlier chapter. This network will not just happen. We must plan for it and set goals accordingly. Jan Sutherland sets aside time in her schedule to make two calls each week on other professionals, dentists, physicians, dental technicians, and others in the health-care professions, as well as setting aside time for one call a week on businesspeople, such as small business owners and personnel managers of large businesses. Also called on are other community leaders, such as the City Manager and the Mayor. Although the time spent on this activity each week is not great, over the years Jan has developed an excellent set of friends and an effective community network.

SETTING GOALS FOR OTHERS IN THE PRACTICE

After we have set goals for ourselves, we must then set goals for others in the practice.

After we have set goals for ourselves, we must then set goals for others in the practice. This is where the "management by objectives" comes in. Determine which activities for each employee are "countable," and then work with each person to set a goal that *can* be met, but that will require hard work to meet. Examples: if your receptionist makes followup calls to patients, reminding them of the need for an appointment, set a goal for the number of such calls to be made each week, or perhaps each day. Then ask that she make a log of such calls so that you can see that they are being made. A good procedure is to check (√) each name in your appointment book as a call is made.

If you have a technician in your practice who uses a particular material, set a standard or goal for the amount of such material used per patient or per procedure. Then check to see that the criterion is being met. If any measure is not being met, it may be that the employee is not doing a good job. It may also mean that the standard is too high. Only *you* can determine which is the case, and then make necessary adjustments. Last, at salary review time, take this goal performance into account in determining whether to increase salaries — and by how much.

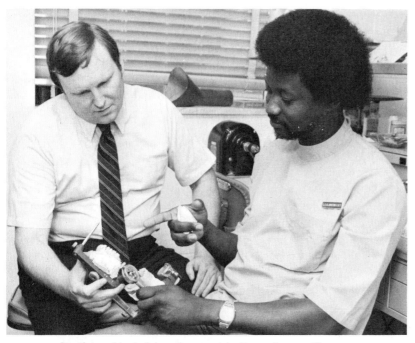

Dentist and technician discuss objectives of a specific case.

GOAL REVIEW AND RESTATEMENT

Once we have set our goals, we aren't finished. In fact, we are never finished with setting them. As the model building diagram presented earlier indicates, goal development is a cyclical process. Each time we set goals and try to achieve them, we then must restate the goals, altering them when appropriate.

When should goals be reviewed and restated? Jan Sutherland has found that an appropriate period for her is every six months. Many of us find once a year more appropriate; some people revise and restate their goals every three months. Whatever time period works for you, use it. However, goals *must* be reworked periodically, and changes must be made based on how well we have accomplished them.

Target dates should be established for each year in any given five-year "plan." On the annual or more frequent review dates, determine whether you are on track in your effort to meet the longer-term goal. You may decide to change your methods or actions for working toward the goal. Or, on the other hand, you may decide that the goal was set unrealistically high — and alter it.

There is a tendency for many people who commit themselves to setting goals and achieving them to lose interest over time. Sometimes we are able to sustain our interest through two or three goal-setting exercises; then our interest flags. To be sure, few of us will admit to losing interest; instead, we claim that we "just don't have the time we used to." If this is what you will do, a case can be made that you shouldn't bother to set goals in the first place — it is too difficult a task for us to undertake if we aren't going to stay with it for the long run. Instead, we must all resolve to set goals religiously on a regular schedule and to periodically monitor our progress toward those goals.

When should goals be reviewed and restated? Many find once a year appropriate; some people revise and restate goals every three months.

Almost as bad as not setting goals and monitoring progress toward them is setting goals that are too high. Certainly all of us deserve(!), or at least would like to have our practice income at a level of $100,000 annually today. Few of us will be able to achieve that at once. We must determine what our income is now and set a realistic increase for the next three-, six-, or twelve-month period, as well as for at least each of the next five years.

WRITTEN GOALS

There is a tendency for many dentists to "plan," to think of the future while doing other things, while shaving or showering, driving, or working on patients. As a result, most of this planning does not get written down and is lost from a person's mind. To be effective, goals and plans have to be written down. They must be referred to frequently and changed when appropriate. To help you start your goal writing, we offer on the pages that follow a set of goal worksheets.

To be effective, goals and plans have to be written down.

CONCLUSION

We have reviewed why setting goals is necessary, what they are, and how they are set. We have outlined for you a number of goals that we have found helpful in our practices. You may well determine other, more appropriate ones for your practice. We encourage you to do so. We hope this chapter has convinced you of the necessity of setting goals and of planning, of the need for specific short- and longer-term goals, and of the need to write goals down and to revise them when appropriate. Only by following these steps will all benefit from planning and setting realistic goals.

Jan Sutherland still does not have all the time she would like for herself, nor all the control over her life and practice that she desires, but things *are* much better now. She has set goals for herself. She has worked with her employees and set goals that are jointly agreed upon for each of them and for the practice as a whole. And, she is reviewing and revising them every six months without fail. "If I keep at it," she reasons, "in time I will be working less and enjoying it more!"

REFERENCES

Abell, D. F., Hannond, J. S.: Strategic Market Planning. Englewood Cliffs, NJ, Prentice-Hall, Inc., 1979.

Domer, L. R., Snyder, T. L., Heid, D. W.: Dental Practice Management, St. Louis, The C. V. Mosby Company, 1980.

Lock, D. J., Farrell, O. C.: Marketing Strategy and Plans. Englewood Cliffs, NJ, Prentice-Hall, Inc., 1979.

NEXUS, 4(2), 1978. Nexus Group, Inc., P.O. Bin 4880, Scottsdale, AZ 85258.

Steers, R. M., Porter, L. W.: Motivation and Work Behavior. New York, McGraw-Hill Book Company, 1979, Chapter 10.

Stinaff, R. K.: Dental Practice Administration. St. Louis, The C. V. Mosby Company, 1960, Chapter 3.

Teethtalk, Ceram-Dent, Inc., 4515 N. 32nd Street, Phoenix, AZ 85018.

PRACTICE GOAL WORKSHEET 1

STANDARDS OF CARE   (write goal as clearly and specifically as possible)

How will this goal be accomplished?

PRACTICE AND PERSONAL INCOME LEVELS

	Practice	Personal
Income last year	$_____	$_____
Goal for this year	$_____	$_____
Goal for the second year	$_____	$_____
Goal for the third year	$_____	$_____
Goal for the fourth year	$_____	$_____
Goal for five years from now	$_____	$_____

How will this goal be accomplished

Completed by _____

Date _____

PRACTICE GOAL WORKSHEET 2

PRACTICE EXPENSE LEVELS

Total expenses last year $_____

Goal for this year $_____

Goal for five years from now $_____

How will this goal be accomplished?

SERVICE TO THE COMMUNITY

Service last year (specific activities)

Service goal this year (specific activities)

How will this goal be accomplished?

Completed by _____

Date _____

PRACTICE GOAL WORKSHEET 3

LEVEL OF FEES	NORMAL FEE IN THE COMMUNITY	MY FEE THIS YEAR	MY FEE GOAL NEXT YEAR
Dental Procedure			
_____	$_____	$_____	$_____
_____	$_____	$_____	$_____
_____	$_____	$_____	$_____
_____	$_____	$_____	$_____
_____	$_____	$_____	$_____
_____	$_____	$_____	$_____
_____	$_____	$_____	$_____
_____	$_____	$_____	$_____
_____	$_____	$_____	$_____
_____	$_____	$_____	$_____
_____	$_____	$_____	$_____

COMMENTS

Completed by _____

Date _____

PRACTICE GOAL WORKSHEET 4

PERSONAL TIME OFF FOR THE DENTIST

Personal time off last year (number of days)

Personal time off goal this year (number of days)

How will this goal be accomplished?

LEVEL OF PATIENT DENTAL KNOWLEDGE

Average correct answers to questions last year _____%

Average correct answers to questions this year _____%

How will this goal be accomplished?

Completed by _____

Date _____

PRACTICE GOAL WORKSHEET 5

LEVEL OF COMMUNITY DENTAL KNOWLEDGE

Average correct answers to questions last year _____%

Average correct answers to questions this year _____%

How will this goal be accomplished?

COMMUNITY NETWORK GOALS

Number of calls on community leaders last year _____

Goal for this year _____

How will this goal be accomplished?

Completed by _____

Date _____

6

Expanding the Scope of Care

Porter and Richard are attending a local dental society meeting. Their practices are both well established and they have virtually identical patient communication skills. One is busy; the other is not. Let's listen to their conversation:

"Hello, Porter, how are things?"

"OK, I guess. Well — not really. Things are down. It seems that the new dentists in town are hurting my practice."

"I understand. I've been holding my own, though. I've been able to do more endodontics since I took that molar course."

"I don't see how you manage, Richard. You're always attending those continuing education courses. I just don't have the time, money, or interest. I hate endo. You can have it! Besides, if you do endo, that means more crown and bridge. I never have liked restoring endo teeth."

"Well, Porter, I've worked hard to add molar endo to my repertoire. I still refer the very difficult cases to the specialists, but I'm doing the simple work now. Did you read the new orthodontics book I sent you?"

"No, I didn't, Richard. You know I don't like pedodontics or orthodontics. I usually refer all that plus routine extractions — let the oral surgeons handle it."

"Porter, no wonder your practice is down. These are new times, man. You've got to expand your practice or shrivel."

Porter has become a referring dentist, offering a minimal scope of care, while Richard is expanding his services. Richard is moving toward becoming a "decathlon dentist," that is, one who offers a wide range of financial and technical services. He doesn't need a large group of patients because he refers few procedures to other dentists. Patients who enter his door are referred out only infrequently.

It has been the vogue in recent years for dentists to restrict their practices to techniques and procedures they enjoyed, felt comfortable doing, and could perform with efficiency. Practice management

Practitioners who once referred out heavily, thus severely restricting their effectiveness, and their incomes as a result, must now re-evaluate their approach to building their practices.

experts told them to concentrate on the procedures that could be done in the least time and yield the most profit. The "experts" also said to refer cases in which speed and monetary return were not as great. Only those patients who accepted *complete* treatment planning were to be kept in the practice; others were to be discouraged.

These may have been effective concepts and they have worked reasonably well until the inflation rate exploded and new dentists flooded the market. The overall effect has been that practitioners who once severely restricted their effectiveness, and their incomes as a result, must now re-evaluate their approach to building their practices.

THE DECATHLON DENTIST

Advantages

The decathlon dentist is trained and skilled in diverse areas. It is, of course, evident that he will have more interest, expertise, and technical ability in some areas than others. Yet the general dentist must have met an overall level of excellence in order to graduate from dental school.

Being — or becoming — a "decathlon dentist" holds many advantages. For example, the wide variety of procedures he performs can be technically and mentally refreshing as well as challenging, and the patient volume may be smaller because more comprehensive treatment is performed on each patient. Patients who already feel secure with a particular dentist usually prefer to have him handle all their dental needs rather than go to an unfamiliar specialist or another general dentist in strange surroundings. It is likely that patient satisfaction is increased by dealing with one dentist rather than with two or more.

From the standpoint of interpersonal relationships, the decathlon dentist and his staff have to deal psychologically with fewer patients than the more limited practitioner. He or she needs a smaller patient population to support his practice, because he does more for less, not less for more. This allows the decathlon dentist to know each patient better, and provide complex care for a limited number of patients. This has its own emotional rewards.

The concept of one dentist treating an entire family also appeals to today's public, who, in the interests of economizing on time and transportation, tend to appreciate "one-stop shopping."

> It is likely that patient satisfaction is increased by dealing with one dentist rather than with two or more.

Assessment of Strengths and Weaknesses

Where should the practitioner begin a program of expansion? In evaluating a practice and constructing a plan to increase its growth, several important aspects must be considered. The initial step is to examine the present scope of care being offered and determine how that scope in itself limits expansion prospects. Are some procedures being referred out that could quickly increase daily receipts if

> Before an expansion of services is considered, the dentist must be competent in the techniques and procedures he currently performs.

incorporated? Would it be economically feasible to discontinue certain procedures that are inefficient timewise and that use expensive materials? Could some entirely new services be added?

In addition, the dentist must truthfully ask if he has the expertise and knowledge necessary for excellence in those services he is already providing for his patients. Are the needed equipment, personnel, and support systems on hand?

Before an expansion of services is considered, the dentist must be competent in the techniques and procedures he currently performs. Does the dentist know the best methods for root canal treatment, for crown preparation, for space maintenance? If weaknesses are discovered, a new start must be made for education and skills improvement, or a determination made as to whether some services should be discontinued. It is a disservice to the public to continue offering procedures in which competence is in question.

The next step is to develop a strategy and program for expansion. The choices are fairly clear: (1) perform more procedures for the patients already in the practice, (2) find more patients, or (3) both. This chapter will deal with the first option, offering more procedures. In assessing strengths and weaknesses in all dental procedures, the dentist should not only look at technical proficiency but should also evaluate the psychological factors involved with each procedure from his or her own viewpoint as well as the staff's. He may be technically superior at fabricating a denture, for example, but be unable to cope

> One way to assess strengths and weaknesses is to list all procedures that are being performed in the practice and rate them according to *technical proficiency, time efficiency, monetary profit,* and *psychological attitude* of both the doctor and the staff.

PROCEDURE	TECHNICAL PROFICIENCY	TIME EFFICIENCY	PSYCHOLOGICAL ATTITUDE Doctor	Staff	MONETARY PROFIT	AVERAGE SCORE
Crown and bridge	4	1	4	3	4	3.2
Endodontics—1 canal	4	4	3	3	4	3.6
Precision partials	4	2	4	4	3	3.4
Examinations	4	4	4	4	2	3.6
Routine extractions	3	3	3	3	3	3.0
Fixed space maintainers	4	4	4	4	4	4.0
Pedodontics	4	4	3	4	3	3.6
Partials	4	4	4	4	4	4.0
Dentures	4	1	2	1	2	2.5
Other						
Other						

Figure 6–1. Current Office Procedures: Assessment of Strengths and Weaknesses. This chart, although only an approximation, will help assess the relative strengths and weaknesses in dental procedures currently offered in the practice. Each one is "scored" by the doctor and staff and an average computed. The larger the relative average score, the greater the strengths; averages of 1 or 2 indicate that weaknesses are present and that changes could be required in specific areas. Excellent (4), Good (3), Fair (2), Poor (1).

PROCEDURE	CHANGES NEEDED	CHANGES IMPLEMENTED
Crown and bridge	More efficient techniques	?
Precision partials	More efficient techniques Slight fee increase	?
Dentures	More efficient techniques Change in staff and doctor attitudes Fee increase	Refer
Other		
Other		

Figure 6–2. Changes needed in current procedures. This chart lists procedures that need some changes. The decision was made to refer dentures elsewhere, since four out of five areas were low. Decisions will now be necessary concerning exactly how to bring about the needed changes.

mentally with the geriatric patient; he may identify with children but be weak in growth and development and space maintenance.

One way to assess strengths and weaknesses is to list all procedures that are being performed in the practice and rate them according to *technical proficiency, time efficiency, monetary profit,* and *psychological attitude* of both the doctor and the staff, as in Figure 6–1. We have used a weighted number system to show scores of from poor (1) to excellent (4). After each procedure has been scored in all columns, the number will indicate to some degree whether a given procedure should be kept, whether more training is necessary, whether fees should be adjusted, and so on.

For example, in Figure 6–1 precision partials show a score of 2 in the *time efficiency* column. It is probable that if efficiency could be increased, profits would also go up. Some procedures, of course, require more time than others and time efficiency can be improved only to a certain point. In cases of this type, especially if profits could be improved, it may be necessary to adjust fees upward.

In the case of examinations, however, where the profit column is low, the dentist may be hesitant to increase fees. This is because he uses the examination as a "loss leader" to attract patients to a first dental visit.

Figure 6–1 also shows that denture services are being provided in the office. After reviewing the numbers, four out of five columns appear to need changes. It may be that in this case it would be better to refer denture patients to another professional so that more time could be devoted to procedures that score higher in all categories. Figure 6–2 lists procedures and changes to be made to upgrade current services.

This scoring procedure will indicate relative strengths and weaknesses for the various procedures. The higher the average score, the more efficiently the office now performs a given procedure. This ranking system is only relative at best but will be a point of departure in considering the strengths and weaknesses of a practice.

If efficiency could be increased, profits would also go up.

PROCEDURE	TECHNICAL PROFICIENCY	TIME EFFICIENCY	PSYCHOLOGICAL ATTITUDE		MONETARY PROFIT	AVERAGE SCORE
			Doctor	Staff		
Impactions	2	1	2	2	2	1.8
Periodontics	1	1	3	3	3	2.2
Endodontics— multiple canals	3	1	2	2	3	2.2
Minor tooth movement	1	1	2	2	2	1.6

Figure 6–3. Referred procedures: Assessment of strengths and weaknesses. This chart, although only an approximation, will help assess the staff's relative strengths and weaknesses in dental procedures being referred. Each one is scored by the doctor and staff and an average computed. The larger the average score, the greater the possibility that the procedure is a candidate for early addition to the practice, with proper changes. Lower scores indicate that several areas need to be changed before the procedures can be added. Excellent (4), Good (3), Fair (2), Poor (1).

After the current procedures have been evaluated to determine the kinds of changes necessary, the next step is to evaluate all procedures being referred in a similar way. Figure 6–3 may be used for this. After scoring has been completed, it is possible that a change in attitude is all that is needed to include some of these procedures in the practice almost immediately. With others, more efficient methods may make the difference in the profitability score. Ethically, the more technically difficult cases should be referred to the proper specialist.

Figure 6–4 lists referred procedures and changes needed in order to incorporate them into the practice.

PROCEDURE	CHANGES NEEDED
Impactions	Continuing education More efficient techniques Change in attitudes Fee increase
Periodontics	Continuing education More efficient techniques Possible fee increase
Endodontics— multiple canals	More efficient techniques Change in attitudes Possible fee increase
Minor tooth movement	Continuing education More efficient techniques Change in attitudes Fee increase

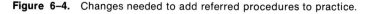

Figure 6–4. Changes needed to add referred procedures to practice.

PROCEDURE	ADD TO PRACTICE	CONTINUE TO REFER
Endodontics— multiple canals	Simple multi-root	Difficult multi-root
Impactions	Bony impactions on young patients Soft tissue impactions	Bony impactions on adults
Periodontics	Grafts Crown lengthening procedures	Osseous surgery
Minor tooth movement	Hawley's for crossbites Molar uprighting for crown and bridge	Full banded cases

Figure 6–5. Order in which referred procedures should be added to the practice.

Next, the procedures can be reranked according to the ease with which they can be added to the practice — that is, with a minimum of training, expense, and adjustment pains. These procedures are limited in scope and well within the capability of doctor and staff (see Figure 6–5).

Procedures requiring more change and commitment by the doctor and auxiliaries can be added later. These evaluations should be made periodically. Each evaluation should indicate whether the additions and changes have worked out as intended.

New Procedures

The next logical step is to investigate the adding of services that have never been performed in the practice, but might enhance its growth. Among these might be nutritional counseling, implantology, management of myofascial pain, or even acupuncture. Related health services that are being offered in some dental offices include hair analysis and applied kinesiology.

Figure 6–6 lists new procedures in the order in which a team might consider adding them to a practice. Your team needs to rank these procedures according to their own preferences. Each one would require specific costs, in money or time.

Order of Expansion of Services

After completing the assessment tasks, several criteria may be used to determine the order of expansion. The addition of services, whether those formerly referred or entirely new ones, can evolve singly or in combination. They may require new equipment and supplies, renovation of facilities, continuing education courses, and/or a change in psychological attitude toward the delivery of

COSTS					
LIKE MOST	PROCEDURE	EXPANSION OF OFFICE	NEW EQUIPMENT OR SUPPLIES	CONTINUING EDUCATION Doctor Staff	ESTIMATED TOTAL COST
	Nutritional counseling	—	$ 300	$ 600	$ 900
	Nitrous oxide	—	3,600	—	3,600
	Emphasis on children/ handicapped	Variable	1,000	1,200	Variable
	TMJ and occlusion	—	1,000	4,000	5,000
	Implantology	—	1,400	1,400	2,800
	Biofeedback	—	600	400	1,000
	Myofascial pain management	—	—	800	800
	IV sedation	—	200	1,200	1,400
	Hypnosis	—	—	1,000	1,000
	Applied Kinesiology	—	—	400	400
	Hair analysis	—	100	1,400	1,500
LIKE LEAST	Acupuncture	—	200	1,200	1,400
	Etc.				

Figure 6–6. Psychological ranking and estimated cost of possible new procedures. In the chart above, note that various new procedures have been ranked first according to preference of addition. After the total cost of each procedure has been tallied, procedures should be selected that will be cost-effective and compatible with the practice. (Costs are not accurate, but are for the purpose of illustration only.)

The addition of services ... may require new equipment and supplies, renovation of facilities, continuing education courses, and/or a change in psychological attitude toward the delivery of services by the doctor and staff.

services by the doctor and staff. Some of these changes may involve considerable cost or time, or require additional new patients.

For example, if the doctor wants to provide services to handicapped patients, there is a good probability that some renovations will be necessary, especially if the building is an older one that does not have wide doorways, ramps, and other special facilities for handicapped people. This addition would take considerable time and money, so he must decide if and when to add this service. It would also be advisable to make a public announcement to encourage handicapped patients to patronize the practice.

Another factor is the financial remuneration that can result from a new procedure. The dentist may increase gross income dramatically in a short time through the addition of certain services. A new

```
┌─────────────────────────────────────────────┐
│           DENTAL CARE FOR YOUR CHILD          │
│            (Including the Handicapped)        │
│                                               │
│    Let us help your child have a pretty smile.  Baby │
│    teeth are important -- regular checkups should    │
│    begin at age 3.                            │
│                                               │
│    Start summer right with an end-of-school checkup. │
│                                               │
│       (Dental insurance/Medicaid accepted)    │
│                                               │
│              DR. CHARLES BLAIR                 │
│             Children's Dental Center          │
│           Highway 74 - Kings Mountain         │
│                  704-739-7956                 │
└─────────────────────────────────────────────┘
```

An example of expanding the scope of care: an overt appeal to handicapped people to join this dentist's practice.

low-cost denture service, for instance, may give rise to much more patient traffic (hence income) at the outset than will implantology, which would require a great deal of patient education and may have less application to the general public.

Other procedures may require continuing education courses. The dentist and staff may want or need additional training before adding nitrous oxide, intravenous sedation, acupuncture, and/or hypnosis to the practice. Even if some of these procedures were taught in dental school, the dentist may need a refresher course before incorporating them.

If the custom has been to refer all molar root canal treatment cases, the dentist may wish to start doing these. In terms of equipment or supplies, there would be very little cost involved, but the doctor may feel a need to brush up on endodontic techniques with a continuing education course. If one will be given in a distant city for two days, the dentist must make decisions regarding the time away from the office and the cost of the seminar plus travel and lodging. Often, a small investment can yield big rewards. A long-range view should be taken when one weighs the positive and negative factors of continuing education.

Catering to the child patient could include the addition of a reward at each visit, books and toys for entertainment, birthday cards, picture boards for patient photographs, televisions in the operatories and reception room, and patient education booklets.

An emphasis in basic pedodontic services may require only minor financial and psychological commitments. Catering to the child patient could include the addition of a reward at each visit, books and toys for entertainment, birthday cards, picture boards for patient photographs, televisions in the operatories and reception room, and patient education booklets. All of these can be added at small cost. Special back-to-school days for examinations may bring in new patients. Observation of holidays with office decorations and staff dressed in costumes will capture public attention. The psychological adjustment may involve staff and doctor reorientation to the young child, especially if they have not been accustomed to dealing with children. It may also be necessary for them to review child management techniques, including drugs and physical restraints, and/or dental procedures relating to growth and development.

For some procedures, a rearrangement of supplies and a more efficient delivery system between assistant and dentist can mean a

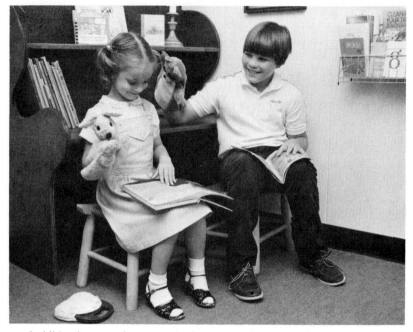

A children's corner in your reception area makes your office attractive to both children and parents.

difference of thousands of dollars over a period of time. All procedures should be assessed for the efficiency with which they are performed. Changes should be made where time and motion are wasted.

Now that many people are concerned with total health and well-being, other health-related services could be incorporated into a dental practice. Some dentists are already offering nutritional counseling, biofeedback, applied kinesiology, hair analysis, vitamin and nutritional supplements as well as health literature in a holistic health center. The dentist who offers these services will attract health-oriented people, because he deals with the whole person, not with teeth exclusively.

Staff Involvement

The staff should be consulted before any changes are made in the practice. Auxiliaries will have excellent observations concerning procedures, and can present them from a different perspective from the doctor's. As highly valued members of the dental team, their opinions mean a great deal, and the dentist would surely request their input and ask for their help. After it has been decided which services and procedures will be added, the receptionist should be very alert to scheduling patients for the new procedures. All staff members should become responsible for telling patients about the availability of the new services.

The staff should be consulted before any changes are made in the practice.

Adding services to a practice will generally help efficiency and quicken the work pace, both of which boost patient flow and receipts.

Whenever the patient load is lighter than normal, the work pace tends to become lackadaisical, resulting in a decline in efficiency. When the entire dental team is excited about being able to fill more needs for more people, amazing results usually follow.

When positive changes develop from the additional work load generated, the doctor needs to consider how to reward the staff for extra effort. Some auxiliaries would prefer a pay raise, some time off from work, and others, perhaps, opportunities for career growth.

Program for Strengthening Technical Expertise

It is obvious that new procedures will produce both economic and psychological rewards. In view of this, the dentist must allot time and resources to becoming technically competent in any new endeavor or more expert in current procedures. The three basic methods for strengthening technical expertise are: (1) self-study, (2) formal continuing education, and (3) interaction with colleagues who are successful in the areas to be improved. Some areas of dentistry can be clearly understood through self-study, others require a more pedagogical approach, and still others a "hands-on" experience. Sometimes a combination of two, or even three, of these approaches works best.

In the area of self-study, the doctor can find not only books and

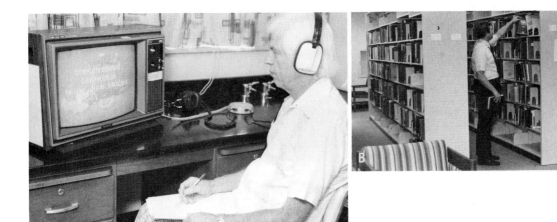

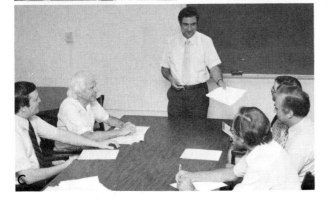

Continuing education, in its several forms (A, self-instruction; B, formal continuing education; C, professional seminars), is vital for the expansion of the scope of care.

other written material, but audio and video tapes as well. Many books are currently on the market in the various technical areas of dentistry. Periodicals often offer tips on improving procedural techniques. Video tapes, which add a new dimension to home self-study, are available from the American Dental Association and Veterans Administration as well as from private companies.

There are numerous formal continuing education offerings from dental schools and private concerns, as well as from individuals, in almost every area of dentistry. Just watch each day's mail for the desired subject or contact the continuing education department of the nearest dental school. Many seminars include demonstrations and participation as well as lectures, and can be valuable in helping the dentist grasp new procedures quickly. Many course offerings, especially those from private concerns, are available on tape. So, if it impossible to attend, you can buy the tapes.

All dentists should be open enough to accept any help that might be offered, and to be willing to share any ideas and techniques that could be helpful to a colleague.

In some cases, a local or area dentist may be particularly strong in a certain procedure and will have no objection to having another dentist observe and learn from him. This method would certainly be less costly than a continuing education course and might well create a feeling of goodwill too. Some dentists are hesitant to ask colleagues questions about clinical problems, possibly because of ego problems. Others seem afraid that another dentist will somehow "steal" their trade secrets. (A dentist outside of the immediate area will almost always be willing to help.) It certainly behooves all dentists to be open enough to accept any help that might be offered, and to be willing to share any ideas and techniques that could be helpful to a colleague. This is close to the essence of professional collegial relations in health care.

RELATIONSHIP TO THE SPECIALTY AREAS

Adding New Procedures

The services provided by specialists should be carefully scrutinized. Traditional areas of responsibility between generalists and specialists have been reached over a period of years. Now it is time for the generalists to examine the various procedures and delimit those that can be performed in their offices versus those that absolutely must be referred to specialists. For example, the general dentist may wish to provide panograph, full series, and oral surgery services for the orthodontist. When pedodontic patients are referred to an orthodontist for growth and development evaluation, the dentist could provide serial extraction, space maintenance, and minor orthodontic appliance services. The orthodontist and generalist would constitute a "team," with the orthodontist performing only the full banding procedures.

Example 1

Ten-year-old Kathy is referred to an orthodontist by her general dentist because of crowded incisors. The orthodontist takes a panograph and full series x-rays, and refers her to an oral surgeon for extraction of first bicuspids. She goes back to her general dentist only for operative treatment and routine recall check-ups.

Example 2

Twelve-year-old Tommy visits his dentist for a check-up and is told that now it is finally time to make that orthodontic visit they have been talking about for several years. The dentist gives a panograph to Tommy's mother to take when he goes. After Tommy's initial visit and diagnosis, the orthodontist sends a letter requesting that the referring dentist perform the following procedures: (1) full series radiographs and (2) extraction of all four 1st bicuspids.

In Example 1, the general dentist does not have the advantage of providing additional services for his patient because the orthodontist takes his own x-rays and then refers her to another specialist for extractions. In Example 2, however, the orthodontist and generalist have a "team" approach in which the patient is sent back for necessary services prior to full banding. This relationship certainly benefits the original referring dentist by providing him with extra services and is a motivating factor in his relationship with the specialist. The same principle would apply to other specialists, such as oral surgeons, periodontists, and endodontists, where some procedures could be performed by a competent generalist.

> The generalist should actively develop close working relationships with appropriate specialists to improve current techniques and learn new procedures.

The generalist should actively develop close working relationships with appropriate specialists to improve current techniques and learn new procedures. This type of relationship generates better dentistry for all patients.

Provision of Services by a Specialist in a Generalist's Office

Few dentists can produce dentistry on an accelerated basis for five consecutive days, and the capital cost of building and equipment is fixed regardless of usage. In light of this, there are several advantages to having a specialist work part-time in the generalist's office. A common example is the orthodontist who works a few days a month outside his own premises.

Example

John Greene is an orthodontist in a medium-sized town that has an abundance of orthodontists. In spite of the fact that he has been fairly aggressive in recruiting patients from general dentists in the area, his workload covers only 2½ to 3 days a week.

His friend, Bob Tyson, has a general practice about

15 miles away in a smaller town. Bob is busy, but doesn't want to work more than four days a week. His overhead has increased considerably in the past few years. One day over lunch, they discuss their problems and decide that since Bob's town has no orthodontist, they could both gain if John would rent Bob's office one day a week.

The presence of a specialist in the office ... helps increase the flow of patients.

They arrive at a mutual agreement whereby John will pay a monthly (or daily) fee, which will escalate with time, for the use of the office space and dental equipment. All supplies will be furnished by John and he will have a telephone installed that will ring at his primary office when he is away from the satellite (a switch on the telephone turns the bell off). His own receptionist and assistants will accompany him on the days he is in Bob's office, and they will bring all necessary records since Bob's storage space is limited.

After two years of this arrangement, both dentists are highly pleased. Both have increased their incomes.

The first advantage of having the specialist in the office is that the rental payment helps with office overhead costs. The presence of the specialist can also add prestige to the practice. Moreover, it helps increase the flow of patients. As orthodontic, periodontic, and other patients become familiar with the location, they will begin to refer their friends and neighbors not only to the specialist, but to the generalist as well. The third advantage is improved access to the specialist in a familiar surrounding. Many patients simply prefer to have all treatment in the same office, probably because of a lessening of the fear factor. In these times of competitive dentistry, every effort should be made to make patients feel as comfortable as possible so they will continue as patients and make referrals to the practice.

Since the specialist is on the premises at specified dates, he is geographically convenient for limited consultation with the generalist. This convenience may enhance the consultative relationship, as well as increase the expertise of the general dentist.

There are some disadvantages within this arrangement both to the generalist and to the specialist. Since the specialist must work in unfamiliar surroundings, his efficiency may suffer slightly at the beginning. The location may be inconvenient for him and his staff. In addition, other local practitioners could be reluctant to refer to a specialist who is working in a competitor's office. Generally, these problems will eventually work out because patients tend to insist on a convenient location when a specialist is available.

There are also some disadvantages for the generalist. The loss of an available day may inconvenience him from time to time when he desires to shift his schedule around. The staff may have to be dismissed on certain days and may resent other people "messing up" their office while they are away.

All in all, however, the advantages generally outweigh the disadvantages. Many arrangements similar to the one just described are meeting with success.

COORDINATION OF SERVICES WITH OTHER DENTISTS

A referring relationship with another general dentist can be an excellent source of new patients or procedures. A favorable situation could exist, for example, when one dentist prefers dealing with children, while the other enjoys endodontics or crown and bridge. If the two practices are compatible, referring may enhance the patient load of each one while providing needed services for patients.

The rewards of this type of relationship are much greater than those between a general dentist and a specialist, because the specialist is more restricted in referring patients to other doctors. If a cooperative spirit prevailed, few patients would need to leave the premises of a facility housing a number of compatible general dentists.

MONITORING AND EVALUATING PROCEDURES

Expanding the scope of care requires periodic monitoring and evaluation. The only way to be sure this exercise is carried out is to set specific time aside for that purpose. As additional services are added, they may need to be reviewed on a weekly basis at first; later they can be evaluated less frequently. Since any change in the practice generates positive and negative factors, standards of quality as well as economic and psychological results should be carefully assessed. It is important that any service be performed at the highest level of skill possible. At the same time, if because of the expansion(s) the practitioner comes under extreme stress or if he finds that the economic factors become negative, he will need to be ready to adjust — possibly by scrapping some of the additions.

> Some of the expanded procedures will simply not work out, so after a sufficient time lapse, necessary corrective action should be taken.

Involving the staff in the evaluation process will not only boost their motivation, but will very probably point out aspects that the doctor alone might miss. The effects of any changes on practice growth are especially important. Some of the expanded procedures will simply not work out, so after a sufficient time lapse, necessary corrective action should be taken.

Many opportunities in dentistry and health-related areas lie ahead to be considered. Thus, failures should be viewed as a learning process, not as a disaster. The constant search for new information and procedures will help to keep the practice outlook young and will ultimately result in more service to more patients — and economic growth as well.

SUMMARY

Many dentists are finding it necessary to expand the scope of their practices because of inflation and the increasing numbers of dentists entering the marketplace. This is causing them to examine their skills and motivations regarding the services they currently do and do not offer. It is also making them aware of the need for continuing education and for keeping in touch with other practitioners in order to stay technically competent in the procedures they perform.

The concept of the "decathlon dentist" is a valuable one to consider in the effort to gain more patients or provide more services for the ones already in the practice. By offering more services to all ages of patients, practice growth can often be boosted. The addition of procedures to an office that is less than optimally busy can also help efficiency significantly.

The staff is a valuable source of input when evaluating a practice and planning for its growth and should be consulted for optimum working relationships as well as for the development of technical superiority.

REFERENCES

Bregstein, S. J., DDS: The Succesful Practice of Dentistry. New York, Prentice-Hall, Inc., 1953.

Billingslea, M. L., DDS: Put nutrition in your practice. Dental Economics, April, 1980, pp 87–88.

Miller, R. L., DDS: Holistic dentistry — Look beyond the mouth. Dental Practice, October, 1980, pp. 36–37.

Rx for the dental office with too few patients. Dental Economics, August, 1980, pp. 34–37.

Sibson, R. E.: Increasing Employee Productivity. New York, American Management Association, 1976.

7

Publicity and Personal Contact

Doug Hoffman is elated. He has just received a letter of notification that he has passed the board. But he also is anxious, since he plans to open his own office. He takes his concerns to Bob Franks, an experienced management consultant, with whom he has developed a friendship.

"Bob, I'm worried about starting my own practice," Doug confesses. "It looks tough with interest rates so high, inflated equipment costs. . . ."

Bob nods and says, "It *is* difficult, Doug. And you've got to be careful. The financial area is riddled with danger. Today's graduate must study the situation. Two other important areas you must consider are, first, your ability to be productive, and second, patient availability. It seems to me, though, that your experience for the past year with the health department proves you have the ability to produce dentistry."

"I gained confidence and speed working for the health department," Doug says. "It also gave me time to evaluate equipment and get a line on some used equipment I can buy at a bargain. I've arranged for a low-interest loan from a relative and that will help some."

"Comparatively speaking," Bob responds, "you're much better prepared to begin practice than many of your contemporaries. You've studied your alternatives. Your major problem will be getting patients. If you can generate patients, everything else will fall into place. You need a plan, Doug, a plan that will draw patients to your practice and keep on attracting new patients throughout your career."

Dentists face problems in the 1980s that were nonexistent in the past. The major problems facing them in the decade ahead are patient load and practice economics. Regardless of a dentist's technical skills, personality, capital assets, and office staff, a practice needs patients to make it a successful one.

In order to attract more patients for any type of practice, most of today's dentists must be willing to promote themselves and their services throughout the community. Regardless of whether your practice is mature or new — or somewhere in between — promotion will make a significant — and favorable — difference.

PROMOTION AND THE MATURE PRACTICE

If you are an established dentist, chances are that you did some promotion when you began your practice, but later you became busy enough to discontinue your PR efforts. If you are now experiencing a decrease of patients, or if you want to expand your practice, you need to move back into that "promotion mode." Think back to your early days of dentistry and try to think of yourself once again as the "new kid on the block." This should help restore you to a promotion-conscious frame of mind.

PROMOTING YOUR PRACTICE

Where do dental patients come from? Where can they be found? Simple questions with simple answers. Patients come from all walks of life, in all areas. Not so simple is trying to open a practice in an area overly populated with dentists or trying to expand an existing practice where patients seem scarce. Like any other business or professional practitioner, the dentist should select as prime an area as possible in which to begin practice.

The new dentist in town will have little success unless the people realize he is there and know the services he offers. How can this be achieved effectively? The most obvious initial method is through the local newspaper. Most editors will publish an article announcing that a new professional service is available. Small-town newspapers are more apt to go into some depth in such articles, including more personal and educational background details and a picture. The articles, generally, will cover the location of the practice, any special services offered, and office hours. They will include information about the dentist's native community, professional education, membership in organizations, marital status, children, and church membership, if the dentist chooses to provide such information. The larger daily newspapers are more conservative with news space, but will announce new practices briefly.

Your first visit to the local newspaper should be viewed as an investment in your future. If you are going to make your home and practice your profession in this community, then remember that the majority of the news of the community will appear in the local news columns. This is a fact of life not only in the small suburban areas, but in the larger urban areas as well. Not only will you get to know people in your chosen community through the local news columns but they will get to know you in the same way.

During your "investment visit" to the newspaper office, try to find a contact person, someone through whom you can work on

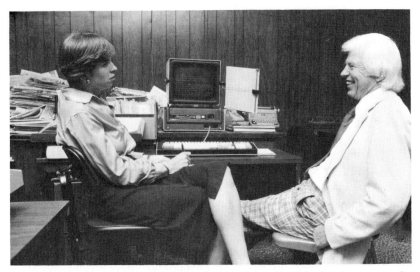

Most newspapers will be happy to publish articles about dentists in newsworthy moments, such as starting or changing the scope of a practice.

publishing future articles in which you or your practice will figure. Of course you must bear in mind that any articles should be of such import as to attract the general reading public. Such stories could include photos as well as text. For example, renovating old quarters or constructing new facilities are natural news items, especially in smaller communities. The addition of personnel to the office staff, especially if they are local, and bringing in other professionals to broaden the scope of the practice, are other examples. (And if the newspaper will not run a certain item as news, you may want to purchase space and run it as an advertisement.)

The unusual also heightens opportunities for media coverage. For example, suppose you are developing a thriving children's practice and to provide an environment esthetically pleasing to them you design and construct a children's game room, complete with decor, reading matter, and toys. Something of this nature, or of a comparable nature for adults, may generate media interest. What's more, you may have some unusual aspect within your practice in technique, services, or accessories. Have you incorporated into your practice the latest dental cosmetic techniques? Could you explain a unique surgical technique or demonstrate how implants are done?

"Going to the dentist, traditionally, is not something the average person looks forward to, Dr. Hoffman," a reporter may say. "What do you do to make the experience as pleasant as possible for your patients?"

"I use nitrous oxide," Dr. Hoffman answers. "You just breathe normally and become relaxed. Many patients then don't focus on discomfort."

Or,

"I use hypnosis."

"Oh? What about a practical demonstration on me?"

"Certainly. Just relax and concentrate. . . ."

". . . . Well? Did you have a nice rest?"

During your "investment visit" to the newspaper office, try to find a contact person, someone through whom you can work on publishing future articles in which you or your practice will figure.

"Yes, I did!"

"Look at your watch."

"Wow! It's amazing how time passed, Dr. Hoffman."

Imagine how interesting it would be to read that in the local newspaper. And imagine how many potential patients, people who — as the reporter pointed out — associate discomfort with visits to the dentist, will read such an article and say, "I think I'll call for an appointment."

While print media coverage is widespread, it is not as exciting and immediate as radio and television coverage. There are numerous opportunities for legitimate and natural exposure in both print and broadcast media. For example, there are increasing numbers of talk shows being produced on both radio and television. Many of the repeat guests on these shows are professionals who can offer demonstrations and informative conversation of interest to the general public. As a dental society representative you could be interviewed concerning changes in the care of patients, new techniques, how government rules and regulations are affecting dental practices and programs, the pros and cons of fluoridation programs, and myriad aspects of the dental profession generally unknown to the public. Many radio stations also offer time for free public service announcements, especially by professional groups such as dental societies.

Civic, Religious, and Fraternal Group Promotion

During the "getting acclimated" time, accept as many social engagements as possible.

Like choosing your community, choosing civic, religious, and fraternal organizations deserves careful evaluation. It is advantageous to visit all such organizations available in your chosen area. Yes, this will take time. But the exposure to large groups of people from all walks of life will be invaluable. You cannot possibly remember everyone you meet. They, however, will be more likely to remember you.

As a new resident, naturally, you will be sought after to become a member of various churches or organizations. Take your time before deciding which groups to join. During this "getting acclimated" time, accept as many social engagements as possible. The engagements will provide you with introductions to great numbers of people in your chosen community.

You may even be invited to speak at some functions. This will open up new challenges — and opportunities. "But what could I possibly talk about?" Dr. Hoffman asked the pharmacist from the Rotary Club who requested that he speak at the next meeting.

"How about the changes that have taken place in dentistry over the years?" the Rotarian answered. "What about some interesting aspects of your job when you worked for the county health department? Have you taken any dental trips to foreign countries? Maybe they practice the profession differently than we do here. Got a hobby? Maybe your outside interests are unusual."

When you decide which groups you will join, ostensibly for the sake of serving your community, you will choose clubs and organizations that involve the membership in community projects. Such

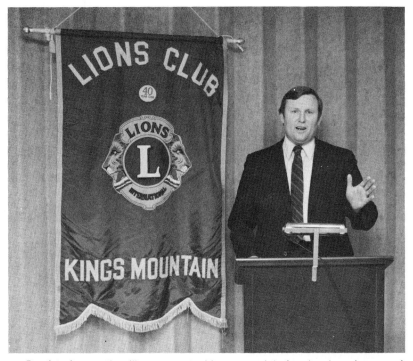

Dentists frequently will get opportunities to speak before local service organizations.

organizations provide members with the opportunity for working closely with other members and with committees from other organizations in the community; the Chamber of Commerce, United Way, American Cancer Crusade, Heart Association, and so on all include a cross-section of people.

Of course there are opportunities to serve the youth of the community through Scout leadership and as a coach for Little League, Pop Warner League, and various club- and city-sponsored athletic and recreational activities.

For more decisive community involvement, the professional may

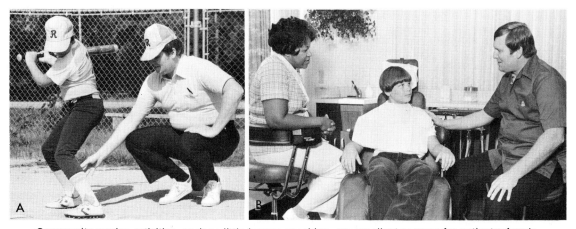

Community service activities, such as little-league coaching, are excellent sources for patient referrals.

want to consider running for a seat on the board of education or as an elected official in the local government. Of course, these offices can tend to be controversial at times, and consequently, may lose you some patients who find themselves in heated disagreement with political stands you may take. Therefore, from a business standpoint, you need to realize that, potentially, there are drawbacks to "high profile" political involvement.

From a business standpoint, you need to see that, potentially, there are drawbacks to "high profile" political involvement.

Other ways of gaining contact with people in the community include participation in groups that jog, play tennis, play golf, ski, bowl, and ride horseback. And there are hobbies: bridge, music, art, and ceramics, to name a few, which can enlarge your circle of contacts.

In the same context, it is important not to overlook the invaluable contributions family members will make during normal community organizational and recreational involvement. The spouse and childrens' services to community organizations, church activities, employment, hobbies and sports are excellent sources for potential patient referrals. Your spouse and children should gladly help in your patient recruitment if they understand how each new patient helps the family budget and lifestyle.

Business Contacts

There are residual advantages to be gained from doing business with the firms in your chosen community. One, of course, is continued exposure to numbers of people. Just as other consumers do, you should comparison shop. You will not only find some bargains for yourself, but you will also establish yourself as someone interested in supporting the community at many levels.

For example, most communites, no matter how large or small, have several of all types of the businesses whose services you will utilize. There are drug stores, service stations, dry cleaning establishments, food stores, clothing stores, and so on. Take each opportunity you can to introduce yourself to the manager and clerks in each establishment. It not only helps the businessman, but offers you the opportunity to broaden your exposure if you initially trade on a limited basis with each establishment.

Which businessperson or professional gets to know new residents first? Well, whom did you get to know first when you moved to town? The real estate broker, probably. Brokers are usually the first local professionals anywhere to know that a new family or business or professional person is establishing in the community. Real estate brokers can offer invaluable service to you.

"Who would you recommend as a dentist here?" a new resident may ask.

"Dr. Doug Jones," the broker answers. "I helped the doctor and his family locate a home and I helped the doctor locate his offices."

You will probably become acquainted with other real estate agents through the church you select, the clubs or organizations you join, or through community projects.

In both your private and professional lives you will need several types of insurance. All communities have numerous insurance companies and agents, so it would be advisable to shop for the best coverage for yourself, your family, and your business. And again, consider distributing your business. Deal with one agent for home owners' insurance, perhaps with another for hospitalization, and with still another for coverage on your business.

The same rule of thumb applies to legal service. One attorney may handle a facet of your business that another is not interested in, and you may require a third to take care of your personal needs.

Keeping your name before the public can also be accomplished through sponsoring a float in the community's annual Christmas parade or a ball club or bowling league and through placing congratulatory or token advertisements in sports programs or cultural events playbills. You will be able to think of others.

Each example mentioned so far deals with large numbers of people from all walks of life on a daily basis. And each can become an excellent avenue for getting your name before the public.

Keeping your name before the public can also be accomplished through sponsorships. . . .

Adult Education Programs

Completing general college and dental school courses may have fatigued you for a while, but don't overlook the advantages of continued education, whether as a teacher or as a student.

The growing importance of community colleges throughout the nation has created an increasing demand for qualified instructors on a wide variety of subjects. The dentist is a natural for teaching in the health areas. As an instructor you will be communicating face to face with the student population, the administration, and your fellow instructors. In addition, most courses are advertised in brochures and newspapers. Your name will be exposed to everyone reading the brochures or advertisements.

And why not investigate the advantages of becoming a student in courses related to your profession, or in courses of personal interest totally unrelated to your work? The results will be the same — education plus personal exposure to more and more potential patients.

Don't overlook the advantage of continued education, whether as a teacher or as a student.

Contact With Other Health Professionals

How many physicians, pharmacists, and other dentists are practicing within a short distance of you? (What constitutes a "short distance" will vary depending on whether you are located in a densely populated urban area — such as Chicago — a suburb, a small city, or a rural area. In Chicago the radius of your visits may be only a mile or so. In a rural area, such as Stokes County, North Carolina, the radius may be twenty miles.) Make it a point to determine the answer, then offer each health professional a personal visit. Get to know them. It may require several visits to meet everyone in a single location, but this is time well spent — another investment in your future. During your get-acquainted periods you can stress your willingness to help in dental matters and to accept new patients. Even if you gain few of these professional people as patients, they may refer others your way if they know you are receptive to new patients.

In talking with physicians and other dentists, especially those well-established in the community, make it clear what type of services your practice offers. If a special area of interest is preventive dentistry for children, the pediatrician will bear that in mind when referring his own patients. Some established dentists are willing to refer their overflow and, after getting to know you, likely will accept your offer to cover for them in emergencies while they vacation or attend conventions.

> Some established dentists are likely to accept your offer to cover for them in emergencies while they vacation or attend conventions.

Volunteer Dental Services

Every community in the country is understaffed in one category: volunteer professional help. No matter how many volunteers are on the rolls, there are never enough professionals willing to do volunteer work.

In the schools, dental screening can be of great benefit to hundreds, even thousands, of students and their families. Such programs will require time and effort on the part of the practicing dentist. This time and effort expended, however, is another bedrock

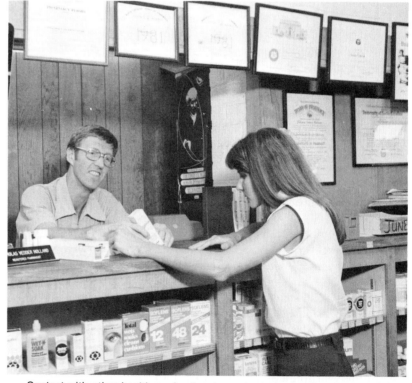

Contact with other health professionals, such as pharmacists, increases your chances for gaining patients.

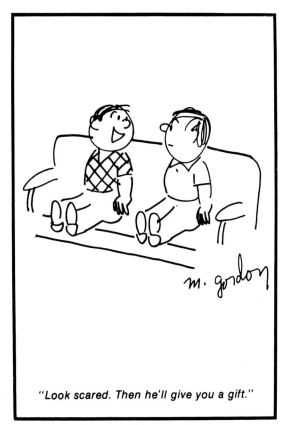

"Look scared. Then he'll give you a gift."

Courtesy of *Cal* magazine.

investment in the future. Another example of volunteer time well spent is in school athletic programs, making impressions for mouth guards to protect the teeth in football and other contact sports.

Volunteer activities are also channeled through ministerial associations, church groups, civic groups, and public health departments. Through these organizations, depending on the time the individual dentist can afford and the strength of his or her practice, discount or gratis dentistry can be offered. Many times the fact that a dentist provides free dental services for needy families will create favorable impressions on other families, who are able to pay, and who, in turn, will become patients.

Other public exposure through volunteer programs could include conducting oral cancer clinics at county fairs, shopping malls, community recreational facilities, or senior citizens centers.

The practicing dentist must, however, be very careful in committing time and energies to volunteer programs because the demand will always far outweigh the dentist's supply of time. Only you, yourself, can decide how much time away from your practice and family you can afford. Check out the possibilities and decide which programs will offer you (1) the best exposure and (2) the best outlet in which your skills can benefit your community. The two can be compatible. (You will recall that Chapter 5 discussed how you might determine the amount of volunteer time to contribute, and, in general, how to set such goals.)

Selective Fee Discounts

Fee discounts to dental auxiliaries can pay off handsomely in patient referrals.

Fee discounts can be argued pro and con. There has been a trend, especially in the more urban areas, away from the practice of giving fee discounts to other health professionals. In the smaller communities, however, fee discounts are still offered to other dentists, physicians, and pharmacists and their families.

On the plus side a discount can potentially build a good relationship with fellow health professionals. As a result they may boost your practice by referring patients to you.

There are several negative factors, though. Professionals and their families who receive discounts may be reluctant, or embarrassed, to call on you, reasoning that they are taking your time away from fee-paying patients. Also, they may tend not to complain about dental problems or less-than-perfect results for fear of seeming ungracious.

There is also a trend away from offering the time-honored ministerial discount, but each professional must make his own decision regarding this. Fee discounts to dental auxiliaries such as lab employees, office personnel, and dental assistants and hygienists can pay off handsomely in patient referrals. Discounts, when offered, usually vary from one procedure to another.

Dental Auxiliary Groups

Dental auxiliaries constitute one of the better sources of patient referrals. As often as you can, provide educational and professional programs for these groups, because it is advantageous to familiarize yourself with personnel from other offices. This can be especially helpful in attracting to your practice patient overflow or emergencies the other offices cannot handle.

Getting to know dental lab personnel could assist you in achieving a greater command in technical areas that can be applied to your practice. Laboratory personnel can also become another patient referral source. They, more authoritatively than anyone else, can say, "Dr. Hoffman is the best dentist for what you need."

TECHNIQUES TO GAIN ADDITIONAL EXPOSURE

It is good to develop rapport
with the local and county
health departments, social
services, welfare department,
Veterans Administration,
Headstart, and similar agencies.

To increase your availability as a professional to the public, why not offer your services for emergency dental treatment through the local hospital or investigate the possibility of being appointed to the hospital staff? Another approach would be to notify health agencies and area hotels and motels of your availability in emergencies to their clients and guests, especially if you have extended business hours.

It is a good and worthy practice to develop meaningful rapport with the personnel in the offices of the local and county health departments, social services, welfare department, Veterans Administration, Headstart, and other similar agencies. Get to know them; offer to help them. In a low-key way let them know about your practice and availability. (Some of these organizations often have difficulty finding a dentist who is interested in and capable of serving their clients or members.)

Develop contacts with management in local industries in which employees are provided with dental insurance benefits. Make it known to the management and to those in the employee insurance office that you would appreciate being able to provide dental services to their employees. Offer whatever help you can, especially to the benefits person. Taking the time to become proficient in processing insurance paperwork is an investment that can pay large dividends in patient referrals. Management may even publish your name in the firm's newsletter or newspaper.

An inexpensive item you may wish to consider is the printed referral slip. This small pad with printed directions — map, street names, and so on — can be left in conspicuous places, such as all of the business and professional and agency offices mentioned throughout this chapter. Most motels, too, would be happy to have you leave referral slips at their front desks in case any of their guests need emergency dental treatment.

An inexpensive item is the printed referral slip, which can be left in conspicuous places.

Just picture your practice building day by day through scenarios such as the following:

"Maybe you could help me," says the man to the secretary at the county health department. "Can you recommend a dentist who will take a new patient?"

"Certainly. Dr. Hoffman is always happy to have new patients," answers the secretary. Then she tears a slip from the referral pad and hands it to the man and adds: "This map will guide you straight to his office. If you should get lost, there is his name, address, and telephone number, so you can call. He's a very good dentist and is well known in town." (See sample referral slips.)

LAY ADVISORY PANEL

As Proverbs says, "There is wisdom in many counselors." Thus, a lay advisory panel is something to consider after you have become better established in your chosen community. By then, you will have a good idea as to whose advice is sound — and whose is less than sound. With this insight, consider approaching a cross-section of people whose judgment you value about serving as your personal lay advisors.

After you have become better established in your chosen community, consider a lay advisory panel.

Service on your advisory panel needs to be on a quid-pro-quo basis. Lay advisors deserve some compensation, which may vary according to their circumstances. For instance, a secretary or medical student might be delighted with $15 a meeting, whereas to a veteran insurance broker this would be inconsequential, though he might, instead, value being the agent for your business and peronal policies.

Once your panel is established, schedule meetings as regularly as you feel necessary, and as your advisors' schedules will allow, to gain advice on your practice policies, which areas of community needs are not being met, and how you might go about filling those voids.

PRACTICE LIMITED TO ORAL SURGERY   TELEPHONE 704-865-7603

MICHAEL J. LEWISTON, D.D.S.

COX ROAD PROFESSIONAL BUILDING
471 COX ROAD
GASTONIA, NORTH CAROLINA 28052

PATIENT'S NAME _____

RIGHT   **PERMANENT**   LEFT

RIGHT   LEFT

DECIDUOUS

RADIOGRAPHS ENCLOSED YES_____ NO_____

PANOREX RADIOGRAPH DESIRED YES_____ NO_____

REMARKS

_____

_____

_____

REFERRED BY DR. _____

EMERGENCY — 24 HOURS ANSWERING SERVICE 865–7603

PAMELA BLACKSTONE, D.D.S.
COX ROAD PROFESSIONAL BUILDING
471 COX ROAD
GASTONIA, NORTH CAROLINA 28052
TELEPHONE 704-864-8896

_____

Introducing_____for Root Canal Treatment.

Appointment Time:_____

Referred by Dr. _____

Comments:_____

_____

_____

_____

_____

_____

_____

_____

_____

DENTISTRY

J. ROBERT GROVES, D.D.S.
WEST GATE PROFESSIONAL CENTER
HIGHWAY 74 WEST
KINGS MOUNTAIN, N. C. 28086

TELEPHONE
(704) 739-7956

_____19_____

THIS WILL INTRODUCE _____
FOR PEDIATRIC DENTAL TREATMENT.

RADIOGRAPHS ENCLOSED   ☐ YES ☐ NO
TREATMENT PLAN ENCLOSED ☐ YES ☐ NO

COMMENTS: _____
_____
_____

REFERRED BY DR. _____

APPOINTMENT: DAY_____ MONTH _____ TIME _____

OFFICE POLICY: OUR PRACTICE ACCEPTS ONLY CHILDREN AS PATIENTS. NORMALLY, CHILDREN ARE
RETURNED TO THE REFERRING DENTIST AFTER AGE 12. ALL CHILDREN **MUST** BE
TRANSFERRED FROM THE PRACTICE BY AGE 18, HANDICAPPED CHILDREN EXCEPTED.

☐ PLEASE SEND ADDITIONAL SLIPS.

(Please see other side for directions to office)

"You're doing a good job with children, Dr. Hoffman," the banker on your panel may say, "and the young and middle-aged adults seem to be getting adequate care. But our elderly do not receive enough attention. I mean the senior citizens living on fixed incomes. Perhaps you could work out a special program for them. Such a program could help your practice in terms of goodwill and more patients."

The fact that you appointed such a panel, putting your trust in your fellow citizens, so to speak, will also favor your practice. Such open-mindedness on the part of a professional is not found very often. The fact that you heed the panel's advice will give you a definite marketing advantage because you have thereby demonstrated your committment to meeting the community's dental needs as perceived by more objective observers.

SUMMARY

Before you can practice dentistry, you must view yourself as a package, your skills as a product. When a patient has purchased the package and the product, the result should be satisfaction for that patient. Once the first patient has been satisfied it will become less difficult, as time goes by, to sell the product.

To aid in creating an effective marketing program, the dentist is at liberty to utilize whatever positive programs the imagination can create. The raw materials available, in a manner of speaking, are local newspapers and radio and television stations; other professional and health-related agencies, both private and public; commercial businesses, civic clubs and organizations and industry and educational institutions; fraternal organizations and recreational programs.

For such a sales-promotion-public relations program to be successful, the dentist must make a serious commitment. It is a commitment to submerge self and family into the very heart of the community and to become an integral part, a viable, functioning member of that community. It requires the dentist to make a substantial investment in the community in time and energy.

How well the dentist's fellow professionals perceive him may be judged by many things, but how well the community at large perceives him will be judged solely on how well he applies his professional skills for the benefit of patients. All of the most effective self-promotional schemes known to man will carry the dentist only so far. Then professional skills must support the promotion. In other words, no matter how attractive the package may be, the quality of the product will be the primary reason it continues to sell.

You should view yourself as a package, your skills as a product.

REFERENCES

Ball, Frank M., DDS: Adventures in advertising. Dental Management, July, 1979, pp. 47–51.

The Business of Dental Practice (by Editors of Dental Management), Stamford, CT, Professional Publishing Corporation, 1969.

Dental Practice Information: Building Your Practice. American Dental Association, 1979, pp. 17–1 and 17–2.

Howard, William O.: Dental Practice Planning. St. Louis, C. V. Mosby Company, 1975.

Loeb, L. H., DDS: Reach your public with a radio message. Dental Practice, Feburary, 1981, pp. 62–64.

Management Aid for the New Dental Practice. Building Your Practice. Professional Budget Plan, 1960.

Rx for the dental office with two few patients. Dental Economics, August, 1980, pp. 34–47.

8

Media Advertising

Ted Joyner paused in the midst of a treatment plan he was reviewing. Within the next hour, he was going to have to make a decision on whether or not to participate in a radio advertising program proposed by a local station. There were many contradictory thoughts going on in his mind. On the one hand, Ted had always believed, and he thought others believed as well, that advertising was contrary to good ethics in the dental profession. "Oh sure," he said, "I know that the ADA removed advertising from its list of no-no's some time ago. But, it still doesn't seem right to me." On the other hand, Ted was aware that some of the other dentists in the area were advertising, and they didn't seem to be looked upon as unethical. Some of them even seemed to be prospering! "Perhaps," Ted thought to himself, "I had better learn more about advertising before I make this decision."

WHAT IS ADVERTISING?

Frequently, the terms advertising and sales promotion are confused.

Advertising may be defined as any form of nonpersonal presentation and promotion of ideas, goods, or services paid for by and identified with a sponsor. The key words here are "paid," "nonpersonal," and "identified." If it is not paid for by the dentist, if it is addressed to a specific person, or if it is not clear who is paying for the publicity, then it is not advertising.

Frequently, the terms advertising and sales promotion are confused. In its broadest sense, sales promotion includes advertising, personal selling, and any other promotional activities. In a narrower sense, sales promotion refers to those activities that supplement advertising and personal selling. Such activities would include displays or exhibits (at school or county fairs, for example), demonstrations, and other nonrecurring selling activities.

One frequently hears the term "word-of-mouth" advertising. As we define advertising above, there is no such term. However, such person-to-person communication, which is perceived as noncommercial, does exist; it can either hurt or help us. Because word-of-mouth advertising is perceived as noncommercial, it is usually seen as an unbiased source of information. It is necessary, then, for us to make certain that all of our relationships in the community, both personal and professional, are good ones. Then, when "word-of-mouth advertising" is used, that is, when people talk about us, we can be better assured that we are well spoken of. Remember, though, that word-of-mouth is something on which we can have little short-term influence. Good reputations come from doing a good job in the community, both in our personal and our professional contacts.

Do Dentists Advertise?

Before we discuss the details of advertising, we should try to estimate how many dentists are advertising currently, and how many plan to at some later date. Two recent surveys give us a percentage range within which to make our estimates. In 1980, the newsletter *The Advertising Dentist* surveyed its subscribers and found that 30 per cent of the respondents said they advertised and 64 per cent said they planned to advertise at some point. Obviously, this was not a sample representative of all dentists; in order to be included in the sample, they had to be subscribers to *The Advertising Dentist*. In other words, this sample favored those with an interest in advertising.

The "true" percentage of advertising dentists . . . is still unknown. Perhaps it falls somewhere between 12 and 30 per cent.

Another survey, by *Dental Economics,* revealed that in 1980 a sample of 2500 general practitioners indicated that only 12 percent advertised and an additional 16 percent either planned to advertise in the future or would consider it if a majority of their colleagues advertised.

The "true" percentage of advertising dentists, of course, is still unknown. Perhaps it falls somewhere between 12 and 30 percent. It would be difficult to make a precise estimate at this time, but perhaps as good a rough guess as any would be to take the mid-point of these two surveys, or 21 percent. Assuming that 21 percent is somewhere near the actual percentage of advertising dentists, what can we conclude? First, we can conclude that many more dentists now advertise than did previously. Considering the relatively short period in which dentists have been "allowed" to advertise, it would not be too much to conclude that advertising is here to stay and that we all must seriously consider whether or not we want to advertise. It is likely that some day advertising will become commonplace among dentists.

Who Advertises?

In the surveys by *The Advertising Dentist* mentioned above, half of all respondents generate between $100,000 and $250,000 in fees annually. Nearly 7 percent generate annual fees of $250,000 to $500,000. Nearly two thirds of the respondents were between 25 and 35 years of age. This group also had the largest percentage of advertising dentists, more than 36 percent. The advertising dentist, then, is young and has a relatively high-grossing practice.

The advertising dentist . . . is young and has a relatively high-grossing practice.

Advertising Appeals Used

When many of us think of dentists who advertise, we are inclined to believe that the appeal is to price — after all, why advertise if you cannot demonstrate lower prices and cost savings to the patient? The survey by *The Advertising Dentist* belies this conclusion. The advertising appeals reported by survey respondents are reported below, and *quality of care* was the most reported appeal. Although *dollar savings* was the second most important reported appeal, this was followed closely by several other appeals, including *hours, convenience of locations, professional competence,* and others.

Appeal	Percent Responding
Quality of Care	54
Dollar Savings	44
Hours	39
Convenience of Locations	39
Professional Competence	34
Rapid Service	27
Pain-free Dentistry	13
Cosmetic Benefits	13
Credit Available	7

Authorities say that reasons for not going to the dentist are usually one or more of the following three: (1) lack of awareness; (2) unwillingness or inability to pay for the service; or (3) fear of discomfort and inconvenience. An advertisement reported to be most effective is "We cater to cowards." If advertising is to be effective with the nonuser, the 75 per cent who receive no regular dental attention, the appeal should be based on one or more of the three primary reasons for not going to the dentist. Advertising is likely to be entirely ineffective with the person who seeks regular attention from a dentist he's satisfied with. The cost-benefit ratio for advertising is likely to be favorable in accordance with its success in appealing to nonusers.

CHOICE OF MEDIA

The first type of advertising most dentists think of is the Yellow Pages. Seventy-five percent of all responding dentists report using the Yellow Pages.

O.K., so we have come to the conclusion that advertising is for us, or soon will be. We also realize that if we are going to advertise, we are going to have to pay for it. How do we decide which of the media we should use? The following discussion is a review of the media available, with an indication for each medium of the use by dentists responding to the survey discussed previously.

Yellow Pages

The first type of advertising most dentists think of is Yellow Pages. Seventy-five percent of all responding dentists report using the Yellow Pages. Apparently, this is the medium first thought of, the one most easily accepted by dentists who start advertising.

The Yellow Pages most often are used by consumers after a need has been felt by them and they are ready to select a provider. From a dentist's perspective, this means that when a person has decided that he or she needs and wants to visit a dentist, the reference source most often used is the telephone book. This medium is the only one that is received and retained throughout the year by all people and businesses with telephones.

In addition to space in the Yellow Pages section of the telephone book, dentists may buy **BOLD** listings, the same as the regular white-page listings but set in boldface capital letters, and extra lines of copy in the Yellow Pages section describing features of the practice.

Studies have shown that the Yellow Pages reach about 77 percent of the entire U.S. adult population aged twenty or over with a frequency of about 40 times per year. There are nearly four billion (!) references to the Yellow Pages in a year, with nearly 90 percent of these followed by a telephone call, a visit, or a letter. Over half of these references were made *without a name in mind beforehand.*

It is clear that the Yellow Pages can be and are very important to dentists. It is little wonder that this is the most used medium for dental advertising.

Newspapers

Daily newspapers were the second most reported medium used by dentists, over 40 per cent. Weekly newspapers were the third most important reported medium, nearly 30 percent. Shopping newspapers, sometimes called "free" newspapers or "penny-saver" newspapers were reported as used by 25 percent of responding dentists. In short, newspapers are a very important medium of advertising by dentists.

Newspapers reach an accumulated 89 per cent of all adults over the five weekday period.

Newspapers come in many forms, as the reports above indicate. In addition to the vast majority of United States newspapers, which are of the general editorial type, there are several hundred foreign language newspapers. Also available are religious newspapers, labor newspapers, the college and high school press, newspapers edited primarily for black audiences, and shopping newspapers. The newspaper is one of the media that gives the advertiser extensive opportunities to reach specific audiences.

An advertiser buys a newspaper space for *audience,* and audience is calculated from *circulation.* Further, circulation is the means by which the cost of advertising is determined. Circulation, therefore, should be verified. Many, but not all newspapers have their circulation audited by The Audit Bureau of Circulation. You should ask the newspaper in which you are considering advertising for a copy of its audit report. One item in the audit report that might be helpful is the geographical classification: city zone circulation is that within the city limits; trading zone circulation, perhaps the most helpful for dentists, is that within the retail trading or shopping area of the city; "other" circulation is that outside the city and retail trading area, most often not at all helpful to a local advertiser, such as a dentist.

There are two comparison factors the dentist should consider in buying newspaper advertising. These will be particularly helpful, of course, to the dentist deciding between or among alternative newspapers. The first of these comparison factors is the *milline* rate, the traditional basis for newspaper rate comparison. The milline rate is calculated as follows:

$$\text{Milline} = \frac{\text{Line rate} \times 1{,}000{,}000}{\text{circulation}}$$

In other words, the milline rate is the cost of sending one agate line* of advertising to one million readers. Suppose a newspaper has a line rate of $2.00 and a circulation of 571,000. Substituting,

$$\frac{\$2 \times 1{,}000{,}000}{571{,}000} = \frac{\$2{,}000{,}000}{571{,}000} = \$3.50 \text{ milline rate}$$

It is possible to calculate a milline rate for total circulation of the newspaper; most helpful for most of us will be a calculation of the milline rate for *effective circulation,* that circulation most important to our practices. For some dentists, retail trading area circulation will be effective circulation; for others, only a part of the city's circulation will be effective.

Milline rates are used less and less in newspaper comparisons, in large measure because they are not compatible with the measure used by most other media, cost per thousand. Cost per thousand (or CPM, as it is commonly referred to) is calculated as follows:

$$\text{Cost per thousand} = \frac{\text{agate line charge} \times 1000}{\text{circulation or delivered audience (000 omitted)}}$$

As with the milline rate, the dentist should try to determine *effective* circulation — the circulation that is most likely to be available to his practice. Also, because circulation is the most readily available quantitative measurement, it is the most often used. However, qualitative factors must be considered as well. Any advertiser must ask himself or herself the question: "Cost per thousand what?" In other words, just because a newspaper prints a lot of copies doesn't necessarily mean that it will be a good medium for a given dentist. Find out all you can about the newspaper you are considering using, and make your advertising decision based on both quantitative and qualitative factors.

According to the Newspaper Advertising Bureau, 77 percent of adults eighteen and older read a newspaper on an average weekday. Newspapers reach an accumulated 89 percent of all adults over the five weekday period. In general, 84 percent of all newspaper readers turn to the page, excluding classified, carrying any advertiser's message. It is little wonder that advertising dentists have found newspapers helpful.

One aspect of newspapers we will discuss here is, strictly speaking, not advertising at all, but it may be more effective than advertis-

Commercial services are available to provide dentists with a prepackaged advertising column.

*Agate line is a common term in newspaper advertising, referring to a space one-fourteenth inch deep by the column width.

ing. That is the writing of a newspaper column on a periodic basis. You may decide to volunteer (or members of a group practice may decide to share the work) to write a weekly, monthly, or less regular column for a local newspaper with the headline something like, but certainly not limited to, "Dental Health Tips" or "Improving Your Dental Health."

In this column, you would review in a nontechnical way how people should treat their teeth, how often they should visit a dentist, the meaning of various dental procedure terms, what dentists do and why, what dental auxiliaries do and why, why flossing ought to be done regularly, how to floss, and so on. There are perhaps hundreds of topics that could be covered in a short column. After the basic topics have been covered, in six months to a year, you can start over with the same topic covered in at least a slightly different way. Commercial services are available to provide dentists with a prepackaged advertising column.

You should require that you be given a "byline" on the column (Ted Joyner, DDS). However, this is probably the limit to which you can or should go in promoting your practice. You should never refer to your practice specifically. Nor should you suggest that people visit your office. If they wish to use you as their dentist, so much the better, but you cannot ask or suggest they do so.

Radio

Slightly over one fifth of advertising dentists report using radio advertisements. This is likely to increase in years to come. Modern

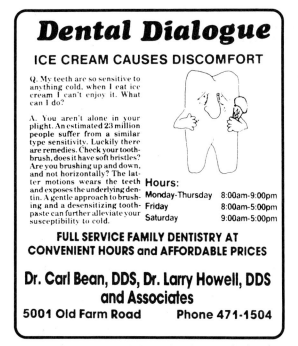

A low-key public service, or informational, type of advertisement.

radio has changed a great deal from what it was prior to the advent of television. Radio has an almost unique ability to deliver advertising to specialized audiences, a made-to-order benefit for dentists. While there is often only one newspaper in a market, there are often several radio stations, each usually delivering a different specific audience. Radio stations can deliver advertising to specific demographically segmented audiences, such as adults, older adults, blacks, farmers, housewives, teenagers, college students, military audiences, and others.

Radio stations can deliver advertising to specific demographically segmented audiences.

Although many dentists will not have a use for a radio station broadcasting in a foreign language, it is interesting to note that in the United States there are stations broadcasting all or part of their programming in Arabic, Armenian, Basque, Cajun, Croatian, Finnish, French, German, Greek, Hindi, Hungarian, Italian, Japanese, Korean, Latvian, Lithuanian, Maltese, Navajo, Pennsylvania Dutch, Farsi, Polish, Portuguese, Pueblo, Romanian, Russian, Serbian, Sioux, Spanish, Swahili, Swedish, Syrian, Tagalog, Ukrainian, Vietnamese, Zuñi, and others.

As with other media, dentists should examine the radio station and its coverage before deciding to advertise. Wide coverage is not necessarily beneficial to the advertising dentist. A *clear-channel* AM station operates at 50,000 watts and will have a very wide coverage, especially at night. In no instance will this be helpful to the dentist. Even regional stations that operate on not more than 5,000 watts, usually covering many counties, will not be of interest. *Local* stations operating 1,000 watts or less (often as little as 5 watts) will most often be the stations of greatest interest to us. The important criterion is that the station or stations be those listened to most often by your current patients and by those patients you most would like to have. The secret to this, if it can be called that, is to ask your patients, usually in casual conversation, which radio station they listen to most. Finding out the station preferences of your desired patients is a little more difficult, but usually can be accomplished in conversation with your friends and the community contacts discussed elsewhere in this book.

Usually radio time is sold on the basis of station break and spot announcement time. Radio rates are usually quoted for one-minute, 30-second, and 10-second announcements. Which length of spot is most effective? For dentists the 30-second spot perhaps works best — long enough to get your message across, not so long as to seem too "high-pressure." However, this might vary from market to market. You should discuss your needs with advertising representatives from local stations. It is possible in some communities and on some stations to buy a *program,* but that will normally not be of interest to the individual dentist or group practice. However, if the local, county, or state society decides to sponsor a program on dental health awareness, then you may be involved in buying a "program."

Radio rates vary according to the time of day. Time periods are divided into classes, depending upon the station's and the market's estimation of the value of the time period. A few stations have classes identified as drive time, homemaker and weekend time, nighttime, and swing shift time. It is not unusual to find discounts offered to the advertiser who agrees to advertise over a period of time. Ask the station advertising representative for a complete list of advertising opportunities and details.

Television

As might be expected, only 8 percent of the dentists responding to *The Advertising Dentist* survey mentioned previously reported that they do television advertising. Television is very important in American society, but it is also very expensive for the advertiser, and it is normally not very selective in terms of audience coverage. The previously described media can normally be chosen and purchased by the dentist without outside help. If the dentist chooses to use television as an advertising medium, we highly recommend that he turn to an advertising agency for professional help.

Other Media

Twenty-five percent of the responding dentists reported using other media of a diverse nature. We will present and briefly discuss some of these below.

Direct mail is the most personal of the media. It is somewhat surprising that more dentists do not use it. One form of direct mail is

A newsletter sent to patients and community contacts... can not only promote the practice, but can also promote greater dental awareness and dental health habits.

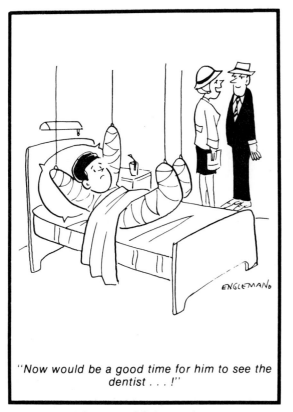

"Now would be a good time for him to see the dentist . . . !"

Courtesy of *Cal* magazine.

simply the announcement letter, announcing such items as services provided, expanded hours of the practice, discounts for senior citizens, and the like. Another form of direct mail is the practice newsletter. A newsletter sent to patients and community contacts periodically, perhaps quarterly, can not only promote the practice, but can also promote greater dental awareness and dental health habits. Many dentists, as you will remember from Chapter 5, have set goals for raising dental IQs among their patients and in the community. Such a newsletter can help achieve this goal. The newsletter should be as light and "chatty" as possible, while stressing better dental health and treatment. Sometimes a cartoon, making fun of dentistry in a friendly way, can help build positive attitudes toward dentistry and help attract to dental offices the 75 percent of the population that is currently receiving inadequate dental care. A direct mail piece as involved as a newsletter can be a very inexpensive yet time-consuming endeavor. It may pay off more than any other advertising in terms of added business versus time and money expended. Much material for the newsletter can be reused from the newspaper column referred to earlier in this chapter, Or, as mentioned, there are prepackaged newsletters that you may wish to purchase and distribute.

Some dentists have chosen to provide to their patients and the community such specialty advertising items as balloons, key chains, emergency number stick-ons for telephones and telephone books, and the like. These can be very effective for very little expense. They are less likely to build the practice than they are to keep the practice in the minds of current patients. Many dentists have been reluctant to engage in such advertising because of the fear, perhaps justified, of appearing too trivial. However, any dentist wishing to investigate the giving of such gifts can usually find local suppliers in the Yellow Pages under "specialty advertising" or "advertising specialties."

HOW MUCH TO SPEND

Advertising should be keyed to results and goals. Arbitrarily allocated sums are keyed to nothing.

Ted Joyner has not yet decided whether or not he wants to advertise at all, let alone whether or not he wants to jump into radio. But one of the topics he knew he needed to address was how much to spend. There are several ways a dentist can decide how much to spend, and some dentist somewhere has tried them all.

The first method we will term "arbitrary allocation." Ted may decide to spend $1,000 for advertising in the first year. He doesn't have much experience or know-how to go on, but that number, or another arbitrary allocation, seems conservative enough for the first year, so he will make that decision, The drawbacks of this method are obvious. Advertising should be keyed to results and goals. Arbitrarily allocated sums are keyed to nothing.

Another possible method is "what the practice can afford." That is, Ted could estimate his total service fees for next year, subtract all likely expenses, including what he would like to pay himself, and if any money is left over, that could be given over to advertising. Obviously, this is even worse than the "arbitrary allocation" method.

A third possibility for Ted is the "percent of fees" method, where he sets an arbitrary percentage of his projected fees aside for advertising. If Ted believes he will gross $150,000 next year and if he believes that 2 percent is "about right" for advertising, then he would plan to spend $3,000 on advertising. This method is not very defensible for a number of reasons, the most outstanding of which is that fees are controlling advertising instead of advertising controlling fees.

Another possible method Ted Joyner might use to determine how much to spend for advertising is "competitive parity." That is, he may try to estimate what his major dental competitors are spending on advertising and then try to spend at least that much on advertising his own practice. This method seems to be pointed in the wrong direction. It does not look at what Ted's practice needs in the way of advertising; it looks at what his competitors' practices need.

The last method we will discuss, and the one we recommend that you use to determine how much to spend on advertising, is the "task" method. In this method, you need to think through and determine what you want your advertising to do. Looking back to Chapter 5, what goals have you set for your service fees for next year, for five years from now? Based on your desired increase in fees, you can translate that into the increase in patients needed. Then, think in terms of how many people you will need to contact with your advertising in order to bring in the required number of new patients. Then you can calculate how much it will cost to reach that number of people with the media available to you.

In the final analysis, money should be spent where it is most effective. Evaluate your program and learn how many new patients each kind of advertising is generating. Depending on what you consider the dollar worth of each new patient, you can rationally allocate budget funds to the various media.

> Think in terms of how many people you will need to contact with your advertising in order to bring in the required number of new patients.

DEVELOPING YOUR ADVERTISEMENTS

It would take a book or two to tell you how to write advertisements. We will not try to do this. Instead, we will give you a few hints. Beyond that, you should use your own good judgment or refer to one of the references listed at the end of this Chapter or to one or more of the several advertising books you are likely to find at your local public library.

Write your ads in terms of *patient or reader benefits*. Make sure there is a central benefit to the patient in your ads. The best benefits are those which promise satisfaction, telling patients "what's in it for them." The text of an advertisement is organized around this patient benefit; the benefit serves as a point of focus. The benefit idea needs to be expressed in just about every important element in the advertisement. It should be obvious in the illustration, the headline, the lead or first paragraph, the text, and in the closing paragraph. It is, thus, announced at the beginning, enlarged on in the text, and repeated in the ending of the advertisement, often in the form of a specific phrase or slogan. Such repetition insures a greater grasp of the idea, deeper penetration, and more memory value.

Let's review some copy considerations. Before an advertisement

> Make sure there is a central benefit to the patient in your ads. . . . The benefit idea needs to be expressed in just about every important element in the advertisement.

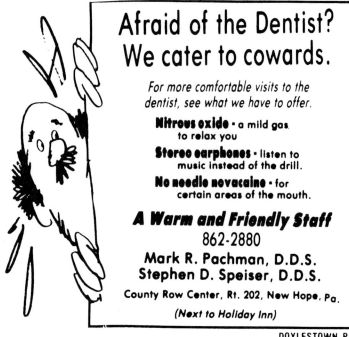

**Afraid of the Dentist?
We cater to cowards.**

*For more comfortable visits to the
dentist, see what we have to offer.*

Nitrous oxide · a mild gas
to relax you

Stereo earphones · listen to
music instead of the drill.

No needle novacaine · for
certain areas of the mouth.

A Warm and Friendly Staff
862-2880
**Mark R. Pachman, D.D.S.
Stephen D. Speiser, D.D.S.**
County Row Center, Rt. 202, New Hope, Pa.
(Next to Holiday Inn)

DOYLESTOWN, PA.
INTELLIGENCER

The headline "We cater to cowards" is considered to be one of the most effective in recent dental advertisements.

can influence and actuate a patient, it must *stop* and *inform*. Basically, the reader wants to know what the service is, what it costs, and above all, what it does to and for him. Two background facts are well worth remembering. One, the typical reader actually knows very little about dentistry and its capacity to provide satisfaction. Two, the reader is not going to study, to strain, to work hard in order to understand the advertiser's message. These two facts recommend that every advertisement be full enough of information to tell the exact story the advertiser wants to tell and full enough so that the reader will not have to make any inferences or assumptions.

Unless people find copy *interesting*, they will not read it. Until the advertiser captures the reader's mind and gets him to think about the possibility of having dentistry performed for him, the advertiser has not made much progress. People are readers before they are dental patients, and great numbers of them will leave the advertising message literally at the end of every sentence unless the copy is good reading — pleasant, enjoyable, even entertaining. Copy that is dull, boring, and monotonously like competitor's copy is passed over in favor of copy that is unusual, fresh, and sparkling.

We have just recognized that if copy is to be read, it must be interesting. We now observe that if copy is to influence, it must be *believed*. Belief is an individual personal matter, resting more on emotion than on reason. The prospective patient's background and experience are strong influences. People tend to believe what they want to believe — about how to become beautiful, or healthy, or wealthy. They tend to believe what others believe, friends, authorities (such as you and other dentists), even "everybody." Claims that are vague and general instead of specific and factual invite rejection. Copy that is insincere, extravagant, or excessively competitive is accepted by few consumers as truthful.

Your newspaper advertisements, needless to say, should reflect taste and thoughtfulness. Try to convey the same image that you convey with your office decor. Esthetics are important. In most cities advertising sales representatives are genuinely helpful in suggesting type styles and wording for headlines and copy. Sometimes you can even have a newspaper graphic artist supply you with sketches of possible illustrations or ad designs.

The last copy consideration we shall mention is that of persuasion. To be successful, copy must persuade; to be persuasive, copy must, most of all, be sincere, a quality most difficult to simulate. When the advertising message is honest and frank, when it is characterized by restraint and simplicity, when its tone is friendly and warm, then readers are inclined to go along with the advertiser's suggestions. Persuasive copy reflects the advertiser's genuine concern for the reader and the interest the advertiser feels in helping the reader enjoy greater success in his undertakings. A straight-forward, direct, obvious approach to helping the reader maximize satisfaction is usually more effective than an oblique, circuitous approach.

Often, the best approach to advertising — or even to the more general spectrum of marketing — is to engage a consultant who is experienced in serving health-care practitioners. (The average advertising or public relations agency may well lack the kind of sensitivity to dental professional ethics and issues that you will need.) Unfortunately, such consultants are still relatively scarce. As marketing becomes more of a necessity among dentists, however, it can be expected that consultants will develop to meet this need.

Claims that are vague and general instead of specific and factual invite rejection.

Here are some other points to note and remember in regard to advertising:

— Don't spread yourself too thin, trying to do too much with too little money. Rather, focus on what seems to you the best medium.

— Advertise regularly. Advertising is no arena for quitters. It will take you more than one or two ads to be effective.

— Keep your patients and their concerns in the center of your advertising campaign.

— Get the best informed help you can in constructing your advertisements. Remember: you're a dentist, not an award-winning copywriter or graphic artist.

EVALUATING ADVERTISING EFFECTIVENESS

One of the most difficult tasks you will have is that of evaluating the effectiveness of your advertising efforts. The basic reason for this is that many, many things will contribute to your practice's success. Among them are your location or locations, the attractiveness of your office facilities, the efficiency and friendliness of your staff, your prices, the quantity and quality of your community contacts, the general level of dental awareness in your community, your personality and personal cleanliness, and, of course, your advertising. Just

Evaluation of specific components of your advertising campaign will be most effective if you keep track of which component generated each new patient encounter.

what part advertising plays in this list of attributes will be hard to determine. You can get some indications of effectiveness by keeping your ears open to patient and community contact comments, by asking new patients how they learned of the practice (instead of just who referred them), and by "keying" direct mail pieces. Keying refers to the practice of offering more information: "For more information on dental health practices, write to Box 59, Your City and Zip Code." In this instance, Box 59 is simply added to indicate to you where the

How Marketing Methods Compare

To get a better understanding of the strengths and weaknesses of various marketing methods, SYCOM had a group of marketing experts and dentists experienced with dental marketing, rate different marketing methods for effectiveness, cost per patients reached and tendency to arouse controversy.

Panel members * were asked to base their ratings on use of the various marketing methods **by a conventional two or three doctor practice interested in increasing patient flow by 30 per cent.** The number 1 ranking represents the methods that are most effective, least expensive and least controversial.

Most Effective	Most Inexpensive	Most Uncontroversial
1. Newspaper advertising & yellow pages	1. Giveaways - distributed to current patients	1. Giveaways (to current patients)
2. Patient education materials (current patients)	2. Patient education materials (current patients)	2. Patient education materials (current patients)
3. Practice brochures (mass mailing)	3. Practice brochures (current patients)	3. Practice brochures (current patients)
4. Newsletters (mass mailing)	4. Patient education materials (mass mailing)	4. Newsletters (current patients)
5. Patient education materials (mass mailing)	5. Newsletters (current patients)	5. Patient education materials (mass mailing)
6. TV advertising	6. Giveaways (mass distribution)	6. Newsletters (mass mailing)
7. Radio advertising	7. Newsletters (mass mailing)	7. Practice brochures (mass mailing)
8. Practice brochures (current patients)	8. Practice brochures (mass mailing)	8. Giveaways (mass distribution)
9. Newsletters (current patients)	9. Newspaper advertising & yellow pages	9. Newspaper advertising & yellow pages
10. Giveaways - balloons, etc. (mass distribution)	10. Radio advertising	10. Radio advertising
11. Giveaways - distributed to current patients	11. TV advertising	11. TV advertising

However, these ratings give only a general idea of the strengths and weaknesses of different methods. To actually select the best approach for a given situation several variables must be considered:

1. The location of the practice. Whether the practitioner is located in a large or small city or a rural area will affect his media choices.

2. The "target audience". Is the practitioner looking for an "upscale" or lower economic audience? A high volume-low fee or low volume-high fee practice?

3. Specialty. If the doctor has a specialty that depends upon patients knowing where to get the service -- rather than from referrals from other practitioners -- he will have to use mass media like radio, TV and large circulation newspapers.

4. The "positioning" of the practice. The individual practitioner should analyze the competition in his immediate area and determine what unique patient needs and desires he can best fulfill.

* Irwin Braun, Braun Advertising, Inc.; Robert Crawford, SYCOM;
Ralph A. Heiser DDS, Institute for Marketing Professional Services, Inc.;
H. Paul Jacobi DDS, GoodCare Dental Centers, Inc.

Courtesy of SYCOM, West Beltline Highway, P.O. Box 7947, Madison, Wisconsin 53707.

person writing in learned of the information. Some advertisers help determine effectiveness by placing in their ads, "Ask for Mrs. West." In this case, "Mrs. West" is simply an indication that a person calling for an appointment was stimulated by a particular advertisement campaign. None of these methods is particularly foolproof, but they do help us determine to some extent just where we should put our advertising effort.

Some authorities say advertising of professional services is ineffective. Given its relatively short history, this is not surprising. The evolutionary process will surely result in more effective advertising. If you decide to advertise, you can refine your program gradually by evaluation of your successive efforts.

Evaluation of specific components of your advertising campaign will be most effective if you keep track of which component generated each new patient encounter. Also confusion will be minimized if you change only one component at a time, e.g., your radio spot or your newspaper ad and determine the effect. The key is to develop a program and monitor the effects of changes you make.

SYCOM, the Wisconsin-based consulting organization, asked a number of knowledgeable people for their opinions of the "most effective," "most inexpensive," and "most uncontroversial" advertising methods. The results of this survey are reproduced in the table on the preceding page. This survey should be most helpful to beginning advertisers. Experience will help you determine your own list.

CONCLUSIONS

Advertising is not for every dentist. Many practices are flourishing, and there are no indications that basic changes need to be made. However, for those of us who have experienced a reduction in numbers of patients, for those of us whose expenses have risen to the point where we definitely need to increase our fee levels, or for those of us just starting out, advertising may be a serious consideration.

There is no question in our minds that the dental practice of the future will have some advertising as an integral part. In the meantime, learning about and perhaps experimenting with advertising may be the best key to long-term success.

REFERENCES

Darling, J. R., Hackett, D. W.: The advertising of fees and services: a study of contrasts between, and similarities among, professional groups. Journal of Advertising, Spring, 1978.

Drilling for new business. Time, December 1, 1980.

Gibbons, P., Chessher, C.: A look at the advertising dentist and the results. Dental Economics. November 1980, pp. 39–40, 42.

Littlefield, J. E., Kirkpatrick, C. A.: Advertising. Boston, Houghton Mifflin Company, 1970.

Littlefield, J. E.: Readings in Advertising. St. Paul, Minnesota, West Publishing Company, 1975.

Mandell, M. I.: Advertising. New York, Prentice-Hall, Inc., 1980.

Smith, R. E., Meyer, T. S.: Attorney advertising: a consumer perspective. Journal of Marketing, Spring, 1980, pp. 56–64.

The Advertising Dentist. P.O. Box 5175, Phoenix, AZ 85010, published as an annual book in 12 current monthly chapters during the calendar year.

9

The Telephone As
A Marketing Tool

In the hands of the right dentist and auxiliaries, the telephone can be a powerful and valuable marketing tool. Improperly used, the telephone can be quite costly. Consider the following two scenarios:

Scenario I

It is Thursday afternoon of a summer's day and Marcia McKnight breathed a sigh of relief. Dr. Russ had recently left for his regular weekly golf game, which he usually scheduled with other dentists who did or could refer patients to him or with a community business or political leader. Even though Dr. Russ held office hours two evenings and one early morning a week, as well as on Saturday morning, Marcia couldn't quite get over the notion that he was "loafing" when he took off work to play golf. This attitude seemed to permeate her behavior when fulfilling her duty of answering the telephone and handling emergencies. Still, she thought to herself, "I'm really glad he takes off on Thursday afternoons. It gives me a chance to call my boyfriend, Ron, who is at a distant army base, and charge it to Dr. Russ' telephone number." In fact, when the telephone rang at 1:20 P.M., she was just getting ready to make the call.

"Hello," she answered, in her most dulcet tone. "Is Dr. Russ in?" the voice on the other end of the line asked. "No!" answered Marcia, her tone changing from sweetness to petulance. Marcia did not believe in wasting any words when the call was potentially taking up her time with Ron. "When will he be back?" the female voice asked. "Not this afternoon!" said Marcia. By now the voice on the phone was becoming exasperated. "Will you tell me where I may reach him?" the woman asked.

"Probably at the 19th Tee — uuh . . . you know, the bar at the Country Club." Marcia didn't like telling on her boss, but she felt as though she had to tell the truth, no matter how ugly. "Well, this is Mrs. Butterworth, and my daughter has a toothache. What do you suggest that I do?" "I'm sure I don't know," answered Marcia, matter of factly, but with little disguise as to her impatience with this caller, by now. "Well, tell Dr. Russ I called," said Mrs. Butterworth, continuing to be patient. "Yes ma'am," answered Marcia, now becoming more polite as she happily realized that finally this woman was going to get off the phone so she, Marcia, could make her important call to Ron.

So for the next 30 minutes, the phone was busy. Ron and Marcia talked happily while three other potential patients tried to call but got a busy signal.

Scenario II

It is the same Thursday afternoon, a few minutes later than when Mrs. Butterworth called Dr. Russ' office. Mrs. Butterworth scanned the Yellow Pages and dialed another number. "Dr. Armstrong's office," the voice answered, "this is May Stevens, may I help you?" "Yes," Mrs. Butterworth said, "this is Mrs. Butterworth, may I speak with Dr. Armstrong please?" "Dr. Armstrong is out of the office at the moment," May answered, "but I expect to talk with him later this afternoon. I can give him a message, but in the meantime, may I help in some way?" "I certainly hope so," said Mrs. Butterworth. "My daughter has a toothache, and she is driving me crazy!" "Are you or your daughter a patient of Dr. Armstrong's now, Mrs. Butterworth?" "No," the woman answered. "In that case, please let me get some information and I'll pass it on to Dr. Armstrong as soon as possible." The following questions, all asked in a sympathetic way, elicited prompt and full responses. "What is your daughter's name?" "What is her age?" "Has she had a toothache before?" "When was that?"

"Do you believe Dr. Armstrong should see her late this afternoon, or would tomorrow morning be soon enough?" was May's last question. "Oh, she'll probably be O.K. until tomorrow," answered Mrs. Butterworth, "what time would that be?" "We could work her in about 9:30, I believe. Would that be satisfactory?" asked May. "Yes, I guess so," replied Mrs. Butterworth.

"Has your daughter ever had an allergy or other reaction to aspirin?" asked May. "No, not to my knowledge," said Mrs. Butterworth. "Then perhaps one or two aspirin every four to six hours would make her more comfortable," said May. "I think you are right," said Mrs. Butterworth, "I have given her aspirin previ-

Good use of the telephone can build a practice mightily; bad use of it can injure the practice, perhaps fatally.

ously when this tooth bothered her. Thanks so much for your kindness." "Not at all," said May. "Now remember, if the pain gets worse, call this number again and either I or the answering service will get in touch with Dr. Armstrong. I know he will want to see her before tomorrow if the pain is severe. Goodbye, Mrs. Butterworth, see you tomorrow." May waited until Mrs. Butterworth hung up first and then hung up the phone.

Meanwhile, Drs. Armstrong and Russ were playing golf together, oblivious of the effect that Marcia McKnight was having on both of their practices.

These scenes may be a bit overdramatized for effect, but their points should not be lost. The telephone is an increasingly important part of the dental practice. Good use of the telephone can build a practice mightly; bad use of it can injure the practice, perhaps fatally. It has been estimated that 85 to 90 percent of all dental office business is conducted over the telephone. Your patients' first contact with your office probably will be by phone and almost every time an appointment is made or a question is asked, it will be by phone. It is imperative that you, the marketing dentist, know just how your auxiliaries are answering the telephone and answering patients' questions. We strongly suggest that you, the dentist, study and practice this procedure, and that you train and retrain your employees in correct telephone procedure. In fact, you may even test once in awhile by having a friend call your office.

TELEPHONE PROCEDURE

When using any telephone, one should speak clearly, enunciate all words carefully, and finish conversations as quickly as possible. Extended conversations with patients or potential patients should, whenever possible, be conducted in one's office, where eye contact can be made and all nonverbal indications of a person's mood or attitude can be spotted.

When using any telephone, one should speak clearly, enunciate all words carefully, and finish conversations as quickly as possible.

Answering the telephone should be delegated to one person, usually the receptionist/appintment clerk/secretary, depending on the size of the office team. Whoever answers ought to handle each call as completely as possible. Only if absolutely necessary should the call be transferred to another individual. You the dentist should be sure that protocol is established as to whom you will speak with. Most dentists will speak to other dentists, physicians, and spouses, unless the dentist is absolutely unable to leave a patient. In that case, the dentist will return the call as soon as possible.

The Greeting

A cheerful, smiling voice that says, "I'm delighted to help you," assists in the establishment of goodwill. Actually smiling into the phone can create a "smiling" telephone personality, one that makes people want to do business with your office. You could even place a mirror in front of your receptionist so she could see her own smile when she answers the telephone. A poorly said, "Hullo," as from Marcia McKnight in our earlier scenario, can discourage patients and potential patients before the first question is asked. No matter how unpleasant a caller is or can be, your office should carry through a definite policy of a friendly reply.

Actually smiling into the phone can create a "smiling" telephone personality.

The telephone should be answered promptly, usually on the first or second ring. An unanswered telephone irritates the caller. Failure to answer promptly is likely to be interpreted as lack of interest, and is no way to build rapport or maintain relationships — so necessary in marketing. A friendly, unhurried greeting should always be used, and the answerer should be ready to take notes on the call.

When the receiver is lifted, something like the following greeting should be used: "Dr. Armstrong's office, May Stevens speaking, may I help you?" Many dentists will have specific phrases they wish their auxiliaries to use, such as "good morning," or "good afternoon." Certainly, these phrases should be pleasant, friendly, and prompt. The greeting will have to be adjusted, of course, depending upon the type of practice. For instance, if the practice comprises more than one dentist, it may be appropriate to have the telephone answered with "Drs. Armstrong and Baker" or "Doctors' Office." In some cases, of course, it may be appropriate to respond to a ring by saying, "Dental Clinic, Miss Stevens, may I help you?"

The hold button should be used sparingly — perhaps frequently but for short periods of time. Ask the caller if he prefers to hold or to be called back. His autonomy ought to be respected. Likewise, a person you are attending at the desk when the phone rings deserves consideration. Rather than keep the person waiting you may need to ask the caller either to wait on hold or if you may call back. Reactions differ as to the use of taped music on hold. If you are thinking of installing it, you might sound out a sample of your patients as to their preference. Not everyone likes it.

The Conversation

Courteous responsiveness is the rule. Do *not* ask the caller's name until you have answered his first question. Otherwise, he will think that the answer differs depending on who asks the question. In establishing the caller's identity, simply say, "May I ask who is calling, please?"

The caller deserves your full attention. Whoever responds should not attempt to do any tasks unrelated to the call during the conversation. Records and charts needed for references should be close at hand. In fact it is a good idea for the receptionist to inform the caller that she is checking records. This reassures him that attention is complete.

Every question deserves a clear and specific answer. As many questions as possible should be anticipated. It is worth the time of the dental team to discuss possible questions and to outline answers that

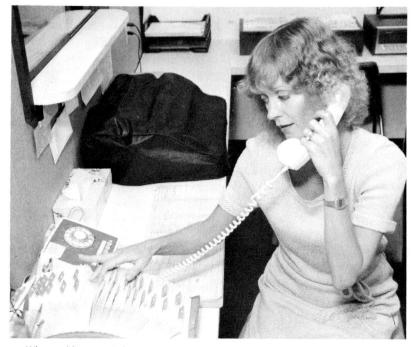

When taking a call from a patient, the capable receptionist will have relevant data at her fingertips.

reflect the office philosophy and image to be projected. One good idea is to record the questions asked and develop the answers for them.

Completeness of each call is the responsibility of the dental team member. Be sure that the caller has obtained all the information he requested before concluding the call. The respondent might say, "Was there anything else Mr. Royce?" This permits the caller to mention any last minute comment or question before being cut off. After the caller has hung up, replace the receiver gently.

Wrong Numbers

If a person not affiliated with the office is asked for, a good way to respond is, "This is Dr. Armstrong's office, 942-7033. There is no one here by that name." Do not respond, "What number are you calling?" This wastes time and is not normally of interest to the responder or anyone in the office.

Sometimes a caller will realize an incorrect number has been reached and will say, not always courteously, "What number is this?" Rather than replying discourteously in kind, it is appropriate to answer, "This is Dr. Armstrong's office, 942-7033." This usually will inform the caller he has reached an incorrect number. However, it will not insult him if later he is looking for a new dentist! Important in all telephone contact is the time saved by a prompt, complete, courteous answer.

Telephone Speaking

The telephone instrument should be held about one inch from and directly in front of the lips. It should not be held under the chin or level with the eyes, as some people sometimes do.

It is seldom necessary to pitch one's voice either higher or lower than normal in order to be heard. If a person has trouble being heard, it is probably because he or she is speaking too rapidly or is not enunciating clearly enough. Speech should be natural and, of course, courteous. Long pauses in speech and "aahs," "uuhs," or "errs," should not be part of the telephone answerer's speech. Of course, chewing gum or eating while answering the telephone or making calls should be avoided.

It is seldom necessary to pitch one's voice either higher or lower than normal in order to be heard.

Placing Calls

The office image is also dependent on the manner of placing calls. It is only courtesy that whoever is to speak to the party being called should be on the line when the party answers. As in answering, the office caller should identify himself or herself immediately and briefly state the purpose of the call, perhaps by saying, "Do you have a few minutes for us to discuss (named subject)?" The telephone is an intrusive device, and we should soften that aspect in every way we can. The time of day for calls should be selected on the basis of convenience for the person being called, if possible.

Messages

Ordinary messages can be conveyed on several different types of message slips. A form for recording the minimum information needed is reproduced on the next page. For unusual names, you could record the phonetic spelling as well as the actual spelling. Information on a patient being given an advance appointment may require a more complex form.

Personal Calls

In the interests of professionalism, telephone lines should be used primarily for business purposes. All team members should understand this and agree to limit personal calls. Your office policy should be clear in its emphasis on the telephone as a primary marketing tool. But if you want a happy staff — and you do, of course — you will need to make at least limited allowance for personal calls.

Telephone Etiquette Summary

1. Answer promptly at least on the second ring.
2. Identify yourself immediately in the conversation — in both incoming and outgoing calls.

```
┌─────────────────────────────────────────┐
│                                           │
│   Telephone Data      _____         │
│                           Date            │
│                                           │
│   _____      │
│   Name                                    │
│                                           │
│   _____      │
│   Address              Telephone No.      │
│                                           │
│   _____      │
│   Child's name         Age                │
│                                           │
│   _____      │
│   Problem                                 │
│                                           │
│   _____      │
│   Disposition                             │
│                                           │
│                                           │
│   _____      │
│   Remarks                                 │
│                                           │
│               _____     │
│               Operator's initials         │
│                                           │
└─────────────────────────────────────────┘
```

Sample message form.

3. Listen carefully to the caller and be sure you understand the purpose of the call.

4. Answer the caller's first question before asking his or her name.

5. Speak directly into the telephone with the instrument about one inch from your lips.

6. Be pleasant. Smile, converse naturally, clearly, and courteously. Avoid slang. Say "please" and "thank you" when appropriate.

7. Give your full attention to the caller. Do not pay any attention to anything else. Use the caller's name frequently.

The telephone provides dentists many opportunities to control their practices.

8. Keep all references such as charts and records handy. Use a pad and pencil to record telephone information.

9. Handle each call yourself as far as possible. Avoid transferring to someone else unless absolutely necessary.

10. Give clear answers to all questions. Predetermine as many questions as possible and outline answers to them.

11. Be sure the caller has the information requested before concluding the call. Replace the receiver gently after the caller has hung up.

12. When placing calls, be sure the party who wishes to talk is on the line when the called party answers.

CONTROLLING THE PRACTICE WITH THE TELEPHONE

Many dentists make use of the opportunities provided by the telephone to control their practices. For example, it might be appropriate for you to have your appointment clerk make a list at the end of each week of all patients who have broken appointments without notice. The telephone reminder can be a good device for decreasing the number of broken appointments. Some practices routinely telephone to confirm appointments. Further, whether you like it or not, the telephone will bring complaints; they must be dealt with successfully. Also, many prospective patients will have questions on your fees; these, too, must be answered, usually by your auxiliaries. And, when surgery or a particularly difficult procedure has been performed on a patient, a telephone call in the late afternoon or evening or early the next day to check on recovery might be soothing and helpful. Unidentified callers are a problem for some dental offices. Each of these will be expanded upon here.

All calls of regular patients should be entered in the patient's record. This will document inquiries and the dentist will know what has transpired. Any patient dissatisfaction should be noted and the dentist notified, if appropriate. The receptionist should understand that if it is important enough for the patient to call, it is important enough for our office to give a positive response, no matter how trivial the inquiry may seem to us.

When surgery or a particularly difficult procedure has been performed, a telephone call in the late afternoon or evening or early the next day might be soothing.

Broken Appointments

When a patient telephones your office to cancel an appointment, and if the call is not handled correctly, your practice schedule can be severely disrupted. Many dentists instruct their appointment clerks

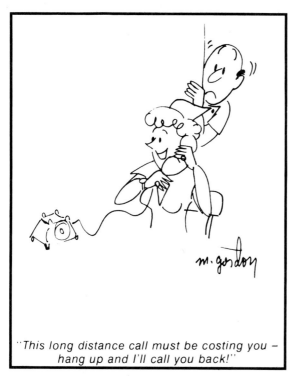

"This long distance call must be costing you – hang up and I'll call you back!"

Courtesy of *Cal* magazine.

Many dentists instruct their appointment clerks to call patients as soon as possible after the missed appointment to set up a new appointment.

to inquire if the appointment could not be kept anyway, and if not, to try to schedule a new appointment immediately. Otherwise, the patient may not call for another appointment until weeks or months later. One way to handle this is to say, "Thank you for calling us, Mr. Jones. If you believe that next week would be better for you, suppose we arrange for next Wednesday at 9:00 a.m.? Will that be convenient for you Mr. Jones?" By this approach, the patient is kept within the practice and commits himself to a definite future visit.

What about a patient who breaks an appointment but does not notify your office that it will be broken? Many dentists instruct their appointment clerks to call patients as soon as possible after the appointment time and remind them that they missed an appointment. They then attempt to set up a new appointment immediately, perhaps in the same manner as when an appointment is cancelled by phone. This informs the patient that his or her treatment is necessary and that the dental practice is interested in and concerned with the patient's welfare. It is essential that such a followup call not be accusing or critical of the patient. We all miss appointments occasionally. It is simply necessary to remind most of us of what we have done to make us more careful in the future. "Punishing" the patient with a phone call merely creates ill-will for the practice.

Appointment Confirmation

It is an excellent idea to have your appointments clerk call all patients one day ahead of the appointment time to "confirm" (not "remind them of") the appointment. Nearly all patients will be pleased to have the appointment "confirmed" and this will cut down greatly on missed appointments. Occasionally the appointments clerk will encounter a patient who does not seem to appreciate such a call. It is an easy enough problem to solve by simply noting "no confirmation call" on the patient's dental chart. The time saved and the productivity improvement for the dentist and all others concerned will be far greater than the time expended on confirmation calls.

Occasionally, a patient will hesitate to confirm an appointment. It is probably better to leave the way open for the patient to call back if he or she wishes to confirm the appointment. If the receptionist or whoever is making the confirmation call becomes "pushy," this may result in another broken appointment. If the patient is not motivated for dental treatment at the time of the call, often no amount of pushing will cause an appointment to be kept.

Telephone Complaints

When a patient or other person telephones the office to register a complaint or dissatisfaction about services, it is advisable not to enter into a long conversation. Many dentists and auxiliaries have found the following procedure appropriate (Reap, 1973, 33–35). First remember that the person feels the complaint is legitimate. Whether you believe it is legitimate or not is not important. Your job is to soothe the caller, and when appropriate, to set up a brief appointment for the angry person to see the dentist or talk to him or her on the telephone.

Step One.   As suggested before, the smile is a most important step. A smile by the person answering the phone will come through to the person calling and will help prevent the answerer from becoming angry and part of the problem. If you find yourself getting angry with a caller, it is advisable to ask the caller if you may return the call in a few minutes. After your have regained your composure, and perhaps discussed the situation with appropriate people in the office, then call back and continue the discussion in a more rational, nonangry way. If a person ever detects anger in you, you have probably lost the "argument."

Step Two.   Listen carefully to what the caller has to say and respond occasionally in as pleasant a voice as possible. Do not make a speech or give a lecture. A series of "yes sir" or "no sir" or "yes ma'am" or "no ma'am" answers usually will suffice. Try to be certain that the caller has been able to "sound off" to the fullest extent he or she wishes. When the person seems to be through with complaints, ask him if there are any other problems, not in a sarcastic or unpleasant way, but in a manner that indicates that you really do care. This tends to disarm the angry person; frequently an apology will be forthcoming. The complainer will tend to backtrack and will tell you that perhaps he or she has overstated the massiveness of the problem. He called to declare war, and found that he was received by a pleasant-voiced person who accepted everything he had to say and asked for more. He had expected an argument, and you have thrown him off balance.

Once you have "gotten the complainer's attention," then you must address the substance of his or her complaints, point by point. Throughout your discussion with him, never indicate that you do not believe his complaint is legitimate. Answer him as best you can, all the while maintaining an air of both professionalism and sympathy. Also, if it is necessary for you to do some research before answering his complaint, give him a specific time by which you will call back and make certain you do call back by that time.

Questions on Fees

How to handle telephone questions of fees has always been a difficult question for dentists. It is sometimes difficult to be civil to people who are obviously just looking for the cheapest dentistry. In many such cases, training, experience, or quality of care is not important, not even considered by the "shopper." There are many possible ways to handle such fee information requests, but handle them you must.

First, for example, you could simply brush-off the request with the statement, "we don't quote fees over the telephone." The prospective patient will then either ask what she must do to get a price quotation, ask to make an appointment for a checkup, or, most likely, go on to the next telephone call asking for fee quotations.

In many such cases, training, experience, or quality of care is not important, not even considered by the "shopper."

Perhaps, the best procedure is to convince the caller that you cannot be truly helpful by quoting specific fees. It should be done in a warm caring manner and not as though you are trying to point out the folly of the question. Suppose the caller asks how much cleaning teeth would cost. You could state that the fee varies according to the difficulty of and the time required for the procedure. Then ask how much subgingival calculus is present. This conversation, if well managed, should convince the caller that it is impossible to quote a fee for adequate treatment. For effective marketing this must be done with empathy, respect, and warmth. You are trying to convince the caller that you can satisfy his needs in every way including the fee. But not by quoting fees on the telephone.

You will find the best way to express the following in your own words, but you need to explain to the prospective patient that each patient and each dental procedure requires a different amount of work, skill, and materials. Therefore, it is impossible for you to state specifically what a "filling" costs, just as it is impossible to state just what any other nonstandard item costs. You should tell the patient that you would be glad to make an appointment for an examination, and at that time it will be possible to estimate what the total dental treatment plan will cost.

In some jurisdictions it has been held that a price quoted over the phone can and has become a binding and legal contract to provide service at the stated price. Even if you *could* quote prices sight unseen, you probably would not want to for this reason alone.

If a prospective patient is not willing to accept your explanation that you must see him and make an examination before knowing what the treatment will cost, he or she may in fact go to another dentist who is willing to quote fees over the telephone. Most patients will not be so turned off by honest and forthright statements such as you have made. The prospective patient, at least, will be impressed with your professional standards, and after "shopping around," may call you for an appointment anyway.

Specific Requests

On occasion, someone will insist that just one tooth needs to be filled or otherwise attended to. Rather than insisting on a full treatment plan, it is probably most desirable to make an appointment to take care of the patient's immediate concern, and then use part of the treatment time to educate the patient in proper dental health procedures. In this way, you will have met the patient's perceived need, and may well have turned the patient into a booster for better dentistry.

Followup Calls

Properly conducted dentistry, of course, sometimes brings about, or at least is accompanied by, pain. Pain is a frightening experience for most people, and causes unneeded anxiety. A followup call, either in the afternoon or evening or the next morning can relieve much of the anxiety, hence some of the pain. The little time it takes can pay handsomely in patient goodwill.

Recall System

Regardless of your recall system, the telephone is likely to be part of it. Arranging all recall appointments by telephone is time consuming but effective. If you send notices asking patients to call for an appointment, you may need to follow up if they do not call. Even if you give an advance appointment at the time of the last visit, you will surely need to confirm that appointment by telephone. Only if you leave the responsibility for maintenance visits entirely with the patient will you not need to use the telephone.

Unidentified Callers

On occasion, a person will call and refuse to give you his or her name or the topic that he or she wishes to discuss with the dentist. Such callers often are salespeople who believe that if their identities are revealed, they will not get an opportunity to speak with the dentist. Your only alternative, it appears, is to answer something like the following: "Dr. Armstrong is with a patient now and has asked me to take all messages. If you cannot tell me who is calling and what you want to talk about, I suggest that you write Dr. Armstrong a letter at _____ (give address). He will give it his full and immediate attention and contact you if he is interested." The caller then has the option of writing or of revealing his name and business. If, in fact, it is something in which the dentist would likely be interested, you then must use your judgment on whether or not to interrupt him.

If you believe that he should not be interrupted, you could suggest to the caller that the dentist will call back and inquire as to a suitable time. Salesmen also should be treated courteously, because each one is a potential referral source.

Telephone Collection Efforts

The telephone is in many instances the most effective form of account collection. In part, this is because the telephone can be faster than a letter or any other type of communication. Often, the faster the contact, the more likely it is that a payment will be forthcoming.

In order to ensure that patients have received previously sent statements, all patients should be called *before* any type of "collection" letter is sent. Such collection calls should be courteous, business-like, and to the point. Use such phrases as "to maintain a good credit rating," "to have a clear conscience," "can I expect cash or a check?" "on what date will I receive the payment?"

Before making a collection call, know all pertinent facts, such as

The telephone is in many instances the most effective form of account collection.

(a) how much is due, (b) how long payment has been overdue, (c) how many statements have been sent to date, and (d) what previous telephone or other contacts have been made. During the call, be brief but persistent. Do not let the patient put you off with vague answers.

Above all, in a collection call be a good listener. Many people do have genuine problems, including economic ones. When you make a call of this type, you must be prepared to listen to a person's problems. Do not argue with the patient. As mentioned before, if you find yourself becoming angry, ask the patient if you may call him or her back. Then after you have regained your composure, call the patient back and start over with the original reason for the call. Last, if it is obvious the person is not listening, stop talking. You will only be wasting your time. There are times when only collection letters or other action is called for. Perhaps you have reached one of them.

Above all, in a collection call be a good listener. Many people do have genuine problems, including economic ones.

TELEPHONE ANSWERING SERVICE

When you or one of your auxiliaries is on duty, you can make certain the telephone is answered properly and promptly. Many dentists find it desirable to have office telephone coverage at least five days a week, even if the dentist is on duty only four to four and one-half days. This gives patients the impression that the office is always open. In most cases, a receptionist can handle the calls, and the dentist can check-in periodically and return needed calls. In some instances, it may be worthwhile to hire a part-time person to take calls when the rest of the staff is off. This part-time person can also perform other needed office functions, such as filing insurance forms, bookkeeping, confirming the next day's appointments, in the spare time between calls. When you or one of your staff cannot be on duty, it is necessary to have someone answer the telephone. Many dentists subscribe to telephone answering services. Some purchase answering machines. Each of these answers to the problem has benefits and drawbacks.

Many dentists find it desirable to have office telephone coverage at least five days a week.

Answering Services

When the telephone rings in the dentist's office or at home, it also rings at the switchboard of the answering service. If the dentist or someone at the office or at home does not answer within a prescribed number of rings, the answering service takes the call. This method is even used by some dentists during regular business hours if there are times when no one can conveniently answer the phone. An unanswered telephone is an extremely poor situation; the answering service allows a little more flexibility in getting the telephone answered promptly. You may instruct the answering service in how to answer. Some dentists ask that their telephone be answered something like: "This is Dr. Armstrong's office, may I take a message?"

You may wish to give your answering service instructions regarding what constitutes an emergency call and what to do in case of an emergency. Unless you can give the service standard instructions which may be used every day, you may have to call the service every evening upon closing the office to tell them where you will be and how they may reach you or one of your colleagues. You will, of course, have to call the answering service frequently, at least every morning, to learn of any messages which have been left for you. These calls will then have to be returned in the morning. In short, the answering service allows the dentist to get "out of the office" in a figurative as well as a literal sense, and still receive calls. All of these points are stated as benefits of the answering service. The main drawback of any answering service is that it is difficult, often impossible, to control fully just how your telephone is answered, once you turn the task over to an answering service.

The solution to this problem, it seems to us, is to test the service regularly, to place calls, or have someone else place calls for you, to determine just how your phone is being answered. If you are not happy with the speed or the manner in which your telephone is being answered, you should have a talk with the answering service and see if they will improve. If they do not or will not improve, you have little alternative except to purchase an answering machine or, if possible, seek another service.

You may wish to give your answering service instructions regarding emergencies.

Answering Machines

Many dentists who have more than adequate answering services available to them still choose to use a machine to answer their telephone when out of the office. In fact, there seems to be a movement away from answering services toward answering machines. Two reasons can be given for this movement. First, answering services, depending as they do on "hand labor," are becoming increasingly expensive. Because an answering machine is a one-time investment, it may pay to purchase one. The second reason why they are used more is the increasing sophistication of such devices. Among other features, machines are now available at reasonable cost which will enable you to call your "machine" and receive your messages from a distant location. Even though you are using a machine, it will pay to check regularly to make certain that it is operating properly and that your patients are getting a friendly and efficient greeting.

NUMBER OF TELEPHONE LINES

In some dental offices, one telephone line for both incoming and outgoing calls will be sufficient. For most offices, however, it will be necessary to have more than one line. Many dentists have a regular telephone line for incoming calls and an "unlisted" line for outgoing calls. These lines, along with others, if needed, can be programmed to handle incoming calls sequentially. That is, if the listed line is busy, the next incoming call comes in on the first unlisted line, the second on the second unlisted line, and so forth.

Insufficient telephone lines to receive incoming calls is a prob-

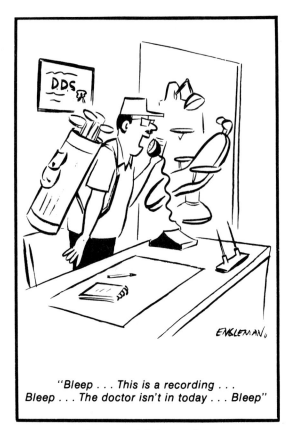

"Bleep . . . This is a recording . . .
Bleep . . . The doctor isn't in today . . . Bleep"

Courtesy of *Cal* magazine.

Patients appreciate a telephone that they can use in your office. The expense of an extra line exclusively for this use is a good investment in the busy office.

lem. To constantly receive a busy signal when calling the dentist (or anyone else) is exasperating. Satisfied customers, clients, and patients will not experience such frustrations. Your regular patients may persist until they get an answer, but persons calling for the first time will probably try someone else.

Ask the telephone company to check your traffic. Company personnel can advise you as to the sufficiency of your lines. They will also be more than happy to advise you on the extension phones and other apparatus necessary to do a good job in your office as well as the types and colors of telephone equipment available to add to the decor of your office.

Patients appreciate a telephone that they can use in your office. The expense of an extra line exclusively for this use is a good investment in the busy office. Otherwise, if your patient volume is low, you can accommodate their need by making your own line available with an extension for their use. This demonstration that you care for their convenience and their needs will pay handsome dividends.

CONCLUSION

The telephone can be an outstanding marketing tool for you, for good or bad, depending upon how you use it. It is necessary for the marketing dentist to do a good and continuing job of training auxiliaries in telephone procedures and techniques. Further, the telephone can be a major factor in helping you to get control over your practice, by using it for patient reminders, followup calls, and the like. The telephone companies around the nation can be a major help in designing the appropriate telephone system for your office. Call them!

Dr. Russ was informed by a patient, although most of us are not, that Marcia McKnight was giving his office a bad name and was turning away prospective patients. After he replaced her with a trained appointment clerk with much better telephone techniques, he found his practice slowly building in volume. He also found the atmosphere around the office to be a more joyful one and more fun to work in!

REFERENCES

Ehrlich, A. B.: Business Administration for the Dental Assistant. Champaign, IL, The Colwell Company, 1972, pp. 3–5.
Ehrlich, A. B., Ehrlich, S. F.: Dental Practice Management. Philadelphia, W. B. Saunders Company, 1969, pp. 61–67.
Frederick, P., Towner, C.: The Office Assistant. Philadelphia, W. B. Saunders Company, 1957, pp. 34–52.
Reap, C. A., Jr.: Complete Dental Assistant's, Secretary's, and Hygienist's Handbook. West Nyack, NY, Parker Publishing Company, Inc., 1973, pp. 32–39.
Stinaff, R. K.: Dental Practice Administration. St. Louis, MO, C. V. Mosby Company, 1960, pp. 186–192.

10

Marketing Through Correspondence

Wouldn't *you* be pleased to receive a letter like the one on the opposite page if *you* were Ms. Stiles and had just entrusted your eight-year-old son to the as-yet-unknown quantity of an unfamiliar dental practice? Does not such a letter bespeak the personal, caring touch that any of us would want from health professionals treating our own flesh and blood?

Correspondence is crucial to the success of your practice, now more than ever before. It ranks in importance alongside the telephone or personal contact. Letters, notes, even bills generated through your practice are extensions of yourself. They will either help or hinder the growth of your dental enterprise. Through each letter you are communicating to a patient just as surely as if you were speaking to him or her directly. Therefore your correspondence needs to be: clear, concise, considerate, concrete, complete — and friendly.

The language used in correspondence should be suited to the reader. Medical terminology and technical jargon would be lost on most patients. Professional terms can be used with fellow professionals, but plain English is preferable for the lay person.

Correspondence ranks in importance alongside the telephone or personal contact.

IMPORTANCE OF CORRESPONDENCE

A dental office generates and receives an abundance of correspondence: letters to the office about the practice, welcome letters to new patients, notes reminding patients of appointments, and thank you notes to those who refer patients. The bulk of correspondence to other professionals is about patient concerns and/or consultations, although there is also some personal correspondence.

Correspondence is also generated to other businesspersons, not

E. RANDOLPH WILKINS, DDS
New Hope Dental Clinic
8 Ravenscroft Circle
Springfield, MA 01119

July 5, 1982

Ms. Roberta Stiles
416 Regency Park Apts.
Springfield, MA 01118

Dear Ms. Stiles:

Thank you for beginning your son, Matthew, in our total treatment plan for youngsters.

He listens well and shows promise of becoming a very health-conscious young man, which I am sure you are pleased to hear.

My assistant, Sally, my hygienist, Jeanne, and my receptionist, Maryann, and I all look forward to helping Matthew in every way possible.

Should you or any other member of your family or circle of friends require any dental care, either on a regular or an emergency basis, I hope you will not hesitate to call upon our dental team.

With warm wishes.

Sincerely,

E. Randolph Wilkins

---

necessarily profession-related: letters about community affairs involvement, letters to fellow club members or organization committee members, and thank you notes for past favors or project assistance.

Third party correspondence is important because it is directly related to your dental practice. This correspondence with dental insurance carriers and accident insurance companies concerns treatment of patients covered by such policies. You also need to correspond with various state and federal programs such as Medicaid, School Health Funds, Headstart, Veterans Administration, and Vocational Rehabilitation. The better your facility in processing such correspondence is, the greater will be your potential for receiving prompt payment for services rendered and for expanding the practice by attracting more patients with third party coverage.

COST OF CORRESPONDENCE

Consider how much ineffective business correspondence may cost you in practice development.

How much does correspondence cost? Realistically, the cost will be wedded to the type of equipment and the quality of the supplies in which you invest, and the labor involved. Labor is the most costly item. Ever-present inflation, over which neither you nor any other single businessman has much control, will continue to bedevil us all.

The cost of producing personalized correspondence is more than that of preprinted form letters. Yes, of course, there are numerous matters that can be taken care of with low-cost form letters requiring only your signature and the costs of mailing. However, rather than monetary concerns, you might well consider how much ineffective business correspondence may cost you in practice development.

Much of the correspondence generated within a dental practice calls for a personal approach. In some cases, though, form or preprinted correspondence can be used very effectively. Form correspondence to third parties — dental and accident insurance companies, governmental and private industry agencies, educational programs offices — is not only effective, but will also provide a business savings. An example of this is shown in Chapter 17.

EQUIPMENT AND SUPPLIES

When equipping a dental office you should place as much care and consideration on purchasing business machines as on dental equipment. Today's dentist may choose from a similar range of office equipment as professional equipment. Literally dozens of makes and models of typewriters compete on the market, from portables to standards, from manuals to electrics. Although the capital outlay may seem sizable, selecting a top quality correcting typewriter will pay dividends in the long run. A sophisticated model will offer a choice of type styles to provide your correspondence with a varied and professionally impressive appearance.

Making carbon copies of all outgoing correspondence is an inexpensive way to have file copies, but every office needs an adequate copying machine for certain types of records. The copier can provide you with flawless copies of insurance forms, patient records, forms for in-house storage and all business, professional and private correspondence, if desired.

Consider also an x-ray duplicator, especially since so many patients now have dental insurance coverage. A set of original radiographs can be sent to the patient's insurance company for examination and predetermination of benefits before treatment is begun. However, after treatment has been started or completed, the original radiographs should be placed in your own files for future reference. Insurance or Medicaid requests for radiographs of work in progress or work completed can be met by sending duplicates — not irreplaceable originals.

Extra, complementary equipment to generate correspondence is available at significantly higher cost. One example is an office computer with a word processor. Although a word-processor can mass-produce all the personal, letter-quality correspondence you desire, purchasing a computer just for letter writing purposes is not yet cost effective. However, a word-processing package for automatic letter writing would be a natural if you already own a computer. All that is required from you or your personnel is an address and signature. Word processors, currently, are rather expensive. But as the number of makes and models increases, along with more and more refinements, the cost per unit is expected to decrease.

Also important is the quality of paper that will carry your correspondence. You may wish to consider several different stocks for different needs. While you would naturally want a high-quality paper for patient and professional letters, a less expensive stock should be considered for correspondence that does not need to be impressive. While considering the quality of stationery, also examine color. Choose a color that will be soothing to the reader as well as reflect good taste and professionalism. The same care and consideration should be exercised when choosing type styles and art work for your letterhead. Strive for a balance between professionalism and esthetic attractiveness.

For your stationery, choose a color that will be soothing to the reader as well as reflect good taste and professionalism.

MAIL SORTING

The effective dental practice generates a continuous flow of correspondence. If you have an effective and growing practice you will need an efficient, timely method for processing all incoming mail. Never underestimate the importance of this aspect of the business. If mail is left unopened, it could cause you to miss priority items that need immediate reply or checks for deposit.

To create an efficient method of sorting, appoint a member of the staff for the job. Make this a daily part of that person's activities and allow that person to create the most effective method. Suggest initially that the sorter separate bills, payments, important correspondence, and third class mail and route each to the appropriate person for proper action.

You may wish to designate the receptionist as recipient of all patient payments, insurance payments, radiographs, insurance forms, business supply catalogs, and correspondence from other dentists concerning patients. If you have a bookkeeper-insurance clerk, that person would receive insurance forms, bills, patient payments, and bank statements. Each type of mail should be routed to the person who is directly responsible for the duty connected with it.

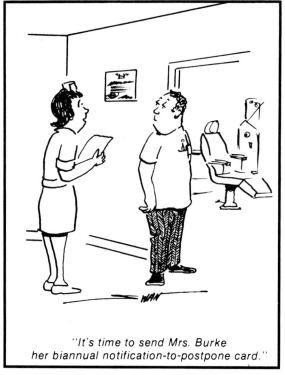

"It's time to send Mrs. Burke
her biannual notification-to-postpone card."

Courtesy of *Cal* magazine.

The dental assistant's packet could consist of all completed laboratory work, dental supply and uniform catalogs, and so on. The doctor's packet would include all personal mail, newsletters, professional publications, and continuing education brochures (maybe even "junk mail").

As important as — or more important than — undelayed processing of incoming mail is timely response of outgoing correspondence. Again this should be delegated to a proficient member of the staff (possibly the same person who handles incoming mail), with the job importance stressed. Some types of correspondence can be handled by the employee; others will require input from the doctor.

The efficiency of a system of correspondence will be reflected in the incoming/outgoing filing system. Such a system will offer quick, easy access to copies of all correspondence. Again, the staff member charged with handling the incoming and outgoing mail may be placed in charge of the filing system.

As important as — or more important than — undelayed processing of incoming mail is timely response of outgoing correspondence.

ROUTINE LETTERS

Philosophically, the new dentist must decide how much promotion he wishes to create through correspondence. In any use of this media, it's a good idea to keep information to the essentials. As patient, business or professional relationships progress, additional information can be dispensed with much greater impact.

New Patient Letter

One instance of a marketing letter is one of welcome to a new patient, such as Dr. Wilkins' letter to Ms. Stiles concerning her child. Just what should the dentist include in such a letter to an *adult* patient? Since this will be the patient's second contact with the dental

First letters, or letters of welcome, should be short, concise, and engaging.

E. RANDOLPH WILKINS, DDS
New Hope Dental Clinic
8 Ravenscroft Circle
Springfield, MA 01119

August 1, 1982

Mr. Richard Moss
2711 Riverside Apts., #3
Springfield, MA 01118

Dear Mr. Moss:

We are so glad that you have chosen our office to provide
your dental care. Sally, my assistant, Jeanne, my hygienist,
and Maryann, my receptionist, and I will do our best to help
you in any way we can.

Our office is located in the New Hope Dental Clinic, which is
shown on the enclosed map. We have scheduled you for a complete
examination on August 23 at 4:30 p.m. This will consist of an
oral examination, necessary x-rays, and cleaning, plus a
fluoride treatment.

If you are covered by dental insurance benefits, please bring
your forms with you, and we will be happy to assist you with
filing them.

If you have any questions prior to your appointment, please call
739-5976. We're looking forward to seeing you soon.

Sincerely,

E. Randolph Wilkins, DDS

ERW/smr

Enclosure

Figure 10–1. Adult welcome letter.

practice (first contact would be the telephone call asking for an appointment), the letter should contain only basic information. Examples of this are: location of the office (you may include a map or have it printed on your stationery), what to expect at the first visit, and possibly the fee for the examination. Of course, there should also be a brief statement welcoming the patient to the practice and declaring your intent to understand and respond to his/her dental needs (see Fig. 10–1).

That first letter is probably not the best place to include your particular office policy or do more than hint at personal philosophy of practice. Studies indicate that people do not absorb information if they are flooded with it. First letters, or letters of welcome, should be short, concise, and engaging. This not only indicates that you are a professional who is ready to render a needed service, but will also instill in the patient confidence in you as a dentist.

Child's Letter

In a welcome letter to a *child* you may be more open and less formal. Remember, the parent may read the letter to the child, but you still have to win the child's confidence. You may wish to build an easy repartee with the child by asking him or her to bring along a photograph or a picture he or she has drawn to be placed on your

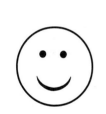

```
                                    Appointment: 9-3-82
                                                 3:30 p.m.




Dear Bobby,

We're glad you'll be coming to see us at Dr. Wilkins'
office soon.  While you're here, you can take a ride
in our special chair, then we'll take pictures of your
teeth with our big "space ship" camera.  Dr. Wilkins will
count your teeth and brush them with a funny toothbrush.
We'll teach you how to take care of your teeth.

Can you please bring us a picture of yourself so we can
put it up with our other friends?  Dr. Wilkins, Maryann,
Jeanne, and I are looking forward to seeing you.

Sally Redmond
Dental Assistant for Dr. Wilkins
```

Figure 10–2. Small child's welcome letter.

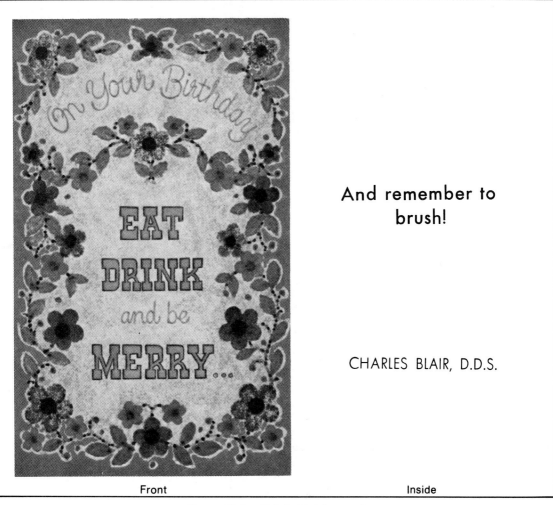

| Front | Inside |

Figure 10–3. Child's birthday card.

bulletin board. You can tell the child what you plan to do during the first visit: count his teeth, take pictures of them and teach him how to brush properly and take care of them (see Fig. 10–2).

A good marketing and public relations technique is to send preprinted birthday cards to your child patients. They feel important when they receive mail, especially on such special occasions. Parents also notice the extra caring that this conveys (see Fig. 10–3).

Treatment Confirmation Letter

Another letter to a patient could be one containing a confirmation of the treatment discussed during a recent visit. You may include a description of the treatment, the total cost, and the payment schedule, all of which were discussed at the appointment. This letter could also emphasize how the recommended treatment will help the patient. While no one wants to unduly alarm a patient, the importance of effecting treatment when examination has indicated it is really needed should not be understated. This point should be made clear to the patient, both during the office visit and in the followup letter.

Completion of Treatment Letter

While no one wants to unduly alarm a patient, it is important to effect treatment when needed.

You might also consider sending a letter upon completion of treatment. In this letter you could restate what you have told the patient regarding the completed dentistry. Praise the patient for good judgment in seeking the finest care, keeping appointments, and meeting financial responsibility on schedule. In this letter you could also point out to the patient the advantage of protecting his investment by having periodic checkups. Such checkups allow for minor additional treatment before newer, developing problems get out of control.

Checkup Reminder

Further correspondence with patients can be in the form of a checkup reminder or "confirmation." With the hectic lives we all lead, patients get busy and often forget to come for checkups unless those checkups are "confirmed." Some dental practices provide a very elaborate recall system while others merely send a card. And some do not utilize any type of system. The old saw — you can lead a horse to water, but you can't make him drink — is reminder enough that an overelaborate recall system is not necessarily effective. A simple postcard, which can be addressed and shown to the patient at the time of his or her last treatment visit, can work wonders. In fact, the patient can be asked to address it. Most people are fascinated to receive a card addressed in their own handwriting. You might inform a patient: "This card will be mailed to you a few days before your next appointment is due, Mrs. Clinton. Then you can call our office to schedule your checkup."

Inactive Patient Letter

A simple card usually will not be enough to get inactive patients to return. Also, the information you want to share with the inactive patient may be too personal for inclusion on a post card. Remember not to scold the patient for failing to return for checkups, but gently remind him or her how long it has been since the last checkup. Remind the inactive patient of the progress you made together and how there is a danger, through neglect, that previous treatment could be jeopardized.

It is advisable to have a standard form letter to send to patients who have been inactive for over a year. Chances are if they have been away that long, they either have moved away or have switched to another dentist. Updating the files can be a profitable activity for the office during lulls in the practice or when the doctor is absent through vacations or attending educational courses or seminars. Then letters can be sent to all inactive patients.

A simple, low-cost method of keeping track of patients is the inclusion of the words "ADDRESS CORRECTION REQUESTED" on all patient correspondence. The postal service charges a small fee for each new address, but it will not only help keep your patients active through recall, but will also aid in collection of delinquent accounts.

Include "ADDRESS CORRECTION REQUESTED" on all patient correspondence.

LETTERS TO OTHER PROFESSIONALS

Aside from general correspondence with fellow professionals on career-related items, you'll need to consider personal letters. You may want to write a letter of appreciation to a colleague for providing, at your request, a lecture to a dental group, social club, or civic organization. Or you may want to send a simple "thank you" for a past personal favor. Actually, this aspect of correspondence has more to do with being a gracious human being than a considerate professional. But even if it doesn't gain you any more patients, you, the sender as well as the receiver, will feel good about it.

Your professional correspondence will include forwarding patient radiographs to a specialist (orthodontist, periodontist, prosthodontist) or radiographs and letter of transfer on a patient who has moved away from your practice.

At times you will also need to forward certain patient radiographs to another dentist. The patient who comes in for radiographs and initial exam and then requests that you send the radiographs to another dentist may be shopping for varying treatment prices. The inactive patient may start back, but with another dentist, and the disgruntled patient may just want to transfer to another dentist, period.

Your professional correspondence may contain requested or completed detailed health histories of patients. When you have examined a patient and prescribed a treatment, but have reservations relating to the patient's history, you need to be sure that the treatment is in the patient's best interest. This practice of seeking additional information protects not only the patient but the dentist as well.

In corresponding with specialists who request radiographs or additional patient data, you may use the specialist's own printed referral slip along with the radiographs in responding, rather than write a personal letter. Many specialists do have such referral slips printed and place them with dentists who might refer patients to them. These slips make it convenient to jot down pertinent notes about the patient rather than composing a lengthy letter. You may want to make copies of such slips for the files, so you will have a record of this correspondence.

If you are a specialist, you may want to write a thank-you to the general dentist for referring a patient. It is an added courtesy to outline the prescribed treatment you have scheduled, and request that he perform certain procedures before you begin (see Fig. 10–4).

Third party correspondence is growing rapidly because more and more companies are offering dental insurance as a benefit to

E. RANDOLPH WILKINS, DDS
New Hope Dental Clinic
8 Ravenscroft Circle
Springfield, MA 01119

September 20, 1982

Charles Taylor, DDS
304 Terrace Lane
Springfield, MA 01118

Dear Charles:

Thank you so much for referring Melody Patterson to our
office. My staff and I really appreciate the confidence
you show in us by your referrals.

Melody's treatment, which is scheduled to begin October
30, will be an extraction case treated by the straight-
wire technique.

Two weeks prior to that date, please extract the following:

                  Left maxillary first premolar
                  Right maxillary first premolar

A few days prior to October 30, please perform a prophylaxis and fluoride treatment.

Thank you again for referring Melody. We're looking
forward to working with her.

Sincerely,

E. Randolph Wilkins, DDS

ERW/smr

Figure 10–4. Thank you from a specialist.

their employees. The forms arriving from insurance companies (dental or accident) or Medicaid, requesting radiographs for confirmation of claimant visit, for pretreatment estimates, and for audit can engender considerable correspondence. Audit inquiries, for example, may indicate that a claim has been made for treatment and the insurance carrier is double-checking to make sure the claim is valid. This is another instance when copies, not originals, should be sent. You don't want the original "lost in the mail."

PROMOTION TO PATIENTS

In recent years health newsletters have grown into a mini-industry. Everyone from financial consultants to recipe clubs write and circulate newsletters. You may want to consider publishing a dental newsletter from your office.

Newsletters

What should you include in such a practice promotion? An obvious answer is dental news. Perhaps you have patients who could benefit from the latest technological developments in the field of dentistry. The trade publications you receive are filled with such articles. Take a few items, outline the basic points, then rewrite them in language the lay person can understand. You don't have to go into as much detail or length as the original article, but just enough to interest your patients with the highlights. (You might want to sharpen your writing skills through an evening college course in journalism or advanced composition.)

Just as obvious for a dental newsletter would be information about various aspects of dentistry: cosmetic techniques for improving appearance, the best treatment for relief of pain, or the importance of preventive dentistry. With a light touch you can do much to dispel the growing myth that preventive dentistry is just another means for the dentist to charge patients for unneeded checkups. And along those lines you could also include information of a nutritional nature — foods that are healthy, and those that are appealing but harmful to the teeth.

There is a wealth of available information about the practice of dentistry, enough to fill hundreds of newsletters. But be practical in planning your newsletter; give the reader some humor, too. Jokes, if you like, and cartoons. Remember the song that goes "a spoonful of sugar helps the medicine go down"? If you don't have the time or inclination for a "do-it-yourself" newsletter, you might consider contracting with a commercial newsletter service.

Everyone from financial consultants to recipe clubs writes and circulates newsletters. You may want to consider publishing one, too.

Handbook

On a more direct informational level you may wish to develop a brochure, booklet, or handbook about your office for your patients.

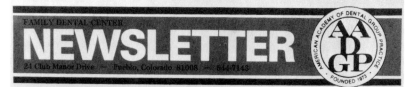

FAMILY DENTAL CENTER CELEBRATES FOUR YEARS OF COMMUNITY SERVICE

Family Dental Center is four years old September 8. The whole staff wants to take this opportunity to thank you, our patients, for your faith, support, and good will all through the past four years. We would also like to let you know what our dentists have been doing in the area of community projects for the betterment of both general and dental health.

Dr. James Baum serves as Secretary for the Colorado Academy of General Dentistry. The AGD is a nationwide organization of general dentists who believe in the concept of on-going education in dentistry. All the doctors at Family Dental Center subscribe to this philosophy and are members of the AGD. The AGD provides for a Fellowship and a Mastership program with rigid requirements for attaining both. As of this time, Dr. Osburne, Dr. Baum, and Dr. Tekavec have fulfilled the Fellowship specifications and are currently working on the Masterships. Of the 120,000 dentists in the United States, 3,000 have attained Fellowship status and less than 100 have attained Mastership.

Dr. George Beck is very active in the dental community. Currently he is serving as President of the Pueblo Dental Study Club. This study club brings in outside dental instructors and experts to provide continuing education for its members.

Dr. Robert Heun is Chairman of the Pump-A-Life Program in Pueblo County. This program provides instruction in CPR (Basic Lifesaving) to the general public and is available to anyone for the cost of the American Heart Association Manual (around $6.00).

Dr. Jack Osburne, long active in Pueblo community affairs, has also been a primary contributor to the functioning of the dental community. A past mayor of Pueblo, Dr. Osburne has also served as President of the Colorado Dental Association and is currently working with the University of Colorado School of Dentistry in a student externship program. This program places senior dental students in private offices for training in the "nuts and bolts" of actual practice. Family Dental Center has sponsored many such students.

Dr. Mel Tekavec is currently serving as Vice President of the International Analgesia Society. This society is a worldwide organization of dentists dedicated to the use of conscious sedation as a means of providing comfort for patients during dentistry. Dr. Tekavec and Dr. Baum were co-founders of the Rocky Mountain Analgesia Society, which grew from eight members in 1967 to over 2,000 before it merged with the international organization last year. Dr. Tekavec lectures across the United States in this field and that of dental practice administration, and he is also a consultant to the Nebraska University Dental School.

Dr. Dee Williams, a periodontist, practices both in Pueblo and Denver. Until last year he was a member of the faculty of Colorado University Dental School in Denver where he was Chairman of both the Occlusion and Dental Morphology Department and the Crown and Bridge Department. A well-known lecturer, Dr. Williams now divides his time between teaching in continuing education and the private practice of periodontics and occlusion.

"PEOPLE HOURS" NOT OFFICE HOURS

Family Dental Center announces that the office will now be open Wednesday evenings until 10:00 P.M. and every Saturday until 1:00 P.M. for the

Figure 10–5. A handsome dental practice newsletter published by an up-to-date Colorado group.

In this medium you can give the patient and potential patient such information as your office telephone number and any emergency numbers you may maintain, office hours, and clear, concise information about the types of services you render, the range of fees (if you like), and possibly payment schedules.

Either included in the handbook or distributed to each patient separately (or both) could be explanations of dental procedures. These would contain specific information for the patient pertaining to what was done and what to expect upon returning home after treatment, such as bleeding, sensitivity, or pain. The data should include what the patient can do to counteract these effects.

Of course patients are always told what to expect and what to do

> You can't always count on patients to remember all of what is said. Written information will supplement the verbal.

immediately after office treatment, but you can't always count on them to remember all of what is said. After all, according to the degree of the treatment, patients are going to have other things in mind, such as coping with pain. It is well known that people remember less than 50 percent of what they hear. The written information will supplement the verbal, and often prevent unneeded calls to you after office hours.

The handbook or office publication is also a superior communication vehicle for providing dental insurance information. You can explain clearly and concisely exactly how your office handles dental insurance. You can also indicate which forms the patient is to bring along to the office on each visit and instruct the patient on how to fill out his portion of the form.

Explain about "deductible" policies, what the term means, and how it directly affects the patient. You may wish to explain that should your professional services fee be less than the deductible, the patient must pay the entire fee — even though insurance forms were submitted.

Be straightforward in explaining that normally dental insurance does not provide one hundred percent coverage of the fee. You may even wish to go into further detail, showing how much the payments can vary from company to company for the same treatment plan. Advise the patient that he or she will generally have to pay a portion of the fee.

Make it perfectly clear to the patient that no matter how much dental insurance coverage a person may have, it is first and foremost the individual, not the insurer, who is responsible for payment in full for services rendered. The subject of third party insurance coverage will be dealt with further in Chapter 17.

Under the "special letters" category, consider seasonal correspondence at Thanksgiving and Christmas. Such correspondence can be handled effectively through a more personalized but mass-produced card or letter of your own design.

> Make it clear to the patient that no matter how much dental insurance coverage a person may have, it is first and foremost the individual, not the insurer, who is responsible for payment in full.

SPECIAL PROMOTIONS

A special way of expressing your sincere appreciation to patients for having sent you one or more friends who became patients is through a personalized thank-you letter. "Personalized" means it is in your words, but in this instance you may use the "canned" or "preprinted form" letter and sign your name on each one. Because you have had such a letter printed by the hundreds does not make it less sincere an expression to a patient for aiding you in building a thriving practice. The same type of letter can be utilized in thanking a colleague — physician or dentist — for referring patients to you.

It is always advisable to be more personalized in dealing with the "missionary" patient (one who sends you many referrals). Besides letters or hand-written notes (see Fig. 10–6), your office may wish to say "thank you" by sending flowers, by taking the patient out for dinner or by having a social for a group of such patients. The latter lends itself well to promoting your practice publicly (see Chapter 7).

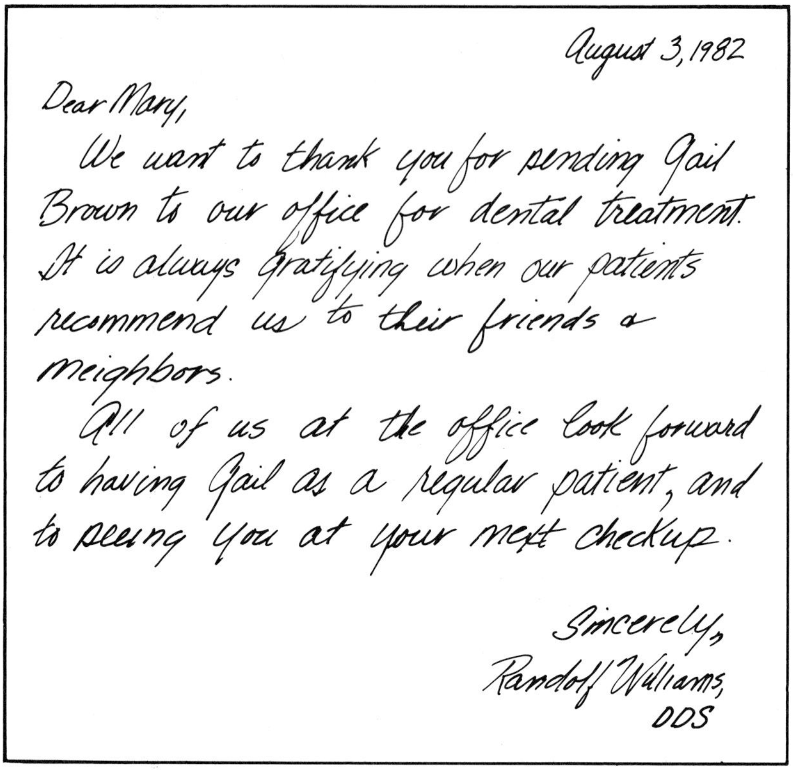

August 3, 1982

Dear Mary,

We want to thank you for sending Gail Brown to our office for dental treatment. It is always gratifying when our patients recommend us to their friends & neighbors.

All of us at the office look forward to having Gail as a regular patient, and to seeing you at your next checkup.

Sincerely,

Randolf Williams, DDS

Figure 10–6. Handwritten thank-you note.

Another great way of keeping in touch with people is connected with watching the newspapers. Is that man who was just voted "Jaycee of the Year" a patient? Is he a friend? What about the woman just promoted to a higher position in business or industry? How about the young person who received a full college scholarship for scholastic achievement? Or the most valuable player in a sport? Clip out the story and picture, slip it inside one of your letterheads or specially printed cards and send it to the honored person with your own personal congratulations. Besides keeping in touch and possibly gaining a new professional contact, it's an opportunity to recognize an individual for his accomplishments — and that person will appreciate it.

COLLECTION LETTERS

Don't be afraid to devise your own cost-effective system for collecting overdue accounts.

It would be wonderful if this subject never needed mention. We all know, unhappily, that it does. For collecting past due accounts, you will need to think about the very definite need for an effective system. The use of a collection agency, which charges either a set fee or a percentage of the past due accounts collected, may be effectual in some cases. Collection agencies have come under fire in recent years for sometimes questionable methods. Lobbyist groups have even been able to get effective legislation passed against certain collection methods.

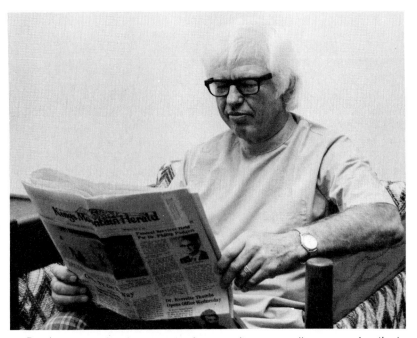

Dentist scans a local newspaper for news items on colleagues and patients. He'll write personal notes recognizing their achievements.

Don't be afraid to devise your own cost-effective system for collecting overdue accounts. If your state permits small claims court action, your staff may be able to handle the accounts for you.

In creating your own system, decide at what point you must begin sending collection notice correspondence. When is the account past due? When is it seriously in arrears? Most accounts are billed late in the month with the due date on the tenth of the following month. These are accounts you have permitted patients in good standing to develop with you. The degree of tardiness in payment will be entirely up to you and you should plan your correspondence accordingly.

Will letters begin after two statements? After a telephone call? (See Chapter 9 for a discussion on use of the telephone for collecting.) Will you send one letter? Two? A third? Again, the decision is yours. Experiment and determine the most efficient method for *your* practice in terms of overhead and results.

Consider these suggestions as to content of your collections correspondence. Such letters must be complete, but brief; straightforward, but courteous. The language should fit the reader so that no doubt exists in his or her mind about why you have written. It is generally preferable to use the telephone for direct contact prior to any collection letter.

In succession, collection letters should become more demanding.

Try to avoid wording and tone that will create anger and hostility within the reader. If you antagonize the person immediately, he or she will not only disregard the letter, but will also make certain that you are the last creditor to get any consideration. Being cute or clever will more than likely create the same feelings in the reader.

Be straight to the point. You may begin your letter by asking if there is something wrong, and give the person an opportunity to air any grievance. You may also legitimately remind the patient of his or her responsibility for payment, the arrangements that were made for payment, and the final date you expect payment to be made.

Above all, be positive in your tone. Conclude the letter with a request for the payment which is rightly due you for professional services. The reason for the latter suggestion is the fact that readers ultimately remember the last thing they read. Succeeding letters should become more demanding. The first letter can be a cheery reminder, but the last should state the consequences of inaction, such as a suit in small claims court (see Fig. 10–7).

E. RANDOLPH WILKINS, DDS
New Hope Dental Clinic
8 Ravenscroft Circle
Springfield, MA 01119

Date

John Doe
100 City Street
Anytown, USA

Dear Mr. Doe:

We are not aware of any reason why your account is unpaid.
Unless payment is received within seven days, the account
will be assigned to Small Claims Court. A prompt response
will stop further action and help you to maintain a good
credit standing.

Please mail or bring payment of $_____ to our office within
one week.

Sincerely,

Randolph Wilkins, D.D.S.

Figure 10–7. Collection letter.

SUMMARY

Correspondence is a very important marketing tool for a dental practice. The dentist can use various forms of correspondence as promotional devices with patients, other dental professionals, and business associates. The cost of producing personalized written communication must be weighed against the benefits derived from the positive public relations it might generate.

Letters or notes should use language that is appropriate to the receiver, whether patient or professional. In certain instances, a personal, hand-written note is the best choice. In other cases a preprinted form letter will be appropriate. At still other times, specific information will be required and a dictated typed letter will work best.

All dental offices need an efficient, timely system of sorting and dealing with incoming and outgoing mail. This is crucial to avoid delaying items of priority.

The use of a dental newsletter to patients may be incorporated as a practice builder, and an office handbook is helpful in providing timeless information to patients.

Regardless of the form of written communication, it should be attractively prepared, brief, concise, and to the point. Strive to avoid wordiness and unneeded information.

REFERENCES

Brahe, N. B.: Great Ideas for Dental Practice. Vols. 1 and 2. Appleton, Wisconsin, Project D Publications, 1973.

Brahe, N. B.: How to build a patient newsletter. Dental Practice, October, 1980, pp. 44–48.

Brahe, N. B., Conner, D. E.: 15 Days to a Great New Practice. Appleton, Wisconsin, Project D Publications, 1971, pp. 107–118.

Brugger, A. A., Brahe, N. B.: The Dental Letter Book: Communiques From the Dental Office. Appleton, Wisconsin, Project D Publications, 1976.

DeMarco, T.: Put it in writing! Dental Economics, May, 1977, pp. 77–79.

Howard, W. W.: Dental Practice Planning. St. Louis, The C. V. Mosby Company, 1975, pp. 133–153.

Lesikar, R. V.: Report Writing for Business. Homewood, Illinois, Richard D. Irwin, Inc., 1977.

The Business of Dental Practice. By the editors of Dental Management. Stamford, Connecticut, Professional Publishing Corporation, 1969, pp. 63–67.

Unger, W. D.: A newsletter as a practice builder. Dental Mangement, March, 1981, pp. 22–24.

11

Getting to Know
the Patient Well

Dr. Jim Logan is reflecting at the end of a frustrating day. Mrs. Lucy Morgan came in for a treatment planning conference and left without agreeing to any further treatment. "I just can't understand it," Jim thinks. "We do a thorough examination and medical and dental history just like they taught me in school. We do a complete set of radiographs and make study models. Then I spend over an hour studying her dental problems and develop a thorough plan to restore her dental health. She admits that she has neglected her teeth. She says she always hated to go to the dentist, even though she liked her dentist who had recently retired.

"But she just doesn't seem to understand how serious her problems are; nor does she appreciate what I had in mind for her. I guess she just has a low dental IQ. Sometimes there's not much you can do for people who are not interested in their teeth. She did say she would probably lose all her teeth anyway. But I really do need to figure out some approach to this problem. I can't go on failing to convince people that they need dental treatment."

THE PROBLEM

Patient Attitudes

What attitudes do patients bring to our offices? Let us hasten to observe that dentists are not individually responsible for these attitudes. Given that most of us have had little training in psychology, we have coped quite well with these unfavorable feelings associated with the mouth and by extension with the dentist. However, we should acknowledge that many people have had unpleasant experiences in dental offices, and that collectively we have some responsibility for experiences people have had.

As Barkley observed, about 90 percent of all adults have been to dentists, but less than half of these return with any degree of

Many people have had unpleasant experiences in dental offices, and we have some responsibility for these experiences.

158

regularity. Perhaps, the ones who do not return have the deepest attitudinal problems, but those are the very problems we need to deal with, if we are to extend our market.

R. T. Martin found people to be indifferent, apathetic, pessimistic, fearful, and distrustful toward dentistry. They regarded dentistry as painful, expensive, and ineffective. They made statements such as "Injections are worse in the mouth," "There's pain in the pocketbook," and "I'm going to lose them all anyhow." They believed that teeth are important only for cosmetic purposes, especially with the opposite sex, and that teeth are not related to general health. Criticism of dentists was voiced in statements such as the following: "Dentists don't trust patients and they don't treat them as individuals. They don't explain — they're straight into business. Don't let you relax. Not able to do much about dental problems anyway." The dentist was seen as an aggressor, one who cuts, numbs, and causes pain and guilt.

Dentists reflected these perceptions. They felt psychological stress from having to cause pain. Complaints were that they had to spend so much time operating at the chair and had little time for more relaxing activity, such as consultation, as physicians had. Dentists were disappointed with patients' lack of interest in their own dental health and lack of appreciation for dental treatment. They were frustrated by their failure to achieve satisfactory communication with patients.

Dentists feel psychological stress from having to cause pain.

All these things seem to constitute a heavy burden, but again, we should not dwell on guilt. We should simply accept our patient's feelings as real and proceed to deal with them more effectively.

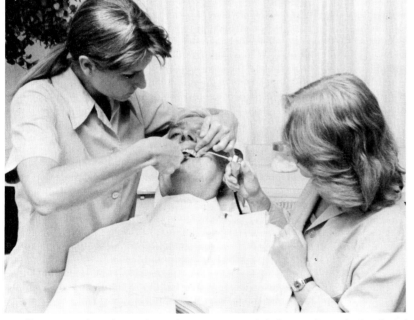

Because patients know that pain can be part of their experience in the dental office, they frequently bring anxiety with them. Dentists need to help patients overcome this feeling.

Psychological Significance of the Problem

The oral cavity is a highly charged emotional area. Infants derive pleasure through it by feeding and sucking. And they suffer pain in the mouth when teeth begin to erupt. In the words of Harold Wirth, the mouth continues to be central in peoples' lives:

> The mouth in its entirety is an important and even wondrous part of our anatomy, our emotion, our life; it is the site of our very being. When an animal loses its teeth, it cannot survive unless it is domesticated; its very existence is terminated; it dies. In the human, the mouth is the means of speaking, of expressing love, happiness and joy, anger, ill temper, or sorrow. It is (a) primary sex contact; hence it is of initial import to our regeneration and survival by food and propagation. It deserves the greatest care it can receive at any sacrifice.

Clearly many deep problems center in the mouth. Apparently most of our regular patients are able to resolve these satisfactorily. They seem well adjusted and appear to cope with dental problems and problems of visiting our offices. However, researchers know, and in fact we all know, that one of the major reasons people do *not* visit the dentist is fear. If we are to reach the 75 percent that we frequently refer to as our market, we need to deal effectively with people's fear.

Robert Froelich tells us that when people are seeking help with a new problem from someone they don't know, they most likely will be anxious. They feel trapped. They have to interrupt their routine to go to the dental office. They may feel a loss of youth, well-being, power, and even wholeness.

Jim Logan may feel that it's unfair that he gets saddled with problems of this kind when he is a dentist, not a psychiatrist. But reality, not fairness, is the issue here. Had Jim even suspected that Mrs. Morgan might be at all distraught, he probably would have approached her differently. If Jim is to increase his success rate in treatment conferences, or case presentations as some of his friends call them, he needs to develop a better understanding of people and improve his communications.

One way to start is to decide that he is not responsible for the states of mind of people who consult him. We dentists did not create the mouth with all its charged symbolic emotional aspects. We can't help it that people associate a very early painful experience, teething, with manipulations in the mouth. Nothing we can do would prevent people from feeling impaired and angry because they have a dental problem. Surely we dentists should not personalize people's feelings about dental problems, which do extend to dentistry and dentists in general.

We have to involve the patient in the solution to dental problems.

Traditionally we have seen ourselves as experts in treating dental problems and not as counselors or helpers. Consequently, we dentists in the United States have developed great expertise in technical dentistry to the point where America's is the best in the world. We can be justly proud of our fine dentistry. And we should continue to develop better methods and materials for treating dental problems. Certainly our patients deserve our best. However, many people have not availed themselves of our fine dentistry. What elements have we left out? How can we reach those who have not sought our services?

For about a decade dentists put their faith in the preventive dentistry movement. Then they became aware that dental disease was still recurring because people did not carry out the relatively simple routines of disrupting plaque from all surfaces of their teeth. Now, it was apparent that we faced a behavioral, not a technical, problem. We found we had to involve the patient in the solution to dental problems.

Personality Development

How do personalities such as Lucy Morgan's develop or how do people become what they are?

Personality is the product of experience. The stimulus-response psychology known as behaviorism says that life is a constant responding to all the stimuli to which we are subjected, and that the consequences of our behavior have great impact on future behavior. Thus we stop at red lights, shake hands with people who extend their hands, answer the telephone when it rings, ad infinitum. Our unique experience of response to stimuli and the consequences of our responses cause us to form habits and develop patterns of coping. In other words we behave in our individual ways, which become well known to friends, relatives, and associates. People who know us well can pretty well predict our behavior; they understand our personalities. Clearly Jim Logan does not know Lucy Morgan this well.

Psychologists and psychiatrists tell us that much of our behavior can be explained on the basis of very early development. As Marvin Weckstein says, the unconscious portion of the mind retains all the experiences we ever had. However, the unpleasant parts cause us to act irrationally. These are acts we cannot explain, but it takes concerted effort for us to act differently. Our reaction to someone we meet for the first time may be dislike, not because of any reason to dislike that person, but because that person calls up an unpleasant association from our unconscious. The same effect may occur with any new experience such as a food we have never tasted or an activity we have never engaged in. A first visit to a dental office is surely a new experience for both the patient and the dentist. If either has an unpleasant association in the unconscious, which is stimulated by the other, the visit may be hard on both parties.

> Much of our behavior can be explained on the basis of very early development.

People

People are knowable, Naomi Brill and others assure us. Our minds enable us to know ourselves, our world, and others. We all share a common biological heritage. Our similarities include basic physiologic needs and some need to enhance our individual situations. All humans hope for a better life.

Cause and effect relationships exist in all our lives. Our personalities, our beliefs, and our values are the result of our experience overlaying our genetic core. Nothing is pure happenstance. The causes are multiple and operate simultaneously. Some of the causes are internal; some, external; and there is an interplay among these. Causes are both fundamental and precipitating; some are ongoing, others immediate, and they interact.

Although the biological heritage is universal, cultural heritages differ. Perception of pain has been shown to vary from one culture to another. Americans of northern European ancestry are more stoic than are those of southern European heritage.

And individual heritage is unique. Although siblings grow up in the same home, eat the same food, and apparently live by the same rules, they are all different. Thus, each individual has a different personality based on unique experience. Clearly each individual has his or her own perceptual field or perspective.

Our problem as helpers is to understand that perspective as well as possible. We need to remember that we can never perceive exactly the same way as another person does. Capability for change, which we all share, enables us to understand each other well enough so that we can function together. Fortunately human beings are sufficiently resilient to adapt. We need not regard our patients as fragile, nor should we expect ourselves to always do and say the right thing. Indeed, we can view our helping relationship as growth; we and our patients will come to know each other better. Our maturing partnership for better health will enhance all of our lives.

The Dental Problem

Each dentist needs to be aware of how the patient's unconscious or subconscious may affect the dental situation.

Neither the dentist nor the patient possesses total information about the patient's problem. Let's turn our attention to this fact using the Johari Window (Figure 11–1) as an aid to our understanding.

In window *1* is information that both dentist and patient are aware of. Such information may consist of such simple facts as that a tooth has decay or is discolored. When the patient first sits down in the chair, this simple body of facts is all that they share as relevant information.

How do patient and dentist communicate to the other the information that each alone possesses? The dentist can diagnose or develop information (window *2*) that the patient needs in order to participate actively in solutions to dental problems. Likewise, the

1 Known by both dentist and patient	2 Known only by the dentist
3 Known only by the patient	4 Known by neither (subconscious)

Figure 11–1. Johari Window.

patient may relay to the dentist information that the patient alone possesses (window 3) and that the dentist needs in order to be truly helpful.

Window *4* contains information that neither initially knows directly — which the patient's subconscious harbors — but that may well have some effect on treatment. Each dentist needs to be aware of how the patient's unconscious or subconscious may affect the dental situation. A dentist who is very skillful in "reading" individuals may be able to make some working assumptions about the material in the patient's Window *4*. This psychocybernetic process should be undertaken cautiously.

Dentist's Knowledge of the Problem

Dental school and much of continuing education provides exquisite understanding of clinical dental problems. Dentists' diagnostic ability is well developed. And well it should be. Diagnosis is said to be the most professional task in which dentists engage. Only the dentist — not anyone else on his team — can provide the diagnosis to the patient.

However, the language containing the diagnostic information must be understandable to the patient. Explanation of dental problems in technical terms does not qualify as information, as we are describing it. Many dentists find it difficult to describe dental problems in plain language. Small wonder. Our body of knowledge is given to us in dental school and other educational settings in technical language. And for good reasons. Accuracy and brevity characterize technical language. When we translate to lay language, we lose accuracy and take more words to describe dental problems. But we must remember that our language is jargon to patients. If we are to share information, as we are obliged to do, we must do it in layman's terms.

We must remember that our language is jargon to patients. If we are to share information . . . we must do it in layman's terms.

Patient's Knowledge of the Problem

As we all know but seem to forget at times, patients continue to live with the consequences of solutions to their dental problems. Clearly they have a great deal more at stake in their dental treatment than do their dentists. If the dentist proceeds to manage the dental problem without adequate input from the patient, he or she is failing as a helper. To succeed as a helper the dentist must obtain appropriate input from the patient.

What is this appropriate input? More specifics will be given in Chapter 12, but at this point, suffice it to say that whatever the patient knows that affects the dental problem or the dental treatment should be shared with the dentist.

The burden is on the dentist as helper to facilitate this sharing. In the past many dentists have been so busy that they have had insufficient time to coax forth this information. In many very busy offices this has been done most effectively by auxiliaries who were

truly helpers and whose skills were well developed. Many dentists
report that the reduced demand for their services permits them to
become better acquainted with their patients. And they find this de-
lightful.

If as some patients allege, dentists are "straight into business,"
dentists are unlikely to learn from patients what they really need to
know in order to help effectively. Sufficient time is necessary. It takes
time to get patient input. And it takes communication skills. If the
helper seems to be in a hurry, the helpee is reluctant to take time to
provide information. Additionally the patient has no way of knowing
what information the dentist needs. It is up to the dentist or auxiliary
to ask questions.

L. D. Pankey has said that patients will tell you anything you want
to know that they think is in their best interests. Effective helpers can
ask questions in such a way that patients will feel that the information
is in their best interests. Again, this is an art that neophyte helpers
must cultivate if they are to become effective.

HELPING

Why Emphasize Helping in Dentistry?

Dentistry needs more complete incorporation of helping skills.
Only dentists with helping skills will be able to understand and attract
the majority of the population who do not already value dentistry as a
means of enhancing their lives.

Many dental consultants now maintain that dentists would do

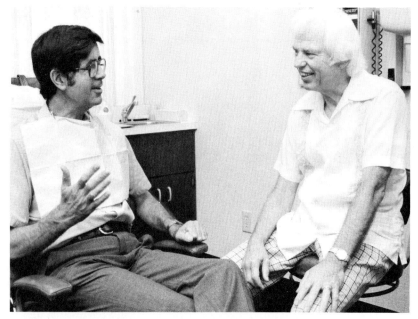

Dentists need to listen — intently — to their patients, to find out information
known only to the patient.

better to abandon the medical model. We have never really been successful in convincing people that we are essential in their lives even though they call us doctor as they do the physician. Maybe people have a more realistic view of us than we have of ourselves. It is time for dentists to perceive themselves as helpers, not as physicians. Of course it will always be necessary for some highly trained dentists to function in hospitals and provide service for medically compromised patients in much the same way physicians do. However, most dentists treat healthy patients and can function more effectively in the role of helper.

> Only dentists with helping skills will be able to understand and attract the majority of the population who do not already value dentistry.

What Is Helping?

Social workers, psychiatrists, psychologists, and many others have been helping people with problems for a long time. Many dentists are finding answers from the helping professions. "Helping" is an enabling act; that is, a helper *enables* someone to accomplish a goal in which they both believe. It is helping others to grow and that requires the helper to work with the person seeking help until that person develops and acquires the skills to accomplish his own goals. Learning by the helper as well as by the helpee is a dynamic two-way relationship. Bringing about change is always the goal of a helping relationship. Usually the change is desired by the person seeking help. You can readily see that we have a problem in dentistry because we, not the patient, are aware of a need for change. Everyone who describes helping as a profession does so in terms of active involvement. In no case is someone doing something to or for another person who is passive.

Dealing with the Problem

Freud and the psychoanalytic school say that analysis is necessary to deal with deep-seated problems. Much time and a high degree of training are required for psychoanalysis. Although some of the dental problems, as we have learned, are deep seated, psychoanalysis does not appear practical except for the most severe problems, and would then have to be done by a psychoanalyst, not a dentist.

Perceptual psychology as described by Combs is a sound basis for approaching the problem. The basic concept of perceptual psychology is that "all behavior of a person is the *direct* result of his field of perception at the moment of his behaving." This is looking at behavior through the eye of the beholder. Individual behavior is particularly dependent on perceptions of self and circumstances in which the person is operating. The word "perception" is used here to mean more than seeing. It connotes meaning of the experience for the individual. The frame of reference is internal, not external. A dental visit is different for the eight-year-old boy than it is for the middle-aged dowager. In fact, it is different for all people even if they are members of the same group.

Resolution of the Problem

Before you ask for a decision by the patient (and the patient always makes the decision), you must be sure that you and the patient have sufficient information. You obtain this by a combination of taking a health history, conducting an examination, and asking the patient to relate his or her knowledge of and attitude about the current dental problem. After studying these data, you can recommend actions to be taken.

At this point, if your information is adequate, the patient will agree with your recommendation. If your information, like Jim Logan's, is inadequate, the patient is not likely to make the decision that you try to encourage. Then by obtaining more information you and the patient can negotiate a decision both of you feel right about.

Generally at this point the helpee must help himself. The helper then functions as a consultant. Dentistry differs from some of the other helping professions in the next stage. A dentist consults first, then treats. Unless there is no dental disease, the dentist usually has to do some procedures to restore faulty dental tissue or to return it to a state of health. In other words he is a doer, not a consultant, at this point. Dentists have become so expert at these technical tasks and have taken such pride in them (and justifiably so), that they have seen dentistry as performance of technical tasks. As a helping profession dentistry is more. Dentists or other team members are continuing consultants to their patients. As psychiatrists continue to be consultants to their patients about how they are getting along in helping themselves, so do helping dentists.

Successful resolution of the problem requires that dentists and patients cooperate with each other. That each does what only he can do. And that each assist the other to do a better job.

Before you ask for a decision by the patient, you must be sure that you and the patient have sufficient information.

HELPERS

Value System

Depending on your cultural background you are likely to have certain values that affect helping ability. If you see certain groups as undeserving, you will find it difficult to help them. Persons in whom you recognize little potential are not likely to receive effective help from you. America, the melting pot, encompasses a wide variety of value systems. We need to consider whether certain groups underutilize dentists because our value systems make little sense to them and theirs to us. Indeed, we need to recognize that value systems, both ours and our patients, get in the way of effective helping. It is characteristic of helping that the helper does everything possible to eliminate the barriers posed by different value systems. This responsibility is ours and not our patients'. If we discharge it effectively, our patients are likely to meet us perhaps not halfway but somewhere in between where we were and where they were.

Health is not as highly valued by everyone as by us. We need to realize that others may be content with a lower standard of oral health than we are. They may value esthetics apart from function or vice versa. For example, Mrs. Fielding may be content to ignore missing posterior teeth so long as anteriors are attractive. If we are to be helpful, we certainly must satisfy their values and in sharing our values we will attempt to persuade them toward our point of view.

Relationship to Others

Relating to others can be broken down into three basic modes: passive or nonassertive, assertive, and aggressive. In our culture males are expected to be rather aggressive; at least they can get by with that kind of behavior. And females are expected to be passive. Neither of these modes is useful for helpers. Aggressive relating requires one person to be dominant and one to be subservient. Helping relationships do not grow and thrive unless both parties participate on the basis of equality as individuals. Of course, helpers have certain skills that qualify them to help people. The helpee probably does not possess the skills but has unique abilities, which are essential if helping is to be effective. Passive helping is an obvious contradiction in terms.

Assertiveness is essential to the helping process. It can be defined as the honest expression of thoughts and feelings to others without belittling them and in order to obtain from others your basic human rights. Assertiveness is a skill that we all develop to varying degrees, apparently depending on modeling and feedback we experience. Honesty and consideration for others with insistence on one's own rights characterize the assertive person. Although we emphasize sensitivity to others' needs, the effective helper must at appropriate times confront others. Failure to confront when necessary compromises the helping process. Assertiveness is very much a two-way street. Dentists and patients alike have rights such as those in The Bill of Assertive Rights. We need to remember that *we and our patients* are entitled to these rights.

Failure to confront when necessary compromises the helping process.

BILL OF ASSERTIVE RIGHTS*

Everyone has the right to:
— Receive consideration and help from others
— Be treated as an adult and not be patronized
— Receive consideration and respect for opinions
— Tell others what one's needs are
— Use judgment in deciding one's own needs
— Make mistakes
— Ask others to change their behavior
— Make requests of others
— Refuse requests from others without feeling selfish or guilty
— Feel and express anger and other emotions
— Not have others impose their values on one

*Adapted from Brill (1978).

— Take time to sort out personal reactions at one's own convenience, not someone else's.

Perception of Others

How do I think and feel about others? As perception of self affects how well one does, perception of others affects how well one does in the helping situation. As King says "We now know, based on a vast amount of empirical data, that the person who has a high ability to help other people perceives them differently than the person who has a low ability to be a helper." Combs has discovered that all successful helpers share common perceptions of others. Effective helpers perceive other people as able to solve their own problems; friendly and well intentioned; worthy — having dignity and integrity; dependable; helpful; and internally motivated. If these are your assumptions about people, you are likely to find that most people live up to them. You will also find that you will be able to help people. Assumption of the opposite traits is no way to start a helping process.

The question arises 'Can Jim Logan change his perceptions of people?" Some would say that the leopard cannot change its spots; nor can Jim Logan change his basic perceptions. As we said in Chapter 4, change is difficult, but it is not impossible. Of course, it is not likely to be rapid unless one undergoes a very dramatic, perhaps shattering experience. We believe that all of us, as we examine our assumptions, may conclude that they are not written in stone. We may see that we can change a little bit at a time, and, as we do, we can change still more. Success breeds success. As we try out new skills and new ideas in our attempt to be more helpful, we are likely to discover that we like them and will commit ourselves to them. Gradually, we can change our assumptions and become more effective helpers.

As we try out new skills and new ideas, we are likely to discover that we like them and will commit ourselves to them.

Self-Perception

"How do I think and feel about myself?" is the first question Brill suggests that we ask ourselves. Regardless of one's physical appearance, age, intellectual capacity, wealth, and almost any other characteristic you can think of, one can usually succeed in life and relate quite well with others if one likes oneself. Feedback from peers and authority figures such as parents and teachers in the formative years seems to be the strongest determinant of this self-esteem. Adolescence with its quest for identify is a hazardous time. Self-esteem is not static, and may change later in life depending on one's experience.

In Combs' language of perceptual psychology, persons with high self-esteem see themselves as worthy, but low self-esteem is characterized by feelings of uncertainty and inadequacy . Positive perception is based on: (1) recognition that everyone has strengths and weaknesses; (2) tolerance of imperfections in self and others; (3) capacity to recognize and deal with negative attitudes; (4) acceptance of the fact that one need not like oneself all of the time.

Need for Growth

Beyond the need for security is the need to grow. The growth or development of our potential appears to depend upon stimulation of experience and internal impulses relating to experience. Balance of growth occurs if experience is balanced. Timing is also important. People who were never stimulated as children to develop coordination may find it very difficult to do so as adults. Growth in the area of helping skills may be difficult for someone who has had little stimulation in that area. However, everyone has untapped potential that can be developed. If Jim Logan is stimulated to develop his latent skills, he surely can progress significantly.

Traits of Helpers

Courage

Risk of failure surely requires courage. Failure can be of several kinds. One may fail to handle a specific interpersonal exchange effectively. It takes courage to try, knowing that it may not work out well, but helpers must try, or fail to help because they do not try. If our patients do not carry out their part of the bargain, failure results. We may get in over our heads with the technical dental problem before we realize it. The problem may be much more difficult than we realize. Helping is risky and risk requires courage.

Allowing oneself to be used constructively without star billing is characteristic of an effective helper.

Humility

Humility is desirable. Willingness to acknowledge the autonomy, the responsibility, and the active role of the patient allows and encourages the patient to be active rather than passive. Allowing oneself to be used constructively without star billing is characteristic of an effective helper. Of course, *you* are also active not passive, but you are not dominant with the patient being subservient. Humility in a helper is really the acknowledgement by the helper that he or she is instrumental, not omnipotent.

Nonjudgmentalism is an obvious manifestation of humility. One who judges others is unable to help them in the sense we are using "help." Judgmentalism is belittling of others; and, aside from the effects on perception of both patient and dentist, tempts the dentist to make decisions that the patient should make. It robs the patient of his autonomy (his ethical right) and reduces the quality of the helping relationship.

Recognition that others could help as effectively as oneself is another facet of humility. Human beings tend to look on themselves as uniquely qualified to perform the tasks they consider their most important ones. Certainly, we dentists are justified in taking pride in what we do well, but each of us needs to remember that there are many others who could do as well and some who could do even better.

We could enhance our lives and those of our patients in some instances if we more freely asked colleagues for help.

The fact is we could enhance our lives and those of our patients in some instances if we more freely asked colleagues for help. Patients are likely to respect us more and like us better if we assist them to get more effective help than we ourselves can provide. Dentists have traditionally done this in referring to specialists for complex clinical problems. We are suggesting that you consider referring for other reasons. This might seem to fly in the face of our espoused principle of expanding your market by enlarging your scope of services. But satisfaction of patient needs is the overwhelming purpose of marketing and it may better be achieved in this manner. Bread cast on the waters is not lost. Dentists need to be realistic about how they can best help people.

Concern

We need to differentiate *concern* for people from *liking* people. Dentists, or any other helpers, cannot be expected to like every patient, but they *can* be expected to be concerned about every patient. The fact that one does not like an individual does not mean that one cannot help that person. Of course, one may choose to refer the individual to someone else. However, that is not always possible. The well-qualified helper is able to overlook the absence of attraction or liking and help the individual out of concern for the person as another human being. Helpers, by definition, are concerned about others.

We need to differentiate concern for people from liking people.

Other qualities mentioned or described in the helping literature include:

friendliness	sense of humor	tact
pleasantness	calmness	kindliness
poise	stability	patience
objectivity	sincerity	fairness
tolerance	broad-mindedness	neatness
social intelligence		

At this point we leave you with your own thoughts about how you as an individual might enhance your helping skills. You can find help in many of the references at the end of this chapter. It is possible that you may decide to seek professional counseling.

COMMUNICATION

Communication can be defined as any interaction of two or more persons. In Combs' language it is the overlap of perceptual fields. We all communicate within the context of our perceptions. Helpers must be aware of this and attempt to communicate with people they are helping in terms of those persons' perceptions. In other words, helpers must take the responsibility for the success or failure of communication.

Developing and Maintaining Communication

A constructive attitude and open feelings are essential for both dentist and patient. A hidden agenda on the part of either will create problems. Many of us, as young dentists, discovered that our desire to impress patients interfered. Also, some dentists balk at discussing money matters because they feel insecure about their own fees. Of course, patients may also face communication barriers. Some may feel guilty because they have neglected their dental health. Some may feel insecure because their finances do not permit them to take care of their teeth the way they would like. As a helper the dentist should clear the air as much as possible so that real communication can take place.

Similarities and differences of the dentist and patient must be taken into account. Anthropologists refer to the culture of the technician as a problem of communication between dentists (and many other professionals) and lay persons. Social class differences exist between dentists and the majority of their patients. Most dentists are better educated and earn more money than most of their patients. It is not the responsibility of patients to bridge these gaps; rather, it is the dentist's.

Capacities to use verbal and nonverbal communication media and to interpret symbolic communication; being trained in logical methods, most dentists are inclined to rely too heavily on the meanings of words rather than what people mean by the words. We need to recognize the limitations of verbal communications, both in ourselves and in others. Our understanding of others will be heightened by developing our skill in reading nonverbal communication as a means of checking the accuracy of the verbal. Nonverbal communication is conveyed by personal appearance, tone of voice, facial expression, silence, gestures, posture, body sounds, physical touch, and so forth. Our office is symbolic communication to our patients. Is it for their comfort or for our convenience — or possibly for both? Dress and manner of the dental team will communicate something to patients — either caringness and professionalism, or their opposites.

> Helpers must use feedback. This is our only means of being certain that patients understand information we give them.

Helpers must use *feedback* when necessary and know how to interpret it. This is our only means of being certain that patients understand information we give them. The difficulty of understanding technical information has already been acknowledged. Telling people something is no assurance that they will understand it. The only way to be sure is to ask them to tell us what their understanding is. If you have any doubt that your meaning has been understood, ask your patient for feedback; otherwise painful misunderstandings may occur.

> The appropriate tempo for speaking is likely to be slightly slower than that of the patient.

The patient's level governs the *tempo of communication*. Helpers must guard against the tendency to provide information too rapidly. Although they have shared the information so many times that it seems elementary, it may be the first time for this particular patient. Even highly intelligent people are unable to absorb dental information at some rates that may seem slow to us. Patients who absorb information slowly must be given plenty of time. To go too fast is a waste of time, because everything you say must be repeated if it is to be understood. The appropriate tempo for speaking is likely to be slightly slower than that of the patient. Too slow a tempo is boring and distracting to the patient; too fast a tempo is at best frustrating, at worst, unintelligible.

Interviewing

Interviewing is a time for sharing information, not merely obtaining it. It is a two-way process. Again, the environment for the interview ought to be reassuring, nonthreatening, and comfortable for the patient.

The stages of the interview are *initiation, exploration, and closing.* Initiation is best accomplished with some small but not inane talk. It could well be about the ease or difficulty with which the patient found the office. This may be useful information to you and it conveys concern for the patient. Exploration, which is the body of the interview, can be eased into next. This can be done by inquiring in some way as to the patient's purpose for coming. Closing signifies to the patient that the interview is terminated. Usually a short recap of what has been said and an indication of what comes next is appropriate. Also, body language, such as standing and ushering the patient to the door or to the next person with whom they will interact, signals the interview's end.

The interview is the first part of a *therapeutic contract* as described by Robert Froelich. Dentist and patient in the interview contract by implication with each other to relate and to exchange information. The third part of the contract, which follows the interview, is to provide and to receive treatment. These three elements of the contract are necessary for a relationship satisfactory to patient and to dentist.

There is a tendency among busy Americans to ask questions and pay very little attention to the answers.

Exchanging information is accomplished by questions and *answers to which the questioner listens.* If the patient needs initial information from the dentist, the questions may be asked first by the patient. Otherwise the dentist (or auxiliary doing the interview) may wish to share information about the office philosophy and then ask questions to obtain the information needed from the patient. Specific information to be obtained from the patient will be covered in Chapter 12.

Questions are of two kinds: *open-ended and limited response.* Open-ended questions ask for information and specify the content in general terms; they cannot be answered by "yes" or "no." General information can be obtained and attitudes ascertained by open-ended questions. "How did this happen?" stimulates information. "How do you feel about this?" stimulates an expression of attitudes. Limited response questions, which can be answered by yes/no or by a response to the question "when," enable you to elicit very specific information. (Such a question would be "When do your gum tissues hurt?") The limited response questions can be used as followup to open-ended questions. More time is required and more information can be obtained by open-ended questions than by limited response questions. Helpers will find it necessary to use open-ended questions to get acquainted with patients.

There is a tendency among busy Americans to ask questions and pay very little attention to the answers. This is grist for the mills of humorists but not useful for helpers. As helpers we need to discipline ourselves to listen to the answers, not think about our response to the answer or our next question.

Active Listening

This kind of listening has been referred to as *active listening*. Thomas Gordon tells us that "active listening" enables us to listen for what the patient means, not merely what his or her words mean. We can utilize it to restate and clarify what we understand the patient to be saying. With this feedback patients have an opportunity to restate and clarify for us what they mean. Facilitating or coaxing out information and attitudes is also possible. Negative attitudes can be explored in a nonthreatening manner. Resistance by the patient, which may be for the purpose of concealing a problem, can be explored. Patients who are inclined to be too dependent upon you can be helped to become more independent.

REFLECTING: Various levels of responses to patients' statements or questions are possible for interviewers. The lowest level of response above nonresponse is *reflecting,* sometimes called parroting, or simply repeating the patients' words. This is of little help to patients beyond letting them know that the interviewer's hearing is not impaired.

> Negative attitudes can be explored in a nonthreatening manner.

SILENCE with its accompanying nonverbal and symbolic communication can be a higher level response than parroting. Silence can show interest or lack of interest, support, or withdrawal. Supportive or interested silence is useful to the dentist. A facilitative "uh huh," nodding affirmatively, or shifting forward more attentively indicates support or interest to the patient.

FEEDBACK by paraphrase or interpretation demonstrates to the patient your understanding of what he or she has just told you. If you did not understand the patient fully, your paraphrasing will show this. Then the patient can restate and you can, if necessary, repeat the feedback process and signify a clearer understanding.

SUMMATION is paraphrasing of a situation and enables the patient to know that you understand completely. If your summation indicates a less than total understanding, the patient has an opportunity to restate to you for refinement.

From Responding to Helping

The purpose of the higher level responses by the interviewer is to become helpful. The Carkhuff model as described by Avrom King in the *Nexus* newsletter, November 1975 to June 1976, is useful in making the transition to helpfulness, which is the ultimate in getting acquainted with your patient. In other words all of your knowledge about the patient is useless until you begin to help him or her.

Getting acquainted with the patient begins in the foundational mode of the Carkhuff model. This is the time for building rapport (affective relationship), which can grow into an effective relationship satisfying to both you and your patient. Out of an effective relationship come action and change.

The time required for going through these three modes may vary greatly among patients. They should be thought of as a continuum through which you progress in your relationship. Some patients

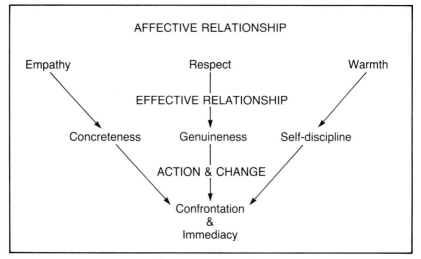

Figure 11–2. Helping.

are capable of moving through very quickly; others will have to go more slowly. The depth of relationship will also vary. Some patients will desire and are capable of deeper relationships than others. Dentists also vary as to their capability and desire for depth and completeness of relationship. Each patient is entitled to progress in the relationship according to his or her own needs, and within the capacity of the dentist.

EMPATHY, as described by Carl Rogers and many others, can be defined as your ability to feel what another person is feeling. An empathic response goes far beyond assuring the patient that you heard. The response is to the feeling, which requires listening with "the third ear." The third ear hears *beyond* the words, hears, that is, not merely what is said but also what is meant. What is *not* said may be as meaningful as what *is* said. Nonverbal communication modes, such as tone of voice, facial expression, posture, also need to be understood.

RESPECT is the positive acknowledgement of another individual's unique personhood. In more common language we speak of treating persons as individuals — not as patients (or worse yet, as cases). The helping dental team has learned that the variety of personalities they deal with makes dentistry more interesting. They don't feel that this variety causes frustration. Variety *is* the spice of life. There's more life and fun in the office where persons are enjoyed, not dreaded, for their individuality.

WARMTH is the ability of the helper to communicate to the patient that the helper cares about the patient's situation. In other words, warmth *communicates* concern.

Warmth cannot stand alone. Empathy and respect are also necessary. The well-liked receptionist who is a perfect hostess may possess warmth but without a sufficient measure of empathy and respect, she will not be able to develop a continuing helping relationship.

Nonverbal communication, such as touching, demonstrates

Nonverbal communication, such as touching, demonstrates warmth. But warmth is more than touching people.

warmth. But warmth is more than touching people. Most people perceive faked warmth. As a friend once said, *"Nobody* can be that *nice."*

CONCRETENESS is the expression of empathy to the total situation, not merely the words. Suppose as she was leaving Lucy Morgan had said to the receptionist, "I just went to the dentist last year, had my teeth thoroughly checked and paid eleven hundred dollars to have them fixed. Will this never end?" The empathic receptionist could touch her arm gently, maintain eye contact and say, "Mrs. Morgan, you must be very disappointed and frustrated, maybe even suspicious. Could you come back on Wednesday afternoon when Doctor Logan does office work and talk this out with him? I'm sure he wants to help you in any way he can."

GENUINENESS (personal authenticity) of the helper is desired by almost everyone seeking help, certainly dental patients. At this stage (intermediate mode in the model) you are beyond the exploration that occurs early in the form of questions and answers. You are digging a little deeper into the helping relationship you are developing with your patient — going from the Affective to the Effective.

> Being authentic, genuine, or real rules out playing games. The genuine helper is able to ask the patient about any problem in their relationship.

Being authentic, genuine, or real rules out playing games. The genuine helper is able to ask the patient about any problem in their relationship. When Lucy Morgan said to Jim Logan, "I'll just have to think it over," he could have pursued the problem directly by saying, "I can see you are taken aback. May I ask what is troubling you?" Had he done this, he might have gotten to the bottom of the problem and been able to really help her. It might not have resulted in her agreeing to his full plan of treatment. However, he might have been able to understand Lucy's problem better and proposed some limited action acceptable to her. This would have helped her and would have maintained their relationship so that he could continue to be helpful.

SELF-DISCLOSURE is the helper's sharing of personal experiences or feelings and assists the patient in accepting the helper's understanding of the problem. The ultimate in self-disclosure is the expression of ideas and feelings that are unique to the helper. Jim Logan's receptionist could have done this with Lucy Morgan. She could have said, "You know, I understand exactly how you feel. I was a patient here before I came to work with Dr. Logan. Just like you, I thought my teeth were pretty good, and when Dr. Logan told me what was wrong and what needed to be done, I could hardly believe it. Anyway, I talked with my husband, who had been a friend of Doctor Logan's since childhood. He convinced me that whatever Dr. Logan said was probably right. I went ahead with some extensive treatment and my mouth has never felt better." When we disclose ourselves, others tend to do likewise and our relationships deepen.

CONFRONTATION occurs when the helper assists the patient to see the discrepancy between what the patient says and what he or she does. IMMEDIACY is the sense of timing by which the helper does the confronting. This sense of timing takes into account what is happening at the moment. The hygienist who is doing deep scaling for the fastidiously dressed person may stop and say something like this, "I've always been impressed at how well you take care of your

> Helpers, to be most successful, must be able to assess the state of mind of the patient and the situation to determine when is an appropriate time for confrontation.

appearance and your general health, but I'm disappointed in the way you care for your mouth." The effectiveness of confrontation depends on how appropriate the timing is and on the quality of confrontation.

Finesse requires a well-developed intuitive sense. Helpers, to be most successful, must be able to assess the state of mind of the patient and the situation to determine an appropriate time for confrontation. Some minimal level of security is necessary for the patient to respond constructively. If the situation is threatening, such as in the midst of a difficult treatment appointment or immediately after distressing information has been presented, the patient should not be confronted. This is the case if the patient is distraught for reasons having nothing to do with the immediate situation. If you wait for the perfect time, it may never come. When you feel that you should confront and there are no apparent reasons why you should not, do so and assess the effectiveness of the response. Sensitivity to the patients' responses will enable you to improve your sense of timing.

How well you do depends on the quality of your confronting as well as on your timing. Quality of confrontation is dependent on all of the prior components — empathy, respect, warmth, concreteness, genuineness and self disclosure. In other words confrontation comes after expression of these components. If life is growth as we believe, you will continue to improve in all of these areas and become more adept at confrontation. Of course, it should be done in the assertive, not in the aggressive mode. Confrontation should come out of concern and this should be evident to the patient.

Confrontation and immediacy require the consummate skills of helping. It is in the practice of these skills that the art of helping is apparent. Some adequate helpers do not acquire these skills to the point where they are well integrated into the helping style. By helping style we mean the manner, the way, the behavior of the helper which is seen as natural. It need not be natural. In fact, with most helpers this technique is very much learned, but can be so well learned that it seems natural, much as a skilled equestrian rides a horse as if he were walking.

All of us who are trying to be better helpers can pick up wherever we are and progress toward our ultimate goal. The goal is ever elusive and we will never attain perfection. But not to try is to fail. To try and fail temporarily is a matter of progressive improvement, frequently (or maybe rarely) punctuated with temporary reversals. In other words, you will never become the perfect helper, but you can continue to improve and enjoy your accomplishments. You can become very well acquainted with your patients, and you will like it.

> Quality of confrontation is dependent on all of the prior components — empathy, respect, warmth, concreteness, genuineness, and self-disclosure.

REFERENCES

Anderson, J. L., et al.: Consumer's Dental Bible. Neenah, WI, Project P, 1974.
Avila, D. L., Combs, P.: The Helping Relationship Sourcebook. Boston, Allyn and Bacon Inc., 1971.
Benjamin, A.: The Helping Interview. Boston, Houghton Mifflin Co., 1974.
Brill, N.: Working with People. Philadelphia, J. B. Lippincott Co., 1978.
Carkhuff, R. R.: Helping and Human Relations. New York, Holt, Rinehart & Winston Inc., 1969.

Combs, A. W., et al.: Helping Relationships. Boston, Allyn and Bacon Inc., 1971.

Combs, A. W., et al.: The Professional Education of Teachers. Boston, Allyn and Bacon Inc., 1974.

Eriksen, K.: Communication Skills for Human Services. Reston, VA, Reston Publishing Co., 1979.

Froelich, R. E., et al: Communication in the Dental Office. St. Louis, MO, C. V. Mosby Co., 1976.

Giblin, L.: How to Have Confidence and Power in Dealing with People. Englewood Cliffs, NJ, Prentice Hall, Inc., 1952.

Gordon, T.: Teacher Effectiveness Training. New York, Peter H. Wyden/Publisher, 1974.

Hollander, L. N., Weckstein, M. S.: Modern Dental Practice. Philadelphia, PA, W. B. Saunders Co., 1967.

Keith-Lucas, A.: Giving and Taking Help. Chapel Hill, NC, University of North Carolina Press, 1972.

King, A. E.: Managing Tomorrow's Dental Practice Today. Cave Creek, AZ, The Nexus Group, 1978.

King, A. E.: Nexus. Cave Creek, AZ, Nexus Group, Inc., 1975–76.

Litwack, L., et al.: Health Counseling. New York, Appleton-Century-Crofts, 1980.

Martin, R. T.: Exploratory Investigation of the Dentist/Patient Relationship. Sydney, Dental Health Education and Research Foundation, University of Sydney, 1965.

Protell, M. R., et al.: Psychodynamics in dental practice. Springfield, IL, Charles C Thomas, 1975.

Rogers, C.: Client Centered Therapy. Boston, Houghton Mifflin Co., 1951.

12

The Examination

First impressions are important. This is so whether a person is on a date with someone new, choosing a car, shopping for a new house, or selecting a dentist. And whether you and your dental team are dealing with an adult or a child — or that out-of-the-blue emergency case — the patients will be deeply impressed, either for the better or for the worse, with what happens to them on their first visit to your office for an examination.*

The examination is not necessarily limited to the first visit; nor is the first visit limited to the examination. Robert Barkley recommended two visits for the examination. The first is for getting acquainted (discovering how the person feels about life, teeth, dentists, and so on) and for obtaining radiographs and study models. The second visit is for a thorough clinical examination by the dentist. Others have made the dental recommendations immediately following examination at the first visit, especially when dental treatment was very simple. The examination is the process of getting acquainted with the patient and of providing an opportunity for the patient to become acquainted with the dental team. It may occur in one or more appointments.

"Examination" can and probably should be done periodically on regular patients. It is an opportunity for patients to bring up any problems that may have been overlooked, although every visit should be such an opportunity. You can take a fresh look at your patient, as a person, and his or her dental conditions more thoroughly than you might on a regular maintenance visit (recall). The periodic interval would depend on the extent of disease and treatment, and also on the effectiveness of the patient's self-care.

BEFORE THE VISIT

As dentists we need to be able to see things from the patient's point of view. Based on perceptual psychology as described in Chapter 11, dentists need to develop the perspective of the patient in order to understand the patient's feelings.

---

*In this chapter the examination is described as a process which for the most part applies to the new patient. The process includes everything that occurs prior to the time when the dentist makes recommendations to the patient about his dental health.

Have you ever thought of role playing a patient? There is a natural reluctance to role play, but it is a mechanism for discovering problems of which dentists may otherwise be quite unaware. There's nothing like sitting down and reclining in the dental chair to see the dead insects trapped in the lamp shade. Likewise, you can get a feel for what it is like to come to your office as a new patient if you role play it yourself.

Call your office as though you were a patient living in a remote part of the community. Pay attention to how the receptionist learns who you are, where you live, and how you will come to the office. Go to that area, ride the bus, drive your car, walk or travel exactly as your patient plans to come to the office, and note the difficulties. If you ride the bus, notice how long it takes to get from the bus stop to the office. Also, if it is appropriate, ask someone (whom you think should know) for directions. Of course, if you're well known in the community, you may not be able to maintain your anonymity. If that is true, you could have a friend ask directions just to learn whether people in your community can direct others to your office. If you discover that persons who should know are unable to direct people to your office, you have an opportunity to correct that.

> You can get a feel for what it's like to come to your office as a new patient if you role play it yourself.

When you arrive at the address, check to see how difficult it is to find your office, if it is part of a complex. You may need more helpful signs and directions at the street entrance. If you drive, check for the difficulty of turning from the street into the parking lot. How crowded is the parking lot? Is it well marked? Well maintained? Does it project the image you would like?

As you enter the office, take a hard look at the entrance. Is it attractive? Does the entry way appear to be in keeping with the kind of dental office you would be comfortable in? Would your patients agree with you? How are you feeling so far about your experience? Is this dental office a good choice?

Now for the entry into the reception room. I hope you haven't seen any signs saying "waiting room." Would *you* want to wait? What happens when you enter? Are you alone? Do you hear any noise in the back? (You will have alerted your assistant to the experiment and will have asked her to run the handpiece as you arrive.) Is there a sign saying "Please ring bell and be seated." Or does the receptionist acknowledge your presence? Does she step into the reception room, introduce herself, and shake hands? Do you feel adequately welcomed to the office?

The reception room connects your office to the outside world. It should open to the outdoors by a window if possible and to the inside — possibly by an open door or inside window. Symbolic communication is subtle and powerful. If your reception room says to patients, "Yes you can look back to where you came from and also into the interior of the office," they are likely to feel reassured. They can maintain their outside world connection and are also able to "see" into the world that is your dental office. Openness engenders trust. Patients coming to your office for the first time should experience a supportive environment, right from the moment they enter your reception room.

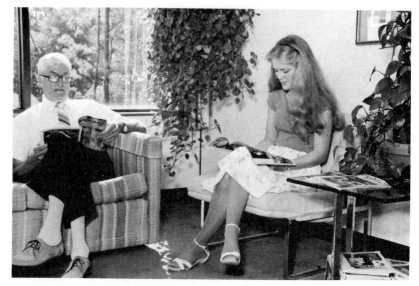

A comfortable, tastefully decorated reception area with contact, via large pane-glass windows, with the world outside the office.

Why not evaluate your reception room as a supportive environment by the following series of questions:

1. Is there a place for patients to hang coats and put packages?

2. Is everything clean — doors, windows, carpet, lights, ceilings, ashtrays?

3. Is lighting adequate for reading?

4. Are magazines current and interesting to patients (and in good condition)?

Patients coming to your office for the first time should experience a supportive environment, right from the moment they enter your reception room.

5. If you treat children, is there a children's corner? Children enjoy it; adults appreciate it.

6. Are there enough individual chairs — arranged so that patients don't have to stare at one another?

7. Is the room properly ventilated — no dental office odors? Not too hot or too cold?

8. Is the style of furnishings and decor suitable for your patients? Is it too plush or too plain?

9. Are there some individual touches — plants, paintings?

10. Does the room seem to connect with the rest of the office?

11. Are there any unpleasant sounds?

12. Is the atmosphere relaxed and home-like?

You can choose to modify the role playing to better fit your individual circumstances. It may be better to have someone else play certain parts of it. You can make it more real for your staff by asking a friend whom your staff does not know to do it. The point is that you can learn a lot about patients' problems in this way and become truly empathetic toward them.

THE PATIENT VISIT

Opinions vary on the ideal procedure for handling the patient's first visit. The purpose of the whole procedure, though, is to center on the patient's needs and to respond to them in a manner that the patient will find helpful.

You may need to modify the suggestions that follow to fit your situation. It may be necessary to do so because of physical facilities and personalities of the dental team. If you modify significantly, ask yourself whether by doing so you are still centering on the patient. Sometimes physical facilities can be altered slightly or merely utilized differently in order to accommodate the patient. For example, if you have been sitting behind your desk to interview patients, you can easily rearrange the furniture to provide a conversation corner.

It takes commitment from all team members to put the patient first. Habits that center on selves rather than on patients may have developed. The dental team ought to take a serious look at itself if it seems necessary to depart from the suggested procedure. It may be helpful to view each patient as though he is the only patient in the practice. If the success of the practice is dependent on only one patient, team members will find it easy to commit themselves to understanding and satisfying that patient's needs.

Greeting the Patient

If Lucy Morgan had been Jim Logan's only patient, in Chapter 11, the receptionist would certainly have had time to step out to the reception room and greet her. We will follow Jim Logan's new patient, Nancy Barron. Jim has decided to take marketing seriously and treat every patient as though he or she were his only patient. Does your receptionist have time to greet your patients in a similar manner? If not, you will have to decide whether time should be made for this. It might require hiring an additional person, or reallocating tasks to free the receptionist for this, or merely convincing the receptionist that this must be done. You may decide not to do this. Your office may be so busy that you don't need to treat each patient as if she or he were the only one in your practice. But if about 20 percent of your patients are moving out of your community each year, the demand for your services will decrease if you do not market to each individual patient.

The marketing mode, as opposed to the production mode, requires that Nancy Barron be greeted immediately when she enters the reception room. The receptionist needs to step into the room, shake hands with her, greet her by name, pass the time of day with her, and inform her as to what she may expect. Close attention to body language will tell the receptionist a lot about the patient. Is Nancy Barron shy, outgoing, nervous, self-confident? This makes a difference in the dental team's approach. The receptionist might ask Nancy if she had any difficulty in getting to the office. Was the bus schedule convenient? Had instructions by telephone been sufficient? Were there any traffic problems? She can thank Nancy Barron for the information and remark that she tries to keep current with such problems so that she can *help* patients. Early on the receptionist plants the idea that *this* dental team is *patient centered* and tries to help people in every way possible.

Nancy Barron can be put at ease by a brief explanation of what to expect. Just as if she were a guest in one's home she might find the

It takes commitment from all team members to put the patient first.

receptionist helping her remove her coat and hanging it on the rack. If anyone has accompanied her, that person, child or adult, should be acknowledged and invited to sit down. If it is a child, the receptionist could show him or her to the children's corner and explain about the puzzles, books, and so on. Attention should be redirected to Nancy Barron. If it is necessary for her to wait in the reception room (and it will not be if she is the "only patient"), she should be asked to do so and an explanation provided of why it is necessary. At any rate, she should be put at ease and not left wondering what she will do next.

She will *not* now be presented with a questionnaire on a clipboard and asked to fill it out. Gathering of information will be done in a more personal and timely manner. Dale Carnegie reported that when he was asked to fill out the clipboard questionnaire, he felt that the physician was more interested in his money than in his health. Marketing speaks first to the needs of the patient. Anything that *seems* to contradict this need should not be done.

Interviewing

The purpose of the interview is to share information. As was pointed out in Chapter 11, the patient has a good deal of information that you need and of course you have information to give the patient. In terms of the Johari Window, what we're trying to do is pull information from window 3 (what the patient knows) into window 1 (what both know). The purpose is to pool knowledge.

Problems of Patient Education

Perhaps dentists have overdone the provision of information *to* patients and need to concentrate on obtaining information *from* patients.

Patient education has been important to dentists for a long time. It still is. But it needs another look. Traditional patient education by films and booklets has been very much a one-way process. It has been an attempt to enlarge shared knowledge by telling the patient what the dentist knows. In many instances it has not worked very well. This is because most patients do not want to be educated, at least not in a patronizing manner. Most of them prefer being listened to, not talked to.

Although patient education is important, so also is the education of the dental team regarding patients' problems. Perhaps dentists have overdone the provision of information *to* patients and need to concentrate on obtaining information *from* patients. This is the primary purpose of interviewing. You will need to substitute for "patient education" a process of "information sharing" about patients' dental problems.

The Interviewer

Who should do the interviewing? Some people are saying that in a busy office it should not be the dentist. Since the busy dentist's time

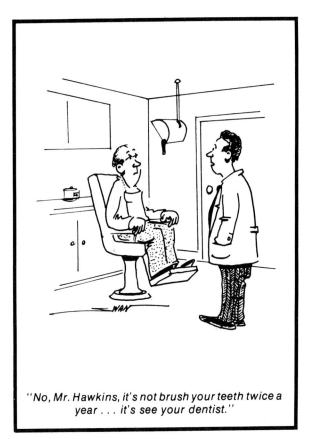

"No, Mr. Hawkins, it's not brush your teeth twice a year . . . it's see your dentist."

Courtesy of *Cal* magazine.

is so valuable, interviewing by the dentist is costly to the practice. Many dentists maintain that even though it is costly, it is so valuable that they choose to do it.

The high value of the interview is implicit in marketing. How else can you understand the patient's needs? Good interviews will make a tremendous difference in the success of the practice.

It may make little difference who does the interview. What does make a big difference is the skill of the interviewer, as described in Chapter 11. If you possess interviewing skills and want to do it, you should probably do it yourself. However, you may decide that it is too costly for you to do. Certainly if an auxiliary has the skills and the interest, delegating the task makes good sense. If you can think of the patient relationship as being with the dental team rather than with the dentist, the most skilled team member should do it.

A variety of persons other than the dentist do interviewing in dental offices. The "communicator," as described by Francis Edwards for orthodontists, will be a female about 35 to 40 who relates easily and communicates well with people. He maintains that this kind of person can more easily establish a trusting relationship with people than can most dentists and that in fact it is not necessary for the dentist to become central in communication with patients. Robert Barkley began to utilize a psychiatric nurse for interviewing several years ago. Many dentists, especially very busy ones, employ a "patient care coordinator" who does the initial interviewing, maintains continual communication with the patients each time they come for treatment, and does followup afterwards, if appropriate. Clearly, it is not essential that the dentist do the interviewing. But it is essential that the interviewer possess the required skill. From now on we will refer to you, the dentist, as the interviewer, recognizing that it may be another team member.

The Place for the Interview

The interview location should be private, nonthreatening, and relaxing. Neither the reception room, nor the business office, nor the treatment room (operatory) qualifies. Some physical rearrangement of the office may be necessary to improve the room for the interview. Such a room can be referred to as the consultation room, the patient lounge, or even the conversation corner.

Social distance of four to seven feet is the distance at which people can most easily get acquainted.

How should this room be arranged? Anthropologists such as Edward Hall use the term proxemics to describe people's interrelationships in space. Social distance of four to seven feet is the distance at which people can most easily get acquainted. Space can be arranged so as to keep people apart or bring them together. *Sociofugal* space, such as waiting rooms in railroad stations, keep people apart, but *sociopetal* space, such as the tables in a French sidewalk cafe, bring people together. In a hospital cafeteria observers have noted that more conversation occurs between two people sitting adjacent to the same corner of the table than in any other position. Although these observations cannot be generalized to all settings, it would appear that

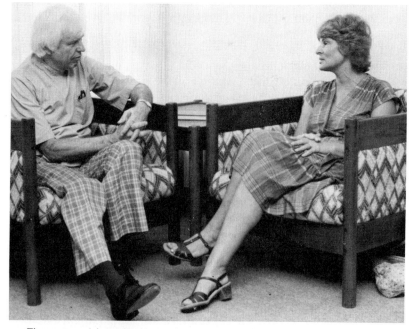

The personal interview is an important marketing and clinical technique. A special "conversation corner" facilitates the process.

we could best become acquainted with our patients if we arrange ourselves at some angle not directly face to face and that we place a small low table between us. Chairs should be identical, such as captain's chairs or office side-arm chairs. Many observers have noted that a large desk between the doctor and the patient constitutes a barrier. In any case, you should arrange your furniture so that interviewer and interviewee are both at ease and as comfortable as possible.

Decor should be cheerful and relaxing. If the room is to be used only for interviewing, relaxing warm colors, such as dull reds, oranges, and yellows, are appropriate. However, if it is also to be used for consultation, where commitment to a dental program is being sought, brighter intensity of the same warm colors will be better. The psychology of color is subtle but powerful. Consultation with an interior designer who is skilled in the communication of color will help.

The interview room should symbolically communicate to patients that here they can relax and that here you are giving them your full attention.

It is essential that the room be orderly. Alfred Benjamin tells us that people tend to feel that they are intruding if the room is cluttered. The low table should have nothing more on it than a lamp, so that if you and your patient are drinking coffee or tea together, you can set cups on the table. No distractions should be allowed. You need the patient's full attention — no dental office odors or noise; ventilation and soundproofing are important. The room should symbolically communicate to patients that here they can relax and that here you are giving them your full attention.

If Nancy Barron had been Jim Logan's only patient, the receptionist would have introduced her to him in the consultation room, or perhaps in the business office, and he would have escorted her to the consultation room. There should be a smooth transition from one team member to another with an introduction to the new team member. Nancy Barron needs to be so courteously treated that she feels as though she were the only patient.

The first few seconds (or at least first few minutes) that Jim Logan spends with Nancy Barron are crucial. He will never get a second chance to make a first impression. At the same time, if he is overly concerned about his first impression, he may make a poor one. If, however, he is simply and genuinely glad to be there to meet Nancy Barron, he is on his way toward success. If he can then devote himself to being as helpful to her as he can, he is very likely to succeed and enroll her as a long-term, regular patient. She will be gratified by his sincere interest in her as an individual.

Initiating the Interview

After Jim Logan has met Nancy Barron, it is his task to guide the conversation so that without interruption or abrupt shifts, it flows into the interview. The initiation ought to be more formal than casual conversation but less formal than the interview itself. Just as the receptionist attempted to be immediately helpful, Jim Logan should do the same. If he knows that the receptionist has asked whether she had any difficulty finding the office, he may choose another opener, such as, does she know anyone else who comes to him for dental treatment? Gradually, he can begin to focus questions on her.

In production-oriented offices the dentist at this point most likely has a questionnaire filled out by the patient. Jim Logan has tried this and it has not worked, so he is committed to a different approach — marketing to each individual patient. He is starting over with Nancy Barron. Each is beginning to learn from and about the other. Having listened to a lecture by Dr. Lloyd Hollander, he decides to try the open-ended no-questionnaire interviewing approach, which is supposed to build trust and confidence. He is now convinced that he has been trying to get the patient to know and to accept him rather than vice versa. He now sees that he needs to ask the patient more questions and pay more attention to the answers.

After inquiring about whether she knew any of his patients, Dr. Logan asks Nancy Barron to tell him about her dental experience. He listens intently to her description of her early years, how she had a lot of decay and had even lost a tooth. He asks if the dentist suggested root canal treatment and she says "no." She goes on to add that had she known there was a way to save the tooth, she would have wanted to do that. They also talk about her family's dental history. Her father still has most of his teeth, she thinks, but her mother has an upper full denture and lower partial. Her mother seems pretty satisfied, but cannot eat steak very well.

Jim Logan and Nancy Barron are conversing in his consultation room, which he has rearranged to put him and his patients on a par. As Doctor Hollander suggested, Jim Logan has not used a questionnaire or even taken any notes. He had misgivings about interviewing without a guide or without taking notes, but he decided to risk it. The outcome was much more satisfactory than he had hoped for. Actually he discovered that he did not need structured questions. Nancy was able to describe her problems in response to general questions. At times he followed the general question with more specific ones to complete the picture. It had been easier than he thought. He is amazed at how much he learned in such a short time. After finishing the interview, he completed the personal data sheet (Fig. 12–1) while Nancy Barron was being seated for the dental examination.

He has learned of Nancy's rather unfavorable dental experience — almost rampant caries as a teenager, loss of a lower molar at age 16, bleeding gums that were worst when she was pregnant with her 3-month-old son, and currently, a sensitivity to sweets on the right side, where there seems to be a loose filling. She has also told him that she is very intent on keeping her teeth and eliminating dental disease if possible. She had almost given up because of discomfort with her teeth and because dental treatment had always been so difficult for her. A friend had told her of having dentistry done by Dr. Logan with nitrous oxide and how pleasant that could be.

Upon further inquiry he learned that as a teenager Nancy had greatly feared injections. In college she had taken some psychology courses and had begun to sense that her fear was more deep-seated than she had realized. Jim Logan agrees with that possibility and assures her that he will do everything he can to make her treatment tolerable — including administration of nitrous oxide. Nancy says

PERSONAL DATA

	Phonetic spelling	To be called	Date
Name			
Concerns:			
Family history:			
Health:			
Health Practices:			
Feelings about teeth:			
Expectations about teeth:			
Pet peeves in dental office:			
Special treatment desired:			
Other:			

Figure 12–1.   Form for noting personal patient information.

that she is sure her dentist had a lot of difficulty doing good work for her because she was "such a terrible patient." And maybe that was the reason he had sent her to the oral surgeon for the extraction.

Financing her dental care will also be a problem. She says that paying for complete dental treatment will disrupt her family's budget unless it could be spread over a rather long period of time. Complete treatment is what she wants, but she believes that it will be necessary to plan it in phases so that they can manage it. If her husband's company or her's should contract for dental insurance, the schedule for treatment can be accelerated, she adds.

Jim Logan has shared some of his feelings about health and dental care and how he as a dentist believes that he can help people. Nancy agrees with his belief that teeth should not be removed if they can be saved. Although she doesn't quite understand how yet, she is delighted to learn that she can control her own dental disease. In fact that she can almost maintain her own health by preventive practices. She appreciates his interest in general health, not just dental health. She doesn't quite understand what he is talking about by "helping." He wonders if rather than having talked about that, he should just have gone ahead and done the "helping." Actions do speak louder than words, he muses.

At this point there seems to be almost perfect congruence in values. Nancy readily accepts Jim's ideas on what the goals for dental treatment should be. Jim has been able to share what he knows and believes very easily without using any films or booklets. However, he may give her some booklets later to be sure that she has complete and accurate written information about specific problems.

Most important of all he has learned about Nancy's experience and attitudes in a way he never dreamed was possible. He is reminded again that "routine" dental treatment is not routine for persons like Nancy Barron. He realizes that there are very good reasons for what might appear to be neglect of teeth. He remembers that in the past he has looked on such individuals as having a low dental IQ and little interest in their dental health. Interviewing Nancy has been a learning experience. Instead of the usual dread of examining new patients, he feels eager to proceed with the dental examination and, later, to talk with her about her dental problems. He feels like a helper.

As Jim Logan has dispensed with any sort of rigid order for his questions, we suggest that you do the same. However, there *are* a number of questions that can elicit information you need. Such questions include the following:

Remember: General questions will require specific followup.

1. Tell me about your experience with your teeth.
2. What about your parents' teeth?
3. What about your experience in dental offices?
4. Why have you gone to the dentist before?
5. Why have you gone to physicians before?
6. What do you do to keep yourself healthy?
7. What do you do to control dental disease?
8. What are your expectations for keeping your teeth?
9. Can you tell me what you like about your teeth? What you don't like? What you would change if you could?
10. How do you feel about your teeth?
11. Is there anything that bothers you about going to the dentist?
12. Are there any special ways you like to be treated in the dental office?

We are not suggesting that you ask all of these questions. Try to think of others. Remember, too: general questions will require specific followup.

The Dental Examination

Rather than describing the clinical dental examination in detail — which is beyond our scope here — let us demonstrate how the interview process continues through the clinical examination in order to heighten patients' awareness of their problems. Most of the attention up to this point has been directed toward learning about the patient's experiences, feelings, and attitudes and having the dentist briefly share his most important dental-related values with the patient. Now we will expand upon the concept of how the dentist learns from the patient — this time from the patient's mouth.

Another transition is occurring for Nancy Barron. When she went from the reception room to the consultation room, she was introduced to Jim Logan. Now when she goes to the treatment room, she meets Jim Logan's chairside assistant. Introduction and identification of team members are reassuring to Nancy Barron. She has noticed that each is wearing a small nameplate with his or her job title, even Doctor Logan. Also she has noted that everyone has been introduced. Rhonda James, the receptionist, seemed very warm and outgoing. Anita Cannon, the chairside assistant, seems pleasant enough, too, if a bit clinical and shy.

Anita accompanies her to the treatment room and asks if she sees anything unfamiliar. Nancy remarks that she doesn't see a cuspidor like her last dentist had. Anita shows her the vacuum system which accomplishes the same purpose. As Nancy sits down in the dental chair, Anita takes her purse and glasses and places them on a small shelf. Anita explains the reasons for the reclined position and reclines her in the chair, which Nancy notices is very comfortable. Although she is reclined farther than she ever was by her previous dentist, she feels at ease, perhaps because she seems to be among friends. At first she thought it strange for everyone to shake hands with her, but, on reflection, she likes it. Everyone seems genuine. She expects to learn more about her dental problems and to embark on a plan to restore her dental health. Having discarded the dread with which she came to the office, she now feels expectant and hopeful.

After washing his hands, Jim Logan sits down on the operating stool and begins the examination. As he had explained that he would, he palpates the neck and lips. Nancy appreciated his explanation of what he was doing and why. Otherwise she would not have been sure that a dentist should do that. His first attention in the mouth is directed to the right side, where he detects a loose amalgam in the lower right molar next to the missing tooth. He told Nancy that he would place a treatment filling in the tooth. After doing that he proceeds in orderly fashion to examine the soft tissue and the teeth. During the examination he asks her several questions.

These questions are carefully designed to make her aware of problems. After he finishes placing the treatment filling he asks her if she is aware that the molar has leaned forward into the space. Also: Has she noticed that the upper molar has overerupted into the lower space? Other questions during the examination include the following:

Questions may be asked to heighten patients' awareness.

1. Has she noticed food packing between the two molars on the lower right?
2. When do her gums bleed?
3. Is she aware of any clenching of her teeth?

They discuss each of these points briefly. Jim assures her that the problems are all manageable. He says he will make specific recommendations next time.

You can think of a number of other questions that might be asked in order to heighten patients' awareness of their problems. Some further examples are the following:

1. Has your spouse noticed you grinding your teeth at night?
2. Has your spouse noticed any mouth odor?
3. Had you noticed this space between your front teeth?
4. Do you have a problem of biting your cheek?
5. Has anyone ever done a mouth odor test for you? Do you mind if I do one?
6. Have you noticed this sore on your tongue?
7. Have you noticed how your teeth are wearing away?

8. Have you noticed the discoloration of these fillings in your front teeth?

9. Have you noticed how your gums are receding?

10. Can you chew equally well on both sides?

11. Are you satisfied with the appearance of your teeth? of your face?

The questions should call attention to potential problems, for which, later on, you will propose solutions.

After Jim Logan has completed the examination, Anita asks him a number of questions from the dental record. These are designed to record general conditions and call Nancy's attention to these conditions in a summary fashion. They are the following:

1. Condition of cervical lymph nodes?
2. Condition of intraoral soft tissue?
3. Condition of saliva?
4. General condition of supporting tissues?
5. General condition of teeth?
6. General condition of dental restorations?
7. Is occlusion satisfactory?
8. Are there missing teeth?
9. Is there abrasion of the teeth?
10. Is there erosion of the teeth?
11. Any other significant findings?

The examination over, Jim Logan begins to conclude with Nancy. He asks if she has any more questions. She replies that all her questions, and many others that she would never have thought to ask, have been answered. He explains that at the next visit he will share with her his findings, including those based on the radiographs and the study models that Anita will obtain next. Nancy thanks him and he leaves the room to meet his next patient.

Written History

After the radiographs have been exposed and impressions taken for study models, Anita escorts Nancy to the business office.

In his lecture Dr. Hollander had said that dentists should not ask patients to fill out forms in the reception room before they even meet the dentist. Rather this should be done after trust and confidence are established in personal interaction. The impersonal questionnaire may create lack of trust in the patient's mind because the patient feels that the dentist does not trust him. Why would the dentist ask social security number, place of employment, credit references, and so on if he really trusted the patient? As Dale Carnegie says, such a routine evidences interest in the pocketbook, not in the patient's well-being.

Certainly the demographic information and health history are very important. Some dentists prefer that the patient take the forms home, complete them there, and return them in a prestamped addressed envelope. Jim Logan has decided to ask patients to complete the health questionnaire in the office unless they don't have time then. In that case, Rhonda gives them the forms and the envelope and asks them to mail or return them by the next day. The

The impersonal questionnaire may create lack of trust in the patient's mind.

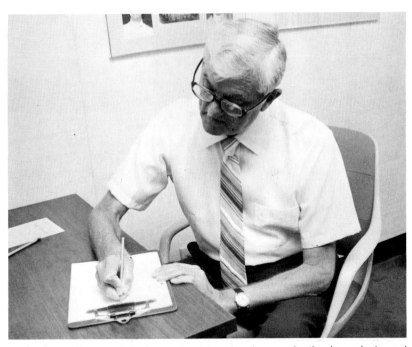

Patient filling out a health questionnaire after the examination in a private spot away from the reception area.

patient may forget about the forms once at home, and for that reason it is preferable that the patient complete the forms in the office.

Nancy Barron assures Rhonda that she has the time (Rhonda had told her to expect to be in the office about an hour and a half). She wondered why it would take so long, but the time has gone rapidly. Of course, Dr. Logan (or Jim, as his name tag says) spent about half of this time with her. Now she realizes what Jim meant by "the dental team."

Rhonda directs Nancy to a small office near hers where she fills out the health questionnaire (see Fig. 12–2). Although she had thought Dr. Logan had obtained all the information from her which he could possibly need, she discovers that a great deal more is asked for. She is even more impressed with the thoroughness with which Dr. Logan's team has gone about assessing her dental and general health. She appreciates the questionnaire, too. Jim Logan had asked for general though important information. The form is more specific and asks questions that Nancy would have found embarrassing had he asked them in person. She feels more confident in her selection of him as her dentist.

After she completes the form she returns to the business office. Rhonda asks her if she has any further questions. Does she know what to expect next time? She assures Rhonda that she has been very pleased with the visit and that she wants to go ahead with her treatment. She expresses again her concern about paying for it, but says that she is convinced that Doctor Logan is very fair and she hopes they can work something out. Rhonda assures her that Doctor Logan is indeed fair and will propose treatment that will be affordable.

PATIENT MEDICAL-DENTAL HISTORY

Date _____

Name _____   Residence _____

Last   First   M. In.   Date of Birth _____

PATIENT MEDICAL HISTORY   Home Phone _____

Physician _____ Office Phone _____

Approximate date of last physical examination _____

	Yes	No
1. Are you under any medical treatment now?	☐	☐
2. Have you had any major operations? If so what?	☐	☐
3. Have you ever had a serious accident involving head injuries?	☐	☐
4. Have you had any adverse response to any drugs including penicillin?	☐	☐
5. Has a physician ever informed you that you had: A Heart Ailment?	☐	☐
6. High blood pressure?	☐	☐
7. Respiratory disease?	☐	☐
8. Diabetes?	☐	☐
9. Rheumatic fever?	☐	☐
10. Rheumatism or arthritis?	☐	☐
11. Tumors or growths?	☐	☐
12. Any blood disease?	☐	☐
13. Any liver disease?	☐	☐
14. Any kidney disease?	☐	☐
15. Any stomach or intestinal disease?	☐	☐
16. Any venereal disease?	☐	☐
17. Yellow jaundice or hepatitis?	☐	☐
18. Do you have night sweats accompanied by weight loss or cough?	☐	☐
19. Are you on a diet at this time?	☐	☐
20. Are you now taking drugs or medications?	☐	☐
21. Are you allergic to any known materials resulting—in hives, asthma, eczema, etc.?	☐	☐
22. Are you in general good health at this time?	☐	☐
23. Have any wounds healed slowly or presented other complications?	☐	☐
24. Are you pregnant?	☐	☐
25. Do you have a history of fainting?	☐	☐
26. Have you ever had any X-RAY TREATMENTS (other than diagnostic)?	☐	☐

PATIENT DENTAL HISTORY

	Yes	No
27. Do you have pain in or near your ears?	☐	☐
28. Do you have any unhealed injuries or inflamed areas in or around your mouth?	☐	☐
29. Have you experienced any growth or sore spots in your mouth?	☐	☐
30. Does any part of your mouth hurt when clenched?	☐	☐
31. Have you ever had Novocaine anesthetic?	☐	☐
32. Any reactions or allergic symptoms to novocaine?	☐	☐
33. Any difficult extractions in the past?	☐	☐
34. Prolonged bleeding following extractions in the past?	☐	☐
35. Trench Mouth?	☐	☐
36. Do your gums bleed?	☐	☐
37. Have you ever had instruction on the correct method of brushing your teeth?	☐	☐
38. Have you ever had instructions on the care of your gums?	☐	☐
39. Do you chew on only one side of your mouth? If so why?	☐	☐
40. Do you at the present time have any dental complaints?	☐	☐
41. Do you habitually clench your teeth during the night or day?	☐	☐
42. When was your last full mouth X-RAY taken? _____ Where?		
43. Any part of your mouth sore to pressures or irritants (cold, sweets, etc.)	☐	☐
If so locate		

Signature _____

FORM 9879 COLWELL CO., CHAMPAIGN, ILL.

Figure 12–2. Health questionnaire. (Courtesy of Colwell Systems.)

Nancy has been worried about whether she has sufficient money to pay for the examination. She has not inquired about the cost, and no one has told her. Jim Logan had decided that he would try not quoting his examination fee unless the patient asked. Some of his friends always quoted the fee before doing the examination but he felt that that was distracting. He believed that trust was necessary and that if it was present, the examination fee would be no problem. Nancy Barron would have agreed with him. Happily, she has sufficient money for the fee, which Jim Logan purposely kept low. He believed that if he tried to make his hourly goal through examinations, the initial fee would be a barrier to many people who would otherwise accept his services gratefully.

After Nancy has made her next appointment and as she is leaving, Jim Logan happens to stop by the desk to tell her goodbye. They both feel that the entire transaction has been very successful and both look forward to the next visit.

THE EMERGENCY PATIENT

The patient in distress has a somewhat different experience in the dental office than the routine patient. The patient who calls in pain should be asked to come in as soon as possible. In marketing terms, a need is evident and an immediate response is in order. If you are not able to work the patient into your schedule immediately, you should see the patient as soon as you can, certainly the same day. It is important that patients sense that your dental team is going to help them as soon as possible.

When the patient enters the reception room, the receptionist should step out and greet him as she does the patient for routine examination. The emergency patient should also be treated as though he were the only patient in your practice. Indeed, many emergency patients do seek routine care from dentists who are helpful. They may be very ready for regular care, but not unless the dental team shows genuine concern for them and their problems.

It is important that patients in distress sense that your dental team is going to help them as soon as possible.

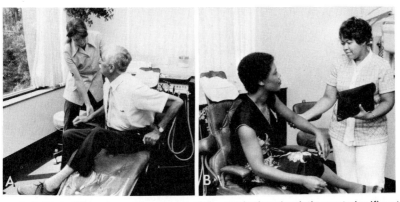

A, B. Two different versions of one of the marketing dentist's most significant moments — helping the patient from the operatory chair. If the dentist is not free to do this, the assistant, at least, should.

Jim Logan's team will treat Earl Pearson, an emergency patient with a severe toothache, and Nancy Barron differently. Rhonda James seats Earl in the emergency dental chair immediately. She informs Jim Logan that Earl has been seated and has a toothache. As soon as Jim inserts the impression material for a crown on his current patient, he asks Anita to hold the tray as he steps into the emergency treatment room. Rhonda introduces him to Earl Pearson.

His purpose now is to quickly learn enough about Earl and his dental problem to get him out of pain. Although Rhonda has informed him that Earl has a toothache, he asks him how he can help him. Earl, who appears to be about 25, tells him that his upper front tooth is hurting. The upper right central is very sensitive to pressure. Jim asks questions such as: (1) what happened? (2) when did it happen? (3) when did it begin to hurt? (4) how would he describe the pain? The questions all relate to the immediate problem. This is not the time to heighten Earl's awareness of his other dental problems. Earl's need for relief of pain is paramount. Jim assures Earl that within just a few minutes he will relieve the pain, but that he now must go back to his other patient and remove the impression. He asks Earl to complete the brief history form (Fig. 12–3, front).

Keep in mind that every emergency patient is potentially a comprehensive care patient.

Jim Logan returns in a few minutes and Earl has completed the brief history form. Upon ascertaining from the history that Earl has no health problems that would interfere with treatment, Jim does vitality tests on the upper incisors. All teeth test normal except the upper right central, which is tender to percussion. Jim tells Earl that the tooth is not vital, probably because of the injury, and appears to be infected. He suggests opening the tooth and assures Earl that it can be done with little or no discomfort even without local anesthesia. Earl agrees to the procedure, which Jim accomplishes easily and quickly with no discomfort to Earl. Jim excuses himself again to check on the temporary, which Anita has been placing for the patient with the crown preparation.

About ten minutes later he returns and finds Earl smiling. The pain, Earl says, has miraculously disappeared. Earl asks if the tooth needs any further treatment. Jim replies that the treatment for this condition is to clean and fill the root canal. Upon being reassured that it would not be painful, Earl agrees to return for the first phase of that treatment. He also inquires as to whether he has any other problems. When Jim suggests that they should go ahead with a complete examination to assess the total dental problem, Earl agrees and remarks that he has dental insurance. Jim assures him that his dental insurance will pay part of the fee, and before they proceed, he will send his recommendations to the insurance company, and the company will inform him as to what they will pay.

Earl agrees to return as soon as an appointment can be arranged for the examination. Now that he has no pain, he feels he is in good hands. He really had not been aware of any dental problems and had had no intention of requesting a dental appointment, even though he knew from friends that the dental insurance would pay much of the fee. Jim Logan has eliminated the pain so expeditiously and effectively, however, that Earl is convinced that he should go ahead and have Jim take care of whatever other dental problems he may have.

PATIENT INFORMATION FORM

PLEASE PRINT

PATIENT

Last Name _____ First _____ Middle _____ Home Phone _____

Address _____ City _____ State _____ Zip _____

How long at this address? _____ Date of Birth: Month _____ Day _____ Year _____

( ) Minor   ( ) Single   ( ) Married   ( ) Widowed   ( ) Divorced   ( ) Separated

PERSON RESPONSIBLE FOR ACCOUNT _____ Soc. Sec. # _____

Address _____ City _____ State _____ Zip _____

Employer _____ How long employed? _____ Business Phone _____

Position _____

Employer address _____ City _____ State _____ Zip _____

SPOUSE OF PERSON RESPONSIBLE FOR ACCOUNT

Name _____ Employer _____

DENTAL INSURANCE

Company Name _____ Local Union No. _____

Whom may we thank for referring you to our office? _____
Has any member of your family ever been treated in our office? (Circle one)   Yes   No

DENTAL HISTORY

Have you been having any specific problems? _____
Last dental visit? _____ Purpose _____ Last Complete Exam _____
Has fear of discomfort kept you from regular visits? _____
How would you describe your present dental health?   GOOD   FAIR   POOR
Do you think you have active dental disease? Decay _____ Gum disease _____
Home Care: Brush _____ Floss _____ Water Jet _____ Other _____
Do your gums ever bleed? _____ Are you troubled with bad breath? _____
How do you feel about ever losing your teeth? _____
Have you had any unusual effects from previous dental treatments? Describe _____

MEDICAL HISTORY: Medical Doctor's Name _____
Date of last physical exam _____ . Women: Are you pregnant? _____ How long? _____
Are you under a doctor's care now? _____ If so, for what reason? _____
Are you taking any medications, pills or drugs? _____ If so, please list _____
Have you ever had any of the following? (please circle):

		Heart Trouble	Arthritis
Heart Murmur	Rheumatic Fever	High Blood Pressure	Asthma
Tuberculosis	Hepatitis	Jaundice	Diabetes
Epilepsy	Prolonged Bleeding	Stroke	Psychiatric Treatment
			By Whom _____

Have you had any other serious illness? _____ What? _____
Have you been hospitalized in the last two years? _____ Why? _____
Do you prefer nitrous oxide sedation (tranquilizing air) during treatment? _____

Date _____ Signature _____

Blood Pressure _____ Pulse Rate _____
Notes: _____

PR 104

Front

Figure 12-3. Patient information form. *Front*, Brief history form. *Back*, Clinical record. (Courtesy of Dr. Mel Tekavec.)

Illustration continued on following page

DATE _____

CLINICAL

_____ X-rays _____ PA's   BW's   Panorex   FMPA

_____ Note any external facial anomalies, swelling, etc. _____

Condition of TMJ

     Present or past pain, clicking, popping? _____

     Any premature interferences? _____

     Any skid or deviation? _____

     Any lateral interference? _____

_____ Cancer Check: Lips _____ Cheeks _____ Palate _____

                     Tongue _____ Floor of Mouth _____ Pharynx_____

Periodontal Tissues

Color:	Normal	ANUG	Marginal Infl.	Chronic Infl.
Contour:	Normal	Swollen Pap.	Blunted Pap.	Hyperplastic
Consistency:	Normal	Edematous	Fibrous	Exudate
Recession:	None	Begin.	Moderate	Advanced	Loc.	Gen.
Bleeding:	None	Light	Moderate	Heavy	Loc.	Gen.
Bact. Plaque:	None	Light	Moderate	Heavy	Loc.	Gen.
Calculus Form.	None	Light	Moderate	Heavy	Loc.	Gen.
Stains	None	Light	Moderate	Heavy	Loc.	Gen.

Muscle Pull_____ Attached gingivae _____

Pockets: #3 DL _____ #12 M _____ #19 DL _____ #27 M _____

Bone Loss: Horizontal _____ Vertical _____

Require complete periodontal exam? _____Yes _____ No   Fetid Oris? _____Yes _____No
•

Periodontal Diagnosis _____

Teeth

_____ Missing teeth

_____ Location of teeth

_____ Anterior teeth: discolored _____ , fractured, _____ , spaced_____ , crowded _____

                     abraded _____ .

_____ Erosion: None   Beginning   Moderate   Extreme   Sensitive

_____ Broken or defective fillings? _____

_____ How are margins of old fillings? _____

_____ Any potential tooth fracture areas? _____

_____ Any food impaction sites? _____

Prevalence of fillings: None   Few   Moderate   Many

_____ Any unerupted teeth?   _____ Any non-vital teeth?

_____ Any overhanging margins?   _____ Recurrent cavities (chart)

_____ Any periapical infections?   _____ New cavities (chart)

Any unmanageable teeth? _____

General condition of mouth _____

State of active disease: Dental decay _____ Periodontal disease _____

State of bacterial control: _____ State of Manageability _____

Children

_____ Habits: Thumb   Fingers   Lip   Tongue thrust

_____ Relationship of first permanent molars: Right _____ Left _____

_____ Relationship of permanent anteriors _____

_____ Orthodontic consultation: No   Yes   Immediately   Later

DIAGNOSTIC MODELS?   Yes   No

Patient's attitude during exam: Interested   Casual   Disinterested

Fears and dislikes of potential treatment possibilities?_____

NOTES: _____

_____

_____

_____

_____

_____

_____

_____

Back

Figure 12–3 *Continued*

Rhonda makes Earl an appointment for two days hence and hands him a booklet about endodontic treatment. He departs pleased.

Emergency patients should be relieved of pain and discomfort as soon as possible and with as little distress as possible. Many dentists have been accustomed to setting aside emergency time and appointing any patients in distress during that time. In the production era, when dentists could hardly keep up with the demand, that may have made good sense. It protected the schedule for maximum production. Now, in the marketing era, the dentist needs to be more accommodating. Slight disruptions of the schedule may occur because of prompt handling of emergency cases, but most dentists find that they can maintain their regular schedule and care for a moderate number of emergencies, too.

Keep in mind also that every emergency patient is potentially a comprehensive care patient. Although some patients under routine care do have dental emergencies, a large proportion of them are part of the 75 percent of the population that shies away from regular dental treatment. They are new patients in the dental care system. With Earl Pearson, Jim Logan had the opportunity to convert a nonuser to a user of the system. Most emergency patients who come to your office present you with this opportunity.

THE CHILD PATIENT

For children, much of the interviewing will be with the parent. But the child should be respected for his or her own intelligence and sensitivities, and brought into the history-taking process.

The greeting in the reception room needs to be both to parent and to child. Neither should be neglected. Rapport with a small child requires that each dental team member greet the child by name and, if possible, at eye-to-eye level. Of course the parent should be greeted in the same manner as the adult patient. Success in the three-way relationship requires that you get off to a good start with both. Introductions should always be made at each transition and they should involve both parent and child.

Rapport with a small child requires that each dental team member greet the child by name and, if possible, at eye-to-eye level.

Your own judgment will guide you best as to how to conduct the interview. If you ordinarily separate the child from the parent for the examination, you can separate them at the interview. While you are interviewing the parent, another team member can be familiarizing the child with the office and the treatment room. Otherwise, you may choose to interview the parent and the child together. The purpose is to learn about the child's dental history and the parent's attitudes toward the child's dental situation. The same open-ended format used for adults with followup by specific questions is appropriate. Possible questions for the child are the following:

1. How do you clean your teeth?
2. Have you been to the dentist before?
3. Why did you go?
4. How do you feel about going to the dentist?
5. What do you like to eat?

The examination can be done in a similar manner to the adult

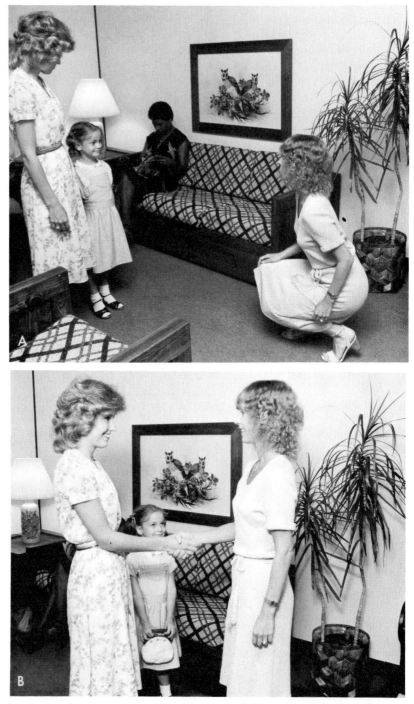

A. Receptionist greeting child at eye level. *B.* Receptionist greets mother.
Illustration continued on opposite page

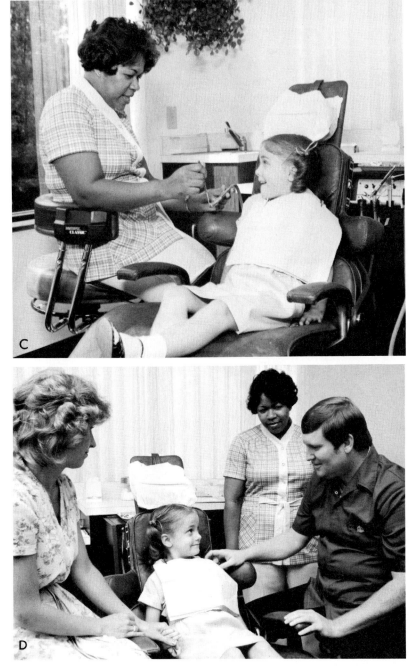

C. "Show and tell." D. The child meets the dentist.
Illustration continued on following page

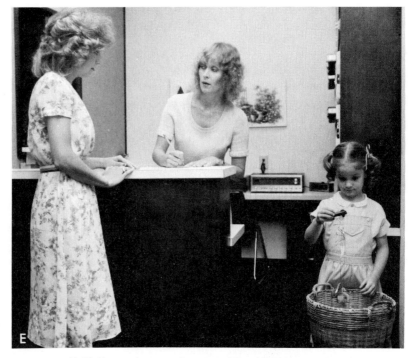

E. Mother makes appointment while child selects a toy.

examination if the parent is present. It is an opportunity to heighten the parent's awareness of the child's dental problems. Possible questions for the parent include the following:

1. Have you noticed how close together the baby teeth are?
2. Had you seen this decay?
3. Has your child bumped this dark tooth?
4. Was a space maintainer ever placed here?
5. Have you noticed how crowded these permanent teeth are?
6. Have you noticed how these teeth protrude?

As you conclude the examination you can ascertain from the parent, and from the child, that understanding prevails. You can explain what has been done during the examination and what they can expect the next time. As with the adult, you should be sure that you understand parent and child, and that they understand you.

Following the examination the demographic information and history can be obtained as for the adult. At this point in Jim Logan's office Rhonda James would ask the parent to complete the form for the child (Fig. 12–4).

As children approach adolescence and young adulthood, some combination of these procedures should be employed. Adolescents are, perhaps, the most difficult to approach in any set way. Ingenuity is required to deal with them effectively — as many dentists can testify.

CHILD'S REGISTRATION AND HISTORY

DATE _____

CHILD'S NAME _____ NICKNAME _____ AGE ____ DATE OF BIRTH _____

SCHOOL _____ GRADE _____ RESIDENCE ADDRESS _____

CITY _____ STATE _____ ZIP _____

FATHER'S NAME _____ MOTHER'S NAME _____

FATHER EMPLOYED BY _____ HOW LONG _____ HOME PHONE _____ BUS PHONE _____

MOTHER EMPLOYED BY _____ HOW LONG _____ HOME PHONE _____ BUS PHONE _____

PERSON FINANCIALLY RESPONSIBLE (IF OTHER THAN PARENT) _____ RELATIONSHIP TO CHILD _____

ADDRESS _____ CITY _____ STATE _____ ZIP _____ PHONE _____

PARENT'S SOCIAL SECURITY NUMBER _____

WHEN DENTAL INSURANCE COVERAGE NAME OF CARRIER _____

WHOM MAY WE THANK FOR REFERRING YOU _____

WHAT IS CHILD'S FAVORITE SPORT _____ FAVORITE TOY _____

FAVORITE HOBBY _____ FAVORITE PERSON _____ FAVORITE FICTION CHARACTER _____

DENTAL HISTORY

Date of last visit to a dentist _____

For what service _____

YES NO

Has child complained about dental problems _____ ☐ ☐

Any unhappy dental experiences _____ ☐ ☐

Any injuries to mouth - teeth - head _____ ☐ ☐

Any mouth habits - thumbsucking, nail biting, mouth breathing, nursing bottle habits, pacifier, etc. _____ ☐ ☐

Any unusual speech habits _____ ☐ ☐

Any lost teeth _____ ☐ ☐

Have missing teeth been replaced _____ ☐ ☐

Orthodontic appliances worn now or ever been _____ ☐ ☐

YES NO

Does your child brush teeth daily _____ ☐ ☐

Do you assist child with tooth brushing _____ ☐ ☐

How often _____

Is dental floss used _____ ☐ ☐

How often _____

Are disclosing tablets used _____ ☐ ☐

Is fluoride taken in any form _____ ☐ ☐

Child's attitude to dentistry _____

Do you desire complete dental service for the child _____ ☐ ☐

Summary (for doctor's use) _____

Form 1022 SYCOM Madison, WI Printed in U.S.A. Front

Figure 12–4. Child's dental history (*front*) and health history (*back*) form.

Illustration continued on following page

HEALTH HISTORY

Child's Physician _____ Address _____ Phone _____

Date of last physical examination _____ Results _____

	YES	NO		YES	NO
Is child under care of physician now _____	☐	☐	Does child have good physical coordination _____	☐	☐
Is child receiving any medication or drugs _____	☐	☐	Are there any emotional problems _____	☐	☐
Is there any excessive bleeding when cut _____	☐	☐	Summary (for doctor's use) _____		
Has child ever been hospitalized _____	☐	☐			
Has child ever had surgery _____	☐	☐			
Is there any allergy to penicillin or other drugs _____	☐	☐			
Are there other allergies: food - pollen - animals - dust - other	☐	☐			

HAS CHILD ANY HISTORY OF OR DIFFICULTY WITH ANY OF THE FOLLOWING:

___ Anemia	___ Chronic Sinus	___ Hearing	___ Mastoid	___ Rheumatic Fever
___ Asthma	___ Convulsions	___ Heart	___ Measles	___ Thyroid
___ Bladder	___ Diabetes	___ Kidney	___ Mononucleosis	___ Tuberculosis
___ Cerebral Palsy	___ Epilepsy	___ Liver	___ Mumps	___ Other
___ Chicken Pox	___ Fainting	___ Malignancies		

SUMMARY: (for doctor's use)

Please describe any current medical treatment including drugs, pending surgery, recent injuries or any other information I should be aware of that we have not discussed.

_____

_____

_____

_____

	YES	NO
May we request release of your child's medical records for our reference _____	☐	☐

This information was discussed with and given by _____

Relation to Child _____

Form 1022 SYCOM Madison, WI Printed in U.S.A.   Back

Figure 12–4. *Continued*

SUMMARY

The examination visit offers you the opportunity to get acquainted with the patient. Role playing as a patient will sensitize the dentist to patients' problems. The patient's impression of the dental team is formed very early by the welcome to the office and initial interaction with your team. During the interview the dentist and patient can share information and attitudes in a supportive atmosphere, which enables each to have a positive experience. Heightening of patient awareness to dental problems can occur in a well-conducted clinical examination. Written forms are best completed after rapport is established in the interview and clinical examination. Appropriate modifications in the procedure are necessary for patients in pain, and for children.

References

Barkley, R. F.: Successful Preventive Dental Practices. Macomb, IL, Preventive Dentistry Press, 1972, pp. 177–208.

Benjamin, A.: The Helping Interview. Boston, Houghton Mifflin Co., 1974, pp. 57–107.

Edwards, F. G.: The marketing of orthodontics. J Clin Ortho, 13:3, March 1979, pp. 163–169.

Froelich, R. E., et al.: Communication In The Dental Office. St. Louis, C. V. Mosby Co., 1976.

Gold, S. L.: Establishing motivating relations in preventive dentistry. JASPD 4:6, Nov/Dec 1974, pp. 17–25.

Hall, E. T.: The Hidden Dimension. Garden City, NY, Anchor Books, 1969, pp. 101–129.

Levoy, R. P.: The Successful Professional Practice. Englewood Cliffs, NJ, Prentice-Hall, Inc., 1970, pp. 115–128.

13

The Treatment Conference

AN EMERGENCY TREATMENT

Dr. Lila Kingsley is looking forward to a treatment conference with James Brighton. James has been in the office twice before — the first time for repair of a broken tooth and a week later for a complete examination. James, age 33, has had little dental treatment in recent years. Large silver amalgam restorations had been placed in his first molars and moderate restorative treatment had been done in his other teeth.

Although the schedule was filled, Lila saw him the same day he called for the first visit. Jeannette, the receptionist, detected a very anxious tone in his voice, even though he said the tooth was not actually hurting. The office policy was that anyone who wanted to come for an emergency on the same day he called would be seen as soon as possible.

James seemed very appreciative that Lila saw him immediately and repaired his fractured tooth. He confessed, sheepishly, that although the tooth wasn't hurting, he was afraid it might begin to hurt. Furthermore, he said he had not sought dental care since he graduated from college — that he actually didn't believe he had any problems. However, after the fractured tooth was repaired, he decided that he should have a thorough dental examination. He told Lila that another reason he had not sought care sooner was that he did not trust dentists. Because she proved her concern for him by her expeditious attention to his immediate problem, he made an appointment for an examination the following week.

That session went well, too. Although Lila had learned a good bit about him on his first visit, she took a few minutes to get to know him better. Later she recorded her findings on his personal data sheet (Chapter 12). James had no other real concerns about his dental situation. His rather suspicious nature was well-suited to his job as the person in charge of quality control in a local manufacturing plant. He had two children, ages 2 and 5. To help the family budget, his wife did substitute teaching in the elementary school. His personal health was good. He exercised about three times a week, bicycling, swimming, and running. Although his mother had lost her teeth to "pyorrhea," his father had retained most of his teeth.

James wanted to keep his teeth and thought he should be able to — at least for a couple of decades. His pet peeve about dentists, based on experiences of some co-workers, was that dentists were arbitrary (almost arrogant) about planned dental treatment. Explanations were lengthy but not clear. And there never seemed to be any choice. It was always, "Joe, this is the treatment you need." Period. Other than wanting to be able to exercise some choice, James did not desire any special treatment.

Some dentists have been seen as arbitrary, almost arrogant, about dental treatment plans.

James Brighton's Examination

Lila did her usual complete examination with radiographs, study models and dental charting. Upon inquiry she learned that James was aware that other restorations were large, but did not realize that some of those teeth might fracture too. He was also unaware of heavy deposits of calculus, although he did admit that his gums bled "once in a while."

Study of the examination findings revealed that James had a moderate periodontal problem and some teeth with unsatisfactory restorations. The lower first molars should be restored with cast restorations; extensive pin amalgams were an alternative. The four other teeth involved were restorable in silver amalgam. Thorough scaling and curettage should control the periodontal problems. Lila believed that her treatment would restore Jim's dental health, which he could maintain with careful home care. She remembered his concern about choice, thinking that there wasn't a great deal of choice available. He could choose to do nothing, which would surprise her. Or he could choose from limited treatment alternatives. Although she hoped he would agree to cast gold restorations for the lower molars, she was prepared to offer him amalgams. Lila felt prepared for the treatment conference.

WHAT IS THE TREATMENT CONFERENCE?

The examination, as described in Chapter 12, is the process leading up to recommendations for treatment. The treatment conference is the process of arriving at agreement for the planned treatment based on those recommendations.

As the examination is not necessarily limited to one appointment, neither is the treatment conference. Nor is the appointment at which it occurs necessarily limited to the conference. Preliminary treatment such as scaling or prophylaxis, or even limited operative treatment, could occur during or before this appointment.

AIDA (Awareness, Interest, Desire, Action), besides being the title of an opera, is an acronym for the process of learning that occurs

A C T I O N
commitment
belief
attitude
self-interest
awareness
unawareness

during the examination and treatment conference. The aim is to promote awareness in patients by means of certain questions. The patient becomes interested in treatment when he perceives that the information presented applies to himself. He then can experience a desire to do something about the problem. Action, the final step, occurs when Robert Froelich's therapeutic contract is completed by the acceptance and provision of treatment. Some people add an "S," making it AIDAS. The "S" stands for satisfaction, making certain the patient is satisfied.

King (in *Nexus*, March 15, 1976) describes the learning ladder, which is divided into smaller increments than AIDA(S). Interest is subdivided into self-interest, attitude, and belief. These three terms indicate an intensification of interest to the point at which a commitment or decision is made leading to action.

While learning is occurring, the patient is undergoing a thought process characterized by "yes" answers to the following questions:

1. Am I susceptible to this disease (disorder), such as caries, periodontal disease, malocclusion?
2. Do I in fact have this disease (disorder)?
3. Are the consequences of this disease serious?
4. Is it possible to intervene effectively?
5. Is the cost of intervention (money, inconvenience, distress) worth it to me?
6. How do I (we) proceed?

While learning is occurring, the patient is undergoing a thought process character-ized by "yes" answers.

The answer to question 1 (and in some instances 2 and 3) has probably been acknowledged prior to the patient's seeking attention. It is up to the dentist to help the patient answer the remaining questions in the affirmative.

The formality and time required for the conference vary. Some dentists may prefer a formal presentation of findings based on the examination and of recommendations based on the findings. Visual aids may be used to enhance the presentation. Such a presentation and discussion may require an hour. Or you may prefer an informal discussion of problems and treatment with little or no use of visual aids. Some dentists require less than five minutes for such a conference.

Regardless of the formality, the time required, whether it occurs at one or more appointments, and regardless of how many appointments have preceded it, the purpose of the conference is the same — to come to an understanding between dentist and patient on what will follow and who will be responsible for what.

PREPARATION

Following the examination, the dentist must prepare for the conference. Thorough preparation does not necessarily require very much time. An experienced dentist needs much less preparation time than the neophyte, even for a complex situation. Each dentist owes to every patient a clear explanation of the dental problem and what is involved in treatment, plus a nonthreatening atmosphere in which the patient can make the choice. Sufficient preparation is required for the dentist to satisfy this obligation. Depending on one's experience and the complexity of the problems, this could range from five minutes to perhaps an hour.

Personal Situation

Effective marketing requires that dentists know their patients well and understand their total situation and feelings relative to their dental problems. Use of the personal data sheet (described in Chapter 12), modified according to your own thinking, will assist you in doing this. Dentists who have been the most effective marketers have gone through this process intuitively. In fact, many have developed their own personal data sheets, as you may prefer to do. Even if you meet several new patients every day, brief notations immediately following the get-acquainted interview will be adequate to remind you of their personal situations so that you can take that data into account as you plan treatment.

Some dentists prefer to deal with patients according to some typology, of which there are many. (One of these classified patients as: passive receptive, passive aggressive, frugal, controlling, paranoid, and impulsive, acting out.) The fact that there are many should suggest that there are hazards in stereotyping. To begin with, you have to learn the various types, their characteristics and how to recognize them. Then you have to learn how to deal with them.

This two-step process is fraught with danger. First you may not be able to decide on the type, because people are not pure types. They are mixtures. To determine the major classification may be next to impossible. Your degree of skill in interacting as you should with a particular type may leave something to be desired, even if you are correct in your diagnosis.

Such prejudging of the patient overly complicates the whole process. We suggest you treat everyone as an individual and respond to his or her needs as you understand them. As you practice being responsive, you will find — and so will your patients — that you are indeed *becoming* more and more sensitive to individual patient's needs.

Remember that the personal situation may affect the planned treatment as much as the dental problem does. It is important that Lila Kingsley consider James Brighton's interest in being able to choose. Every patient has some unique concern or interest. A dentist who ignores or remains unaware of this concern does so to his or her peril and to the detriment of the patient.

Effective marketing requires that dentists know their patients well and understand their total situation and feelings relative to their dental problems.

Dental Problems

Clearly, the dental problems must be thoroughly understood. Inability to diagnose is incompetence, and failure to diagnose is unethical. Diagnosis is fundamental to all dental treatment and therefore to marketing. To develop marketing skills without the necessary skills for diagnosis is unethical. This takes us back to the

Hippocratic dictum of "Do no harm." If, as authors, we failed to put marketing in perspective relative to competence, we would be doing dentistry a grave disservice. Competence, as exemplified by the ability and the practice of the skill of diagnosis, is *sine qua non* in the marketing of dentistry.

Dental Fees

We said in Chapter 2 that there are various ways to *establish fees*. Most dentists have established them according to the *competition*. The going fee in a community for a specific service is where many of us start. True, we may go up or down from there according to our individual circumstances. Or, as Geoffrey Marks suggests, we could compute an hourly charge based on overhead and what we believe should be our personal income. The rationality of this cost-based approach is appealing. Some even use the *market-based* approach, which derives from the notion that people will pay a certain price for a certain service. Testing the market can be done by raising the price to the point where there is resistance, commonly known as "charging what the traffic will bear." A combination of these methods is possible in which one develops a fee schedule according to one method and then checks it by other methods. You could develop a cost-based fee schedule and check it against the competition (going fee) and the market (what you think people are willing to pay for specific services). Few of us rely on a single method, although those who do will enthusiastically argue its merits. Your fee schedule is yours to set depending on your personal inclinations, needs, and philosophy.

Another notion regarding fees is the *value* of the service. L. D.

> The fee should be no less than the value placed on it by the dentist and no more than the value placed on it by the patient.

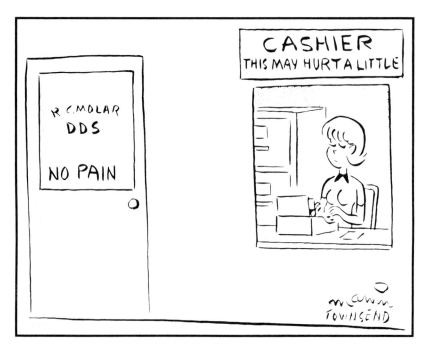

Courtesy of *Cal* magazine.

Pankey pointed out years ago that different people place different values on dental service. Avrom King maintains that the fee should depend on the value of the service to the patient and to the dentist. The fee should be no less than the value placed on it by the dentist and no more than the value placed on it by the patient. Clearly, the dentist who is marketing consciously has to help the patient to appreciate the value of dental care.

A *fee for services* or a fee for specific services may be the basis for the charges. Traditionally, dentists have developed fee schedules for specific services which third party insurers have adopted. Thus, we have a fee for two surface amalgams. PFM crowns, and so on. This piecework type of fee is quite acceptable to some dentists, but repugnant to others.

The dentists who are repelled by fees for specific services compute a fee for total services. The dentist's hourly rate, office overhead, and laboratory expense make up this total fee. King modifies the hourly rate by factoring in the difficulty of the problem and the exquisiteness of the solution. Marks factors in the cooperativeness of the patient. Those who talk a lot, are late for appointments, or may fail to show are charged more. King might even charge less to the patient who is an absolute delight — taking a portion of the fee in "warm fuzzies."

If you are targeting a certain segment of the market, *perception of the fee* by patients in that segment must be considered. A market comprising primarily lower-middle-class and blue-collar individuals may be concerned about fees amounting to more than their budgets can bear. A fee for specific services that can be readily identified, such as prophylaxis or extraction, needs to be kept in the lower middle range for such a practice. Otherwise, the dentist will become known as high priced, and the practice will fail to thrive in this market.

Perception of the fee by patients must be considered.

On the other hand, if the practice caters to wealthy people, fees need to be in the higher ranges. Lower fees are likely to mean to such people that the dentist is not very good. Otherwise he would charge more, wouldn't he? Some people pride themselves on the level of fees they pay for services. Quite likely the dentist will earn a higher fee for a specific service, because such people tend to be rather demanding and in some instances less considerate of the dentist's time. Thus, a fee for service computed with all the factors will be in the high range.

Fairness of the fee should be our goal. A dental student once defined a fair fee as one that allows both dentist and patient to put bread on the table. Marks stresses fairness to both dentist and patient. *You* will need to determine what is fair *for you and your patients. You* decide as to how you will apply the various considerations above.

What about *discounts* of regular fees? First, will you discount any fee at all, and if so, for whom? In the cost squeeze in which dentists find themselves, there is currently less tendency to discount. Furthermore, available government programs that provide dental care to indigents make discounting less necessary than formerly.

Beyond your own staff (whom we shall discuss later), who should be considered? As a marketing tool, you could give allowances to people who refer you many patients — regular patients, especially if finances are a problem, other staff people, certainly those in specialists' offices, or maybe even agency employees who refer heavily to you. Perhaps you could offer some consideration to loyal patients who have fallen on hard times. Other possibilities are loyal elderly patients on reduced incomes, children in large families with modest income, and poor relatives of loyal patients.

How much discounting should you do? That which is done for direct marketing purposes is limited by the criteria by which you select these people. These criteria should be set cost-effectively. The discount to a specific patient should be determined by the amount of business from persons referred by the individual. A budget for the charity-based discounts should be established as a percentage of your collections, perhaps up to 5 percent.

Lila Kingsley computes her fees for specific services, totals the various fees, and quotes the total for the service. She has considered a fee for service based on an hourly rate plus overhead and laboratory charges and expects to adopt that system next year. However, at this time she feels more comfortable with fees for specific services.

Philosophy of Treatment

When Lila Kingsley graduated from dental school five years ago, she was imbued with the technology of dentistry. She had always been interested in people as individuals. But for a time she had begun to view them as sets of teeth. After about a year in practice, a friend who came to her as a patient startled her by remarking that she seemed to be forgetting that he was an individual who happened to have teeth. Since that time, Lila has always reminded herself before every appointment that "this is an individual with whom I can relate as a person and may be able to help with my skills as a dentist."

The marketing dentist, as Lila has been for the last four years, develops a philosophy about people. Lila continues to be concerned about the dental health of the community and of individuals. She is proud of her dental skills. She works hard to ensure her patients of the best clinical dentistry she can provide. She has learned to approach patients first as unique persons who may have some misgivings about dentistry. Her people skills have continued to improve, so that it seems as natural to relate to the person now as it does to perform dental care. She is very comfortable talking with persons who seem to need to talk; also, she is comfortable getting on with treatment for those in a hurry who don't want to "waste time talking." Her philosophy is that *people are most important;* teeth are important, but only as they relate to people, not in and of themselves. Her many patient referrals are proof that the patients accept and approve of her philosophy.

Desirable Environment

As for the initial interview, the place for consultation should be orderly, nonthreatening, and pleasant. Orderliness is important for

The discount to a specific patient (if given for marketing purposes) should be determined by the amount of business from persons referred by the individual.

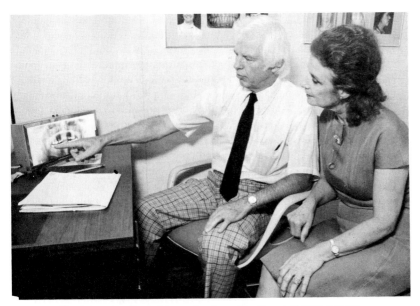

Dentist and patient discuss treatment in the conference room.

two reasons: a cluttered area tends to make a patient feel uncomfortable because he feels that he is intruding into a busy work area. Nor is such an area likely to enhance the patient's confidence in the dentist. It will cause him to suspect sloppiness.

The patient needs to feel comfortable and in control in order to exercise freedom of choice (make the decisions). As the helper can better obtain information in a conversation corner, so can the consultant better offer advice in a similar setting. The symbolic communication is that the advice is being given without threats. In the words of Les Giblin, "One should not lord it over them."

Is the treatment room acceptable or must one use a consultation room? Most agree that a consultation room is preferable, but the treatment room may be quite appropriate on occasion. Certainly for very simple situations requiring minimal treatment, the treatment room may be better. In such instances, using the consultation room may make the patient feel that the dentist is "making a mountain out of a molehill."

If you consult at the chair, try equalizing the situation by positioning the patient upright and slightly higher than you are as you sit on your operating stool. Some dentists feel more at home in the treatment room, but some patients are more at ease in the consultation room, away from the dental equipment. Either dentist or patient may feel somewhat uncomfortable no matter what room is used. Although you should feel comfortable, consider acquiescing to the patient's feelings and conducting the treatment planning conference in the consultation room.

How should the consultation room be furnished? As with interviewing, you need a setting in which you and the patient are seated in similar chairs in an equal relationship. If you view radiographs and models together, you could do this by sitting on the same side of a

The patient needs to feel comfortable and in control in order to exercise freedom of choice (make the decisions).

table of appropriate height. You may choose to vary this to fit your own circumstances and preferences. Try to avoid any symbolic communication that puts a barrier between you and the patient. By all means do not sit in a large chair behind an impressive desk, unless you want to relate in an authoritarian manner, which is not good marketing.

The ideal mood for an interview room is warm and relaxing; for a treatment conference room, warm and stimulating. If you can use separate rooms for each purpose, the decor should be selected on this basis. If not, moderately bright reds, oranges, and yellows should be selected as a compromise. An interior decorator can be a great help.

Organizing the Presentation

All patients are entitled to know the *choices* available and the consequences of each choice.

To be effective, the *presentation* must be organized, but its degree of formality can be controlled. Schemes of organization vary, but generally the elements should include the problem(s), the choices for management of the problem(s), the consequences of the choices, and the responsibilities of both dentist and patient.

The statement of the *problems* or conditions in the patient's mouth (dental diagnosis) is the foundation for the conference. In the problem-oriented record, you would list the various problems of the individual patient in technically correct terminology. However, in the presentation to the patient, use common, easily understood terms.

You can hardly anticipate all of each patient's questions. However, from any patient, you could expect to hear some or all of the following questions:

1. Do I have any dental problems?
2. What is my problem?
3. How severe is it?
4. What can be done about it?
5. How much and what kind of pain and inconvenience will this treatment involve?
6. How long will the treatment take?
7. How much will it cost?
8. What are the various payment plans?

Because no one patient is likely to ask all of the questions, it makes little sense to answer them all until they are asked.

All patients are entitled to know the *choices* available and the consequences of each choice. In the absence of pain, bleeding, or swelling, one choice is to do nothing. Alternative forms of treatment that the dentist is willing to do should be presented. Alternative choices of treatment that you believe are appropriate should be prepared. Try to remember patients' total needs.

The responsibilities of both dentist and patient must be understood. The dentist must explain in understandable terms what he or she will do and what the patient is expected to do, such as keep appointments, follow instructions, and pay dental charges.

Some dentists prepare *written plans* as a basis for consultation. The elements of conditions, choices, and consequences should be included. In most instances fee estimates for alternative courses of treatment would be provided.

Many dentists who believe very strongly that people respond only to felt needs prepare written plans, which they provide to their patients after the examination. Patients are asked to study the plan, written in plain language, and to inquire later if there are questions. The treatment planning conference might take very little time, during which the patient simply asks when treatment could be started. Otherwise, you can deal with specific questions by the patients and waste no time discussing things in which the patient has no interest.

Lila Kingsley sometimes prepares written plans to summarize the conference for patients who are unable to decide. She is considering prior preparation of such plans, but she still feels that she wants to discuss her findings with each patient personally. Her conferences usually take less than twenty minutes, because she has eliminated technical descriptions of conditions and treatment. Instead she discusses with each patient in general terms what the problem is, what can be done about it, and how much it will cost.

Scheduling

At what time of day should conferences be scheduled? Evenings may be best for those patients whose spouses work during the day, if you or the patient desire the spouse to be present. Other times of the day may be best for other individuals. Some believe that people are more accepting in the morning, before possible irritations or reversals of fortune are suffered in the course of the day.

A particular time period, such as Thursday afternoon, can be set aside for the patient conferences. This frees most of the staff for other duties, such as housekeeping or perhaps personal time off.

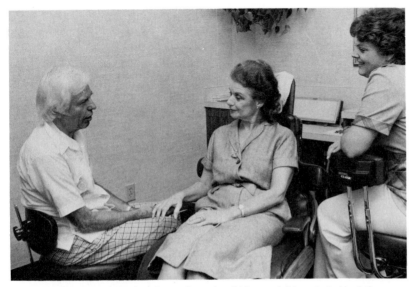

In chairside consultation the patient should be upright and at about the same level as the dentist.

Also, if the conferences do not require all your time, you can use the balance of the conference period as you choose.

Patient convenience must be considered, as for any other appointment. If you ordinarily schedule conferences at a time when a specific patient cannot come, you will need to schedule that patient at another time. Your own personal convenience will generally need to yield to patient requirements.

Financial Arrangements

Even with assignment of insurance payments, firm financial arrangements are necessary for the balance.

As stated in Chapter 2, the purpose of marketing is to satisfy patients' needs at a *profit*. The dentist's income is dependent upon efficient provision of services and collection of fees for those services. There should be no hesitancy about firm financial arrangements and sure followup in collection procedures if the arrangements are not observed.

Fortunately, dental insurance has lightened the financial burden of dental treatment for many Americans. Even with assignment of insurance payments, firm financial arrangements are necessary for the balance. Patients must clearly understand their obligations, and the dentist or some other member of the dental team must clarify them. Although dental insurance eases the financial burden, in most instances it does not remove it.

It is up to you to decide what financial arrangements are acceptable. Good marketing requires you to recognize that credit makes many purchases possible, and without it fewer purchases would be made. If you choose to give no credit, you will limit your market. If you extend credit, you will need to decide by what terms.

Very extended payment plans of a year or more should be considered only in exceptional circumstances. Generally you can (and consultants will tell you that you should) confine credit arrangements to three to six months. In inflationary times, the future value of the dollar shrinks rapidly enough that you will grant longer terms only if you are willing to absorb dollar-value losses.

However, if you add financing charges you can reduce your loss by inflation, and these charges can be added easily by computer billing. Otherwise, computation and posting are troublesome. Truth in lending statements, as required by federal law, must be provided if you charge interest, or even if you schedule at least four payments without interest.

Remember, the purpose of the financial arrangements is to enable the patient to receive the dental treatment he or she desires and you to derive a satisfactory income. You owe it to yourself and to the patient to develop payment plans that accomplish these purposes.

Self-preparation

Dentists must also prepare themselves personally to be congenial to their patients. Lloyd Hollander discusses a number of characteristics of dentists which are blocks to acceptance. They include the following:

1. unpleasant personality
2. unattractive appearance
3. lack of interest in the patient as a person
4. lack of cleanliness
5. roughness
6. habit of talking too much or too little
7. indecisiveness
8. tendency to be too critical

None of us can overhaul ourself completely, but we can all be aware of these problems and present ourselves as favorably as possible.

THE CONFERENCE

Lila Kingsley is scheduled to see James Brighton at 4:00 P.M. Wednesday. She varies the day and time of day to accommodate the patient as much as possible. She prefers 4:00 P.M., which gives the staff plenty of time to put the office in order. Many times she is free to leave at 4:30, so that she has more time with her 3-year-old son.

As she ushers James into the consultation room, she inquires about the tooth that she repaired at his first visit and is assured that it is fine. Jeannette has already placed the radiographs on the viewer and the chart and models on the table.

After they sit down near the table, she asks James, "Have you thought of anything else about your dental situation that you would like to share with me?" James states that he began to realize that he had neglected his teeth and hopes that he has not experienced any irreparable damage. Lila assures him that although there has been damage, all of the problems are manageable.

She is glad that he has brought that up, because she always likes to make a positive statement about the problems. Formerly she had been so intent on making clear to patients the seriousness of the problems, that some of them became discouraged and were reluctant to proceed with treatment out of a sense of futility. For some time now she has avoided that, and statistics have shown that her loss rate of patients has declined markedly.

Jim then asks her what is wrong and how much it would cost to correct. She responds by showing him on the models the surfaces of the teeth outlined in red which need restoring. Since the problems are not readily apparent on the radiographs, she points out those same teeth on the radiographs and tells him that there is no evidence of any disturbance inside the teeth or in the supporting bone. In fact the radiographs reveal a very favorable situation, and she says that the problems are worn-out fillings and heavy deposits of calculus on the teeth, fortunately with no serious gum disease.

At that point, Jim asks what needs to be done. Lila remembers his concern for choice, but decides to recommend cast gold restorations on the lower first molars and silver amalgam restorations in the other teeth. He then asks if he has to have gold in the molars and she replies, "No, it is possible to place large amalgams held in the teeth by small pins, but they might not last." They then discuss the advantages and disadvantages of both the cast gold and the silver amalgam. Jim seems reassured by this open discussion and decides to accept Lila's recommendation.

She then reminds him of the calculus deposits, and says that it would be necessary to remove them by a thorough scaling which should be accomplished in two appointments. He asks what caused the calculus, and she explains about dental plaque and how when it is undisturbed for more than about twenty-four hours, it hardens into calculus. When he asks whether there is any way to prevent it, she explains how adequate home care would prevent it almost entirely. Jim says that he always brushed his teeth, but that he wants to learn how to clean them thoroughly. Lila assures him that they will begin that next time.

Then Lila says, "Now we can talk about finances, and of course your dental insurance will pay part of it." Jim had learned from coworkers that the insurance would not pay the entire fee, and he asks why not. Lila explains that his employer needs to know the cost of the fringe benefit, and that the insurance company limits payment by these mechanisms to something less than the full fee, the remainder to be paid by the patient. Jim seems to be satisfied by the explanation and asks what the total of his portion would be. Lila replies that she would immediately submit the estimate for treatment and should know within two weeks exactly what the company would pay. Meanwhile, preliminary computations based on past experience show that of the $810 fee, the insurance company should pay $565, leaving a balance of $245. Jim is satisfied and states that he could pay the balance whenever she asks for it. They agree that after the company informs Lila of what it would pay, Jim will pay the balance at the next appointment by check. Lila asks Jim if there is anything else that he needs to discuss, and he says no, that he is very satisfied and is looking forward to getting his mouth into good order. She says, "Very good, thank you for coming in and letting me help you with that project. Jeanette will schedule a time for us to begin scaling your teeth. After that, we will restore the teeth that have the worn-out fillings and we should finish within about two months." She shakes hands with him at the desk, and Jeanette schedules his next appointment.

The most common failing in the presentation is the dentist's lecturing to a passive patient.

Initiation

As with any appointment, the patient is entitled to an initiation into the treatment conference. Your bridging back to what has occurred previously reminds the patient that you remember his experience. This reassures him that you treat persons as individuals, not as numbers. Lila's inquiry about Jim's repaired tooth provided a bridge. Her question about anything he might like to share with her led her into the discussion when he asked her what was wrong and how much it would cost.

Discussion

The elements of presentation referred to under preparation constitute the basis for the discussion. The most common failing in the presentation is the dentist's lecturing to a passive patient. Rather than a one-way process, you need *dialog*. In fact you should solicit feedback by saying something like, "Is that clear so far? Any questions?" Be sure not to use a tone of voice that would be intimidating to the patient. You should also encourage the patient to express his own views and feelings.

Although you should be well-prepared for the discussion, you will need to be flexible. During the dicussion you should completely satisfy the patient's curiosity and meet objections. The order of discussion will make more sense to the patient if you respond to his input directly and at that time. The well-prepared dentist can do this and still cover essential points. In fact, examine carefully any points about which the patient has no questions or comments; they may not be essential.

Certainly dentists are obligated to explain patients' problems to them. The explanation should follow some awareness-heightening questions, as described in Chapter 12. Explaining a "problem" which the patient does not perceive as such is not likely to work out well.

A positive tone should prevail. Dentists have tended, as Lila Kingsley once did, to describe primarily the problem's negative aspects. Benefits of treatment should be stressed, but, as Earl Estep says, patients should not be. In fact, a light, if not humorous, touch is appropriate at times. However, use humor cautiously. You could emphasize the positive by saying, "Mr. Abrams, with this treatment you should chew well and have a healthy smile for many years," rather than "You will lose your teeth if you don't have this treatment." Patients deserve hope, not threats.

Your language should be carefully chosen; above all, it must communicate. Dentists, especially those just beginning to practice, tend to use language that is too technical for lay people to understand. Technical language is efficient between professionals, but it is usually ineffective with patients. On the other hand, dentists must guard against talking down to patients, because that makes them feel that they are being patronized — hardly the way to build relationships.

> Technical language is efficient between professionals, but it is usually ineffective with patients.

Presentation of *alternative treatment plans* allows patients to choose the course that best satisfies their needs. Some dentists present the ideal treatment to everyone; others present what they believe is the most appropriate treatment for the individual; still others present various possibilities, tooth by tooth and problem by problem. What to do in this regard is a matter of individual treatment philosophy. In the interest of autonomy, discussed in Chapter 3, we believe that dentists should allow patients to make choices within the constraints of accepted dental practice and the dentist's concept of acceptability. A narrow concept of the span of choices on the part of a dentist reduces the spectrum of patients whom that dentist can attract.

Discussing the alternative plans in the order of your preference enables your patients to select the most preferred treatment they can accept without wasting time discussing all the possibilities. You may prefer to present only one basic plan and suggest to the patients that treatment can be scheduled as they are ready. Whenever possible, choices should be offered.

Consequences need to be described objectively. As we describe consequences, however, we must be careful not to threaten. In fact this is very difficult to manage, because consequences are threatening in themselves. Only choices that have acceptable consequences should be presented. The analogy with automobiles has probably been overworked, but any automobile should get us to where we want to go. Similarly, any dental treatment should provide an acceptable result. Remember that what is acceptable to a particular patient might not be acceptable to you if you were the patient. But you're not.

Audio-visuals and other aids should be employed judiciously. Yes, you may well enhance patient understanding of the problem, but in the process, you may also make the patient feel overwhelmed. The manner in which such aids are presented is critical. If the patient perceives the presentation to be for the purpose of eliminating ignorance, he is likely to be threatened. However, if the purpose is "to help him understand a little better," he is more likely to accept it. We need to remember that patients already feel insecure in our offices and we should attempt to make them feel more secure.

Agreement

If you are convinced that the fee is fair, then you can quote it with conviction and without apology.

The purpose of the conference is to agree on some course to be followed. Whatever else it is, it should by all means be motivating. Informing is not enough; it should be persuasive. There is no reason to be hesitant about persuading a patient to accept a needed course of treatment. Before the patient can agree on a solution, he may need to know the fee. We believe that if you are convinced that the fee is fair, then you can quote it with conviction and without apology. It will be in perspective and the patient will accept it unless he is financially unable to do so. In that case you are back to explaining alternatives for a more feasible solution. As a dentist in the marketing mode, you will negotiate with the patient until you both agree on a helpful course of treatment at a fee that the patient accepts.

After the patient accepts the fee, *financial arrangements* are the next part of the agreement. You may choose to delegate this discussion to another team member. The office policy serves as a basis for this discussion. Financial situations of patients must also be considered. One way to do this is simply to ask the patient "How would you like to pay for this?" If all the previous discussion has accomplished its purpose, the answer will be a reasonable one and might be a more accelerated payment schedule than you would otherwise arrive at.

Another method is similar to presenting alternative treatment plans. You simply suggest the most acceptable method first. If the patient cannot accept that, suggest the next most acceptable and so on until you suggest one that is acceptable to the patient. If you are unable to agree, you are back again to the treatment plan to arrange one that the patient can finance. It may be a matter of doing treatment in phases that the patient can pay for as treatment progresses. Rehabilitation in this way may take years, but will enable the patient to have fine dentistry at a rate he can afford.

Summary

When the dental problem and factors pertaining to it are understood; when all agreed-upon treatment is planned; when the fee is accepted and financial arrangements are made; when an appointment is made to begin definitive treatment, then the treatment conference can be called a success.

REFERENCES

Barkley, R. F.: Successful Preventive Dental Practice. Macomb, IL, Preventive Dentistry Press, 1972, pp. 177–209.

Brahe, N.: We Like These Ideas. Appleton, WI, Project D Publications, 1970, pp. 293–324.

Estep, E.: The Obvious Secret. Athens, TX.

Froelich, R. E., et al.: Communications in the Dental Office. St. Louis, C. V. Mosby Co., 1976, pp. 30–31.

Giblin, L.: How to Have Confidence and Power in Dealing with People. Englewood Cliffs, NJ, Prentice-Hall, Inc., 1956.

Hollander, L.: Modern Dental Practice. Philadelphia, W. B. Saunders Co., 1967, pp. 26–47.

Levoy, R. P.: The Successful Professional Practice. Englewood Cliffs, NJ, Prentice-Hall, Inc., 1970, pp. 115–137.

Marks, G.: How to Practice Successful Dentistry. Philadelphia, J. B. Lippincott Co., 1963, pp. 93–111.

Protell, M., et al.: Psychodynamics in Dental Practice. Springfield, IL, Charles C Thomas Publisher, 1975, pp. 137–157.

14

The Treatment Visit

INTRODUCTION

During the initial examination visit, a bond of trust should develop between the dentist and patient which will result in a mutually acceptable treatment plan. That trust, which should continue to build during each successive treatment visit, can only develop if the dentist and staff members deliver on all promises. If patients discover that they can believe what is said, they are much more likely to complete treatment and to pay for services rendered.

This means there must be effective communication between the doctor, staff, and patient. Accurate statements must be made to the patient pertaining to fees, treatment, and any expected results. In addition, once the patient has returned for initial treatment, the dentist must make every effort to be punctual and professional, and complete the planned session in a painless and comfortable way.

The Patient's Arrival

The receptionist inaugurates the trust-building process by personally greeting the patient by name.

Trust-building between patient and dentist should start the moment the patient arrives for his or her first treatment. The receptionist inaugurates the trust-building process by personally greeting the patient by name. This recognition helps the patient perceive that he is not just a number, but someone who is important. Recognition should not be difficult, since the patient will have previously visited the office for the examination. It is advisable to always use the patient's name in entering appointments in the appointment book. Then the receptionist can check the name against the time of arrival and make the patient feel welcome with a personal greeting. Your office staff should never ignore a patient. Nothing destroys confidence faster than being ignored or being treated impersonally.

"Good morning, Mrs. McGill," the first-class receptionist will say. "It's good to see you again. Dr. Howard is on schedule and will see you in a few minutes. Please have a seat and make yourself comfortable."

The receptionist can also serve to divert the patient from any anticipated unpleasantness by offering reading material; patients sense that you care when they see suitable material in the reception area for all ages and reading tastes. Background music or television can "mask" offensive dental noise or the crying of a child patient in an operatory.

The term "waiting room" can suggest a negative connotation and should be avoided in communicating with the patient. The use of "reception room" or other titles are recommended, because waiting rooms represent places where people are stored until the assembly line needs them.

To relieve obvious anxiety, the receptionist or other staff member should engage the patient in conversation. When patients are treated with concern for their comfort, they will tolerate limited waiting with much less displeasure. Remember: you will never offend anyone by recognizing them and displaying interest in their well-being. Ignore them and you most certainly will.

Every office needs a system that will alert the staff to a patient's arrival. Patient's names are listed on the appointment schedule along with the time for treatment, so as patients arrive, the receptionist can place a check beside each name. Some offices have the patient sign a check-in log with time of arrival, but this is less personal.

Patients accept waiting much more readily if they know the dentist really cares that they have been inconvenienced.

If a "pegboard" accounting system is utilized in the office, an easy way to keep track of arrival times is to have the receptionist jot down the time on the portion of the slip that goes to the dentist. This will let the staff know how long the patient has been waiting; if the wait has been excessive, the doctor should come out and apologize. Patients are much less resentful if they know the dentist really cares that they have been inconvenienced. Another method of notifying the staff of arrivals is through an intercom. But patients under treatment may think the staff and doctor are hurrying to see the next patient. A light system could be incorporated for this purpose, as it may be less intrusive.

Once an appointment has been made and the patient has arrived for treatment, every effort should be made to expedite the visit. There are occasions when appointments of different patients overlap. When this occurs, the second person should be kept informed. If it is necessary that a patient be kept waiting, it should be noted on the chart so that the same patient will not have an extensive wait a second time. Your major goal is patient satisfaction. This will go a long way in building any practice, whether general or specialty. If the dentist is delayed, one technique to help the wait seem shorter and make it easier for the patient to accept is to have the patient stay in the reception room for a period of time and then move him or her to the treatment area.

Moving Patient to Treatment Area

It is conducive to efficiency to have an orderly flow in getting the patient into the operatory from the reception room.

Before a patient is brought back into the treatment area, the operatory should be prepared for the scheduled treatment. Dental instruments should normally be covered with a paper napkin, because even though these are tools of the trade to the dentist, they may heighten fear and anxiety in the patient.

The assistant, properly trained, can do much to calm the patient and make each visit pleasant. Initial conversation should be light without rushing into the dental aspects of the visit. She should always read the patient's chart and check for a topic of conversation (something gleaned from the examination visit and noted in the chart). She should show the same interest in the patient as the receptionist did, always calling the patient by name (first or last, according to the patient's own preference) and being friendly. The treatment should also be reviewed in case the patient has a question concerning what will be done. Another way of extending the courtesy shown in the reception area into the operatory is to have a place to hang coats, hats, umbrellas, purses, shopping bags, and so on in the vicinity of or inside each operatory. Staff members can offer to assist patients in hanging up coats, hats, and personal belongings.

If the patient's treatment is going to be delayed, it is important to have reading material, music, or television to keep him or her occupied even in the operatory. Neglect of the patient at this phase of the visit is especially counterproductive. The patient, at this point, is likely to be very fearful (especially if this is the first treatment visit). Therefore, all effort must be taken to help the patient relax. Generally, the patient should not be left waiting in a reclining position in the treatment chair, as such a position can provoke feelings of helplessness, vulnerability, and anxiety.

Role of Dentist and Beginning of Treatment

During the first minute, give the patient your undivided attention — without washing your hands, viewing radiographs, or examining records.

The confidence of the patient can be won or lost by the manner and speech of the dentist. If he or she does not show self-confidence and a relaxed manner, the patient will immediately pick up on the professional insecurity and will be affected by it.

When you enter the operatory, greet the patient warmly and by name. During the first minute or so of the visit, it is important to give the patient your undivided attention — without washing your hands, viewing radiographs, or examining records. This is a good time to inquire of the patient how things have been going since the last visit. This attention serves several purposes: one, the patient will feel that you are not too busy to take a personal interest in him; two, a bit of small talk will ease any natural anxieties; and three, it will give the patient a chance to feel some control over what he is about to undergo. Topics of interest, hobbies, and so on can be noted on each person's chart for future conversation.

Going back to an inter-office system of communication, the dentist should always be aware of what time the patient arrived and how much time has elapsed. If the treatment has been delayed, some explanation should be offered, because this lets the patient know you take your work seriously and that you are genuinely sorry he or she

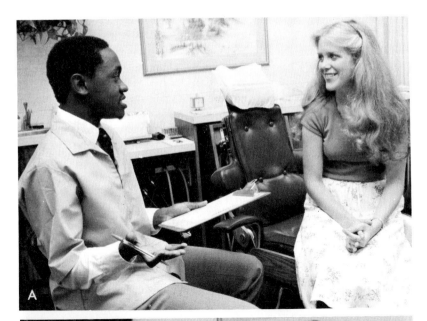

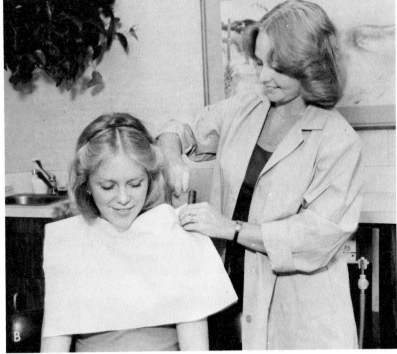

A, Dentist takes a few moments before treatment to chat with the patient. Note patient has not yet been reclined in the chair.

B, Warmth is an important quality for all members of the dental team.

was inconvenienced. You might also take the trouble to explain (if such was the case) that the delay was caused by your having to care for someone else in pain. This will impress upon the patient that you are a dentist who cares about people.

When it's time to focus in on the dental aspects of the visit, approach them in general terms, especially since the vast majority of patients know nothing of the technical terms you employ when talking to a colleague. Explain fully the work that will be done during the visit, which teeth will be involved, and so on. Also let the patient know that should teeth have to be extracted or prepared for crown and bridge, you will not leave any noticeable gaps where the teeth were and will place pleasing temporaries before the visit is completed. Always emphasize the positive aspects of the treatment, not the negative ones. The patient should be encouraged to ask questions pertaining to the treatment because clear communication between doctor and patient is essential in building and maintaining trust. It is good to inform the patient that every effort will be taken to make him as comfortable as possible during the visit. Approaching the patient in a nonthreatening way will help combat real or imagined fears.

In order to motivate people toward total dental health, the dentist must have a genuine interest in them, that is, view them as human beings with problems he or she can help to solve. Patients cooperate in assisting you to help them if they fully understand what you intend to do to their teeth. Approach adults, teens, and children with language selected for their own levels of comprehension. Children's cooperation will be enhanced if you talk to them as you do to your adult patients. No matter which age group you are addressing, do not forget that even though dentistry is simple to you, even intelligent lay people will have difficulty absorbing technical information. Pace your comments. Give the patient time to absorb what you say. A good rule of thumb is to speak slightly more slowly than the patient speaks. If there are any questions, answer them slowly and carefully. By doing so you will promote far better patient understanding of problems and treatment.

Clear communication between doctor and patient is essential in building and maintaining trust.

SELECTION OF TREATMENT FOR FIRST VISIT

For a first visit the dentist should consider selecting easy operative procedures as a means toward creating and developing a deeper doctor-patient trust. The visit should generally be short, relatively low-cost (especially if the patient pays the charge the same day), and involve as little postoperative discomfort as possible. Not only should this visit be designed to increase confidence and trust, but it should also encourage the patient to make successive visits that you deem necessary.

It would generally be imprudent to elect to extract third molars ("wisdom teeth" to the patient) during a first visit because of the potential for postoperative complications. If the patient suffers pain and discomfort at the beginning, you run the risk of destroying the confidence and trust that have thus far been built. It is wise, then, to plan the first visit with the idea of fostering the trusting relationship. Keep the pain potential low.

By beginning with a short, low-cost, easy operative appointment, the dentist can evaluate the patient even further before more complicated procedures are undertaken. You thereby have a chance to note the patient's cooperativeness, anxiety, and tolerance for dental procedures; you can also measure the patient's financial commitment and faithfulness in keeping appointments.

You might tell the patient that you have planned a short visit so you can get to know each other better. At the same time encourage patients to tell you how they feel after the appointment is over, and whether there was any anxiety or discomfort.

On the first visit, keep the pain potential low.

Explain that you want to schedule appointments for the patient's convenience and comfort. Some patients may prefer to have many short appointments because their level of tolerance for dental treatment is initially very low. If you work with these patients and show concern, their tolerance may increase very rapidly so that they may come to place more priority on your getting a certain amount of work accomplished during the visit than on any discomfort they may experience. With the right approach by the dentist, the majority of patients will fall into the pattern that good practice management encourages: long appointments that generate efficiency for the dentist and decrease the number of injections or missed work for the patient.

HANDLING FEAR OF PAIN AND THE UNKNOWN

First-visit patients are very unsure of what will happen during treatment. Much of their anxiety is really a fear of the unknown, which arises from their own experiences and the tales family and friends have told them about dental pain. The dentist, while he is not responsible for the patient's fears, must at least attempt to understand them. This is not always easy, because no two individuals have the same perception of pain. Each person has had unique experiences. The dentist must be ready to deal with patient fears, but should not accept guilt for creating those fears. He should employ his most favorable personality traits to adapt to the changing moods of patients and to carefully explain to them what will happen.

A soothing voice can allay fears and help the patient to relax and cooperate.

The cultivation and use of a soothing voice can be greatly beneficial in allaying fears and helping the patient to relax and cooperate. Since everyone receives some abuse and unfriendliness from the public each day, providing a port of calm in that tempest can be an asset for the dentist who is willing to develop a caring atmosphere in the office.

Sincerely expressed sympathy for fears of pain will go far toward getting the patient to trust you. When a patient conveys tension, it is of particular importance that you be cautious of your response or reaction. Froelich has said, "You cannot change how another human being feels by just commanding or telling this person how he or she *should* feel."

Telling the patient "Just relax," "There is nothing to be afraid of," or "Come on now, that didn't hurt," and so on will gain you absolutely nothing. You will get the same results by telling the patient, "This is going to hurt you more than it will me." Always remember how you yourself feel when *you* are on the receiving end of a needle.

A common-sense approach to explaining the treatment based on the data you have about the patient's personality and age is essential. Children especially fear the unknown and really have very little conception of what is going to happen in the dental chair. They will come closer to understanding what you are going to do if you simply tell them "I am going to take pictures of your teeth," or, "I am going to put your tooth to sleep and fix the hole in it." An elaborate explanation is not needed. With an adult, however, you may say, "We are going to take x-rays of all your teeth so we can determine your dental condition." Or, "After I inject your gum, I will remove the decay and place a silver filling in the tooth."

The needle and handpiece are both viewed by patients with trepidation that will range from mild to quite extreme. Even taking radiographs may create fear, especially in children. Any instruments used in treatment should be prepared and concealed prior to the patient's seating, if possible. If patients never see the instruments even when the dentist begins treatment, they will usually not experience fear.

Dentists should be aware of patient fears and phobias and devise methods to calm them.

A marketing tool widely used today to induce patients to relax is nitrous oxide analgesia, sometimes referred to as "laughing gas." Because of its calming effect, it is especially useful as an aid in giving injections and during treatment. It would be wise to have nitrous oxide available whether or not it is routinely used since many patients will initially inquire as to its availability. Patients may request "gas" during the first visit and from that point on not require it again.

In using nitrous oxide the dentist may find a different set of fears to overcome in certain patients. For instance, it has been documented by Rosenbaum that teenagers are fearful they will confess secret thoughts and feelings while under the "gas." Teens also exhibit fears that they may have some dreaded disease of the mouth, that you will hurt their mouths, and that they will be treated like children.

Dentists should be aware of such fears and phobias and devise methods to calm them. If the patient is particularly nervous, you may wish to prescribe a mild tranquilizer to be taken prior to the first visit. Provided this method is successful, the adult patient may not require this medication on the second visit. Children may also be premedicated to soothe them during the initial treatment.

Giving the Injection

It's true that no one completely overcomes the fear of a hypodermic needle meant for injection into gum tissue. However, the dentist can make it a little less frightening by telling the truth. If you say, "This is going to pinch for a moment or two," the patient will have more confidence in you because of your candor. To go even further in comforting the patient, the dentist should become adept at the use of topical anesthesia. "Painless" injections are great practice builders; people who say they "can't stand going to the dentist" will go, and go gladly, to a dentist who can inject them without causing pain. You should describe as normal the tingling sensation the patient feels in the lips and tongue. Also warn your patient not to chew on gum tissues while they are numb. A cotton roll may be inserted between a child patient's teeth to help prevent damage from chewing.

Prior to the injection, tell the patient that if he or she experiences significant discomfort to either raise a hand or make a sound, so you can stop. The patient will thus feel more in control. Make sure he understands not to move his head or make jerking movements, as this will only tend to increase the pain or cause injury.

With some patients you may simply have to become adept at convincing them that the discomfort from being injected is bearable, and get them to relax and trust you. Patience, a soothing voice, and an easy manner on your part will be your best allies in such an effort.

Many times the numbness following an injection will give the distinct impression that the face or jaw is swollen, and the patient may feel that something is amiss. By your describing the feeling and showing the patient in a mirror that there is no swelling, you will greatly relieve his fears.

After the injection, inform the patient of how long it will take the anesthetic to become effective. Say that you will proceed when the gum is fully anesthetized. Be sure to raise the chair to a sitting position and provide some reading matter, music, or television for the interim period, or else fear and anxiety may again invade the patient's psyche.

During Treatment

Prior to treatment endeavor to make the patient understand that everything that will be done is for his or her benefit. Also tell him that if he is troubled with your technique, to please stop you. If there is no alternative, inform the patient in a kind way that you are aware of his discomfort but could he please bear with it for just a moment longer. Any time discomfort is present, apologize for it but play it down by dwelling on the positives. For instance, praise the patient for his cooperation.

During treatment, informing the patient at each step gives him the psychological advantage of pacing himself.

During the course of treatment it is wise to keep the patient informed at each step. This gives him the psychological advantage of pacing himself. If a bite block is employed, remove it from the patient's mouth every so often to give the jaw a rest. Any time treatment is extensive, let the patient have a break. Suggest that he walk around or visit the restroom. These small tension breakers, like comedy relief in a drama, will be greatly appreciated.

The patient will invariably note your concern for his welfare during treatment. Other little extras such as providing disposable sunglasses to reduce the glare from the treatment light, tissues to remove lipstick, lubricant for the lips, and relief from having the mouth open too long similarly suggest to patients that you really care about them.

DEALING WITH CHILDREN

A very good marketing technique for building a practice is the successful treatment of children. Parents often bring their children to a dentist before they come in themselves. If you prove by the way you handle their offspring that you are a caring and competent dentist, the parents will very likely come to you, too — and recommend you to their friends.

Continuing education courses in the child management area can be important in spurring the growth of a practice. Since operative techniques for children are relatively simple, one of the most difficult tasks is managing the young patients during treatment. To be successful in treating young patients, the dentist needs to have knowledge and training in such techniques as voice control, the controversial hand-over-mouth technique, show and tell, and positive reinforcement. The use of nitrous oxide and adjunct drugs will also be a big help in the treatment of difficult children.

Suppose there is a child in the treatment area who is loud, disorderly, and crying. The dentist decides to employ voice control by leaning close to the child and raising the voice in a no-nonsense way — "Johnny! Stop it!" As soon as the child's attention is obtained the child should immediately be praised for good behavior and cooperation. "Good! Now you're being a big boy!"

A second technique is to simply place a hand over the unruly child-patient's mouth and say, "I won't move my hand away until you settle down." Again, you gain the child's attention, and with an assuring tone of voice, offer a comment of praise when the child calms down.

Show and tell is simply letting the patient see the dental instruments you will use and explaining how they will help the child to have healthy teeth. This can easily be done by an auxiliary.

Getting a child to actively participate in the treatment goes a long way toward making the appointment a pleasant one. It is safe to allow the child to help mix the alginate for impressions, help develop x-rays, and assist you in actual treatment by holding some instrument for you. A potentially negative visit may be turned into an adventure for the child, which makes the job of providing professional services much easier for you the dentist.

Getting a child to actively participate in the treatment goes a long way toward making the appointment pleasant.

END OF VISIT

When the treatment phase of that first visit is over, the dentist must still work at keeping the patient's trust. What occurs at the end of a visit will be what the patient remembers best — even more than some of the unpleasant moments in the operatory. As a speaker can make his important points in closing, so can a dentist cement relationships at the visit's end. This can hardly be overemphasized.

At the end of the visit you will want to review the work that has been accomplished and outline what will be done during ensuing visits. Be sure to inform the patient what to expect from his treatment, such as sensitivity from metal temporaries, deep fillings, pulpotomy, and so on. Explain that temporaries will be in for only a short time and may be somewhat off-color. Add, of course, that the custom crowns being made will be color-matched to the patient's teeth.

The last few minutes of the first appointment are considered

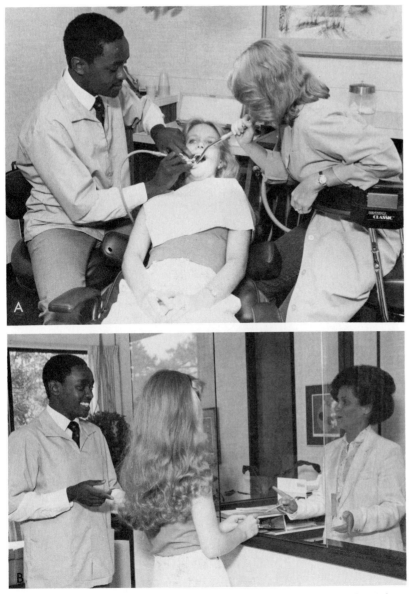

A, While treatment is under way, the good dentist and assistant will always keep the patient's comfort in mind.

B, The dentist sees the patient out to the reception area. This is excellent marketing practice.

Illustration continued on following page

highly important in building a good doctor-patient relationship. In tense moments the dentist should inform the patient of the benefits the treatment just completed will provide, such as more comfort and better appearance. And during this time, thank the patient for his cooperation and laud him for keeping the appointment. He will appreciate you more and, as a result, may refer his friends and relatives to you.

Take this time to inquire if the patient has any questions concerning the treatment. It is bad for your practice if the patient

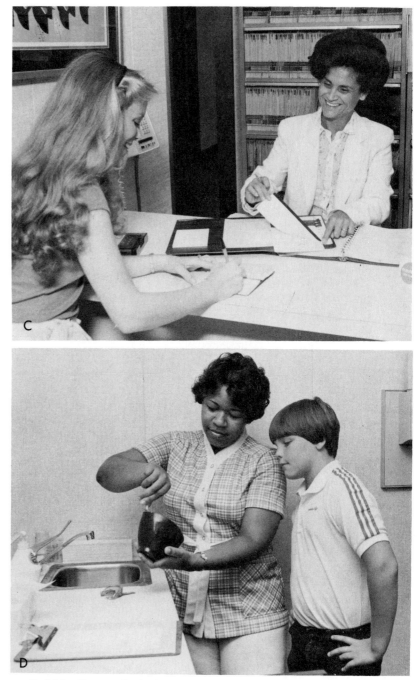

C, A friendly receptionist is vital to the marketing effort.
D, The curious child patient (and which of them isn't curious?) likes to be brought in on how things work.

ever leaves the office feeling uncomfortable, confused, or dissatisfied because of any portion of the treatment or the financial arrangements. As you discuss the treatment with the patient emphasize all the positives. You may even get him to agree that the visit was, overall, a pleasant experience. The power of suggestion can be used in planting "seeds" that will lead to more patient confidence in your ability and less patient fear of treatment.

Briefly, review the work that will be accomplished during the next visit. When the patient is ready to leave, be quick to assist with coats, hats, and personal belongings. If the patient is a woman, direct her to a mirror so that she might freshen her makeup or comb her hair. If the patient is a child, use imaginative-positive devices, such as a sticker on the cheek reading "My mouth is numb — don't let me chew it" or a rubber stamp on the back of the hand stating "I'm a good dental patient."

Postoperative Instructions

Even though you may have carefully explained what to expect following treatment, do not rely on verbal communication alone to get the message across. Remember that the patient has been in an unfamiliar environment and may be unable to retain explicit information. So, have the instructions written out, preferably on a single sheet of paper. Include data about the treatment that was just completed and about what can be expected after leaving the office. It is doubly important to include instruction on how to relieve any possible discomfort. To simplify matters, color-coded instruction sheets may be given for each procedure (see Fig. 14–1). Give any necessary prescriptions at this time.

If the treatment is expected to cause discomfort, so inform the patient and give an assurance that you want him to call if he has a question or unexpected additional discomfort after he returns home. As a result of such counseling, the majority of patients will not call except for a true emergency.

Have postoperative instructions written out.

Charles Marks, DDS   739–7056
STAINLESS STEEL CROWN

Your child has been fitted with a stainless steel crown. After the gums were numb, we removed all decay from the tooth and prepared it for the crown. Then the crown was cemented to the tooth.

Because the margin of the crown was placed below the gum line to help prevent further decay, the gums may be tender for a few days.

Please watch to be sure your child doesn't chew on the insides of the cheek, tongue, or lip while they are numb. The feeling should return within one to three hours. Please call if any problem develops.

Figure 14–1. Postoperative instructions. One sheet of instructions can be given for each procedure performed during the visit.

Responsiveness to Patients

In order to show your concern even further, have the reception-ist prepare a call list of selected patients who have had extensive crown and bridge, root canal, periodontal surgery, oral surgery, or any other procedure that generally has associated postoperative pain. This will require only a few minutes of your time each day. And it could be the single best practice builder you will ever use (see Fig. 14–2).

It is worth your time to return patient calls rather than rely-ing on your auxiliaries.

Instruct the office personnel that when a patient calls with a problem, it should be treated as such and not taken lightly or ignored. If a patient feels strongly enough about something to place a call to your office, that "something" certainly qualifies as a problem. The dental office staff should be instructed to show the same courtesy and interest in the patient on the telephone as they did during the office visit. When responding to a "called-in problem," use as full an explanation as possible. Many times the problem will pertain to something the patient was told would occur following treatment, but which he probably forgot. There are times, however, when the problem is something new that has developed. Patients should be encouraged to call again should new problems occur that were not expected. The dentist should also establish guidelines with the receptionist for when he or she is to be summoned to the telephone to talk with a patient. One case would be when the nature of the problem the patient has described does not jibe with the normally expected results following a given treatment. The receptionist should, in most cases, inform the patient that the dentist will call back "soon." It is worth your time to return patient calls rather than relying on your auxiliaries, though in some instances, auxiliaries can handle a situa-tion perfectly well and satisfy the patient's need for an answer or reas-surance.

In dealing with such things as postoperative pain, honesty is best. If the patient is given a full explanation of what to expect *before* it happens, you will be a hero. If afterwards you say only, "I knew that would happen," the patient is going to think you are making excuses. Remember: the patient will have confidence in you if what you say and do turn out to be true in his own experience.

DATE:		
NAME	PROCEDURE	PHONE
John Taylor	Pulpotomy	482–1675
Marcia Goforth	Perio surgery	587–2377
Susan Miller	3rd molars	739–2211
Sissy Brown	Root canal	487–6258
Tom Ware	Root canal	865–1399

Figure 14–2. Patient call list. This list is made up daily by the receptionist so the dentist can call patients who may experience postoperative discomfort or compli-cations.

SUMMARY

The treatment visit offers the opportunity for the entire dental staff to work toward a deeper development of patient trust. The primary tools in this undertaking are communication, kindness, and concern.

If patients are recognized by name, they will feel important; if they are provided with pleasant distractions, they will feel less anxious; if they receive explanations before procedures are begun, they will be less fearful. If they know you will respond with kindness to their pain and discomfort, they will relax; if they believe you have been truthful in both action and word, they will trust you. And they will not only return for future treatment but they will also send their friends and neighbors to you. Thus, enhancement of patient trust during the first treatment visit is a primary foundation stone in building a dental practice.

REFERENCES

Blass, J. L.: Dentistry as Personal Service. Philadelphia, J. B. Lippincott Company, 1963.

Brahe, N. B., DDS: Great Ideas for Dental Practice. Vol. 1 and 2. Appleton, Wis, Project D Publications, 1973.

Carr, J. H., DDS: How to be a patient's best friend. Dental Practice, June, 1981, pp. 73–75.

Dunlap, J. E., DDS: Do you have a waiting room? Dental Economics, December, 1977, pp. 68–74.

Froelich, R. E., et al.: Communication in the Dental Office. Saint Louis, C. V. Mosby Company, 1976, pp. 65–68.

Hollander, L. N., DDS: Modern Dental Practice: Concepts and Procedures, Philadelphia, W. B. Saunders Company, 1967.

Marks, G., MA: How to Practice Successful Dentistry. Philadelphia, J. B. Lippincott Company, 1963, pp. 162–166.

Martin, R. T.: An Exploratory Investigation of The Dentist/Patient Relationship. The Dental Health Education & Research Foundation of the University of Sydney, October, 1965.

Neuberger, E. J.: Reduce fear with sensory confusion. Dental Practice, May, 1981, pp. 88–90.

Protell, M. R., et al.: Psychodynamics in Dental Practice. Springfield, Ill., Charles C Thomas, 1975, pp. 147–157 and 252–256.

Rosenbaum, V.: Whatever Happened to Those Teen-Age Dropouts? Reprint from Dental Economics, September, 1974.

Stephens, D. W., DDS: How to develop key patients. Dental Management, July, 1981, pp. 28–31.

What Do You Say Before You Say "Goodbye"? AAPA Communicator, May, 1976.

Zunin, L., Contact: The First Four Minutes. New York, Ballantine Books, 1973.

15

Retaining Patients

Even a thriving garden, full of lush vegetable plants, grapes, melons, and flowers, can wither and die in a hurry if left unwatered and unfertilized for very long. Just as living organisms stabilize life processes by homeostasis, so must the vital dental practice maintain at least stability, or grow at a desired rate, or it will wither and die. A vital dental practice does not just happen. It results from planning, hard work, and dedication from the whole dental team. And much of the focus of a healthy practice is on the retention of patients.

Given that approximately 20 percent of a dentist's patients may move away annually, retaining as many patients as possible of the remaining 80 percent is essential (at least as important as adding new patients, really).

POST–TREATMENT CONFERENCE

For a long time dentists have invested time and energy in perfecting the treatment conference. And rightly so. But the conference *after* treatment can probably pay even larger dividends, which become reinvested in the life of the practice. It is at this time that the patient more fully understands the benefits of the treatment, which, at the treatment conference, you tried so hard to describe persuasively. Whatever improvements have been obtained in esthetics are more apparent; in comfort and function, more evident. In other words, the patient is a living example of what you described before treatment. At this time the patient can readily appreciate the previous conditions in his mouth and the treatment for those conditions.

Do all patients need to be scheduled for a conference? No. But be careful about deciding that it is not necessary. Paul Jacobi says such a conference will pay handsome dividends. The tendency is for dentists who have not scheduled a post-treatment conference to doubt its value and feel that the patient would not be interested. Of course, if you have done very minimal treatment or if the patient is the second or third member of the family, the post-treatment conference may not be necessary. Otherwise, why not explain to the patient at the last treatment appointment that you would like to see him and make

Remember: as long as you need patients, you have time (and it doesn't take much) to do post-treatments.

minor corrections if necessary "just to be sure that everything is okay." If the patient balks (not likely if you have related well), you can forget it. Remember: as long as you need patients, you have time (and it doesn't take much) to do post-treatments. If you do not schedule a separate appointment, you should at least recap the experience at the final treatment visit. And ask the patient to "help us do a better job by filling out the questionnaire" (see Fig. 15–1).

The purpose of the conference, other than marketing, is to:
— Find out whether the patient is satisfied and comfortable, and if not, what can be done to make him feel so.
— Review the dental problems, the treatment, and the rationale.

Scheduling

When should this session be scheduled? Especially for persons who have had extensive treatment, set aside an appointment for this purpose only. Otherwise, the impact will be lost in the routine of the final treatment visit. Also, time is needed for the disappearance of postoperative sensitivity, which may occur after surgery or placement of a restoration. Possibly, after final definitive treatment you may need to make very minor adjustments to ensure complete comfort and longevity of the restoration. For most patients an appointment about two to four weeks after treatment will work out well.

The marketing dentist can ill afford dissatisfied patients.

Patient Satisfaction

At this juncture patient satisfaction is essential to the ongoing health of your practice. If for any reason the patient is dissatisfied, you should do everything possible and within reason to gain the patient's satisfaction. What is "necessary" might range from discussion through a minor adjustment on a restoration to replacement of the restoration. The marketing dentist can ill afford dissatisfied patients.

In fact, as Robert Levoy says, beyond being satisfied you want the patient to be enthusiastic about the experience and result of the treatment in your office. Enthusiastic patients refer more people than do merely satisfied patients.

People vary in their capacity to be satisfied, let alone to be enthusiastic. Not every patient for whom you complete treatment will be a big booster of your practice. If you and your staff have been true helpers, however, the patients who are enthusiastic by nature will refer their friends to your office. Others will refer, too, but to a lesser extent.

Soliciting Referrals

Even the enthusiastic patient needs encouragement. Traditionally people have believed that dentists are overworked trying to care for all the people who seek their services. This belief may have been reinforced by dentists themselves, who used to appear to be almost unavailable. Of course, some dentists have truly been overworked and could hardly care for any new patients. With the increasing supply of dentists most dentists are not now overworked and are seeking new patients. In order to obtain referrals, the dentist must ask for them.

How does one go about asking? First, decide whether you do in fact need new patients. Then decide that you are going to solicit referrals from your patients, who are your best source. The degree of directness depends upon your philosophy and your personality. Some are comfortable doing this in a very direct manner by saying something like, "Mrs. Taylor, we have enjoyed doing your dentistry. We hope you've had good experiences here. We would like you to refer other fine people like yourself to our office. We will give them the same quality care that you feel you've received."

If this is too direct for your taste, you can utilize a post-treatment questionnaire such as Doctor Richard Rossi of Rochester, Minnesota does (Fig. 15–1). You can even obtain a business reply permit and print your address on the back of the questionnaire so that the patient can fold and mail it. You may choose to do both. The questionnaire also provides the patient with an opportunity to give you feedback on how he perceived the treatment and to offer suggestions. This will enable you to better understand the total needs of your patients and how you can improve your service.

Dr. Rossi reports that his patients invariably mention the pleasant comfortable atmosphere of his office. Specifically they appreciate the calm, relaxed staff and the use of nitrous oxide analgesia coupled with stereo music headphones.

Regardless of how directly or how subtly you solicit referrals, you will need to express appreciation to your patients. It has been said that business goes where it is appreciated. That is as true, or maybe more so, of a professional service such as dentistry as of any commercial product or service. Patients risk their health, not merely their money, with dentists. It is logical for people to believe that the dentist who appreciates patients will treat them better.

> It has been said that business goes where it is appreciated. That is as true of a professional service such as dentistry as of any commercial product or service.

History of Treatment

By the time extensive treatment is completed, the patient may have forgotten the original conditions. For such patients you may need complete pre-treatment and post-treatment records. Chief among these for impressing patients are before and after photographs, especially if esthetics have been improved. Before and after models will demonstrate the improvement of function by restoration of the occlusion. If you choose to make postoperative radiographs, you may be able to demonstrate the elimination of some disease conditions. However, you should be cautious. Remember that your patient is not a dentist (except in rare cases) and will not have the same appreciation for the technical excellence that you do. As in all discussions with patients, the dentist must avoid jargon (technical

It is our hope that you have been pleased with the dental care received from us. It is also our desire to offer you the best of dental treatment in the future. By working together on preventive care of your mouth, we can keep your dental treatment needs to a minimum in the future.

So we may serve you better, will you please take a minute or two now to answer these questions? We appreciate it.

1. Were you referred to our office by someone? _____ Yes _____ No

   If Yes, who referred you? _____

                                     (Name)   (Title)

2. Have you referred anyone to us? _____ Yes _____ No

   Would you recommend our services to others? _____ Yes _____ No

3. In general, do you feel you are well treated in our office? _____ Yes _____ No

   By everyone? _____ Yes _____ No

   If not, in what way were you not treated well?

   _____

   _____

   _____

4. What do you like most about our treatment?_____

   _____

   What do you like least?_____

   _____

5. Have you any suggestions to improve our service to you in the future?_____

   _____

   _____

6. How do you feel about our preventive attitude and home care instruction?_____

   _____

   _____

NAME (if you wish)_____DATE_____

Please leave this at our office or fold and mail. No postage is necessary.

Thank you very much, have a good day.

Figure 15–1. Post-treatment questionnaire. (Adapted from a questionnaire developed by Dr. Richard Rossi.)

language). Speak plainly. Emphasize the *benefits* that are already evident to the patient: appearance, comfort, and ability to chew. Pay particular attention to benefits relating to any problem for which the patient originally sought care.

The *etiology* ("cause" to the patient) of the original problems should be reviewed. Talk with the patient about how he is doing in controlling those causes and whether there are any particular problems. Is he cleaning his teeth effectively? How about eating habits? Or any other factors? A caring manner on the part of the dentist improves the effectiveness of such discussions. Dentists have acquired the reputation of badgering patients. You almost have to figuratively lean over backwards to avoid coming across as a nagging parent. Nagging, after all, neither recognizes the patient's autonomy nor stimulates patient responsibility.

Free people find their own ways, according to Arthur Combs. Dentists need to acknowledge individuals' freedom, because that freedom is a fact. We cannot control other people's behavior, only attempt to influence it. Our patients deserve our support in their attempts to care for their teeth. They may find it difficult to exercise the discipline necessary for effective home care. We, for our part, can try to be understanding of their problems and assist in any way we can. This helping approach should be reinforced at the post-treatment conference. Otherwise, patients may feel that they must pretend to do what we want them to do, whether they can or not, whether they choose to or not. As Carl Rogers reminds us, a helper is by definition real and cannot help in the face of pretense.

> Nagging neither recognizes the patient's autonomy nor stimulates patient responsibility.

This is a good time to review the rationale ("reason" to the patient) for the kind of treatment done. Especially so if alternative modes of treatment were discussed and the patient agreed to the dentist's first recommendation. Again the highly satisfied patient is a living example of the reason for the particular kind of treatment. For the more logical kinds of people, the reasons for the specific treatment make eminently good sense and give them reasons to refer other patients.

Although *limitations* of treatment must be discussed before treatment, they are much more acceptable to the satisfied patient afterwards. If limitations were appropriately presented before, they may seem less limiting after. However, if the limitations are on the longevity of the treatment, they must at this time be put in perspective. By all means, be honest with people and do not raise false hopes. Exquisite home care by the patient can result from the knowledge that such care can extend the life of his teeth.

Incomplete Treatment

Up to now we have been discussing patients who had complete treatment as recommended by the dentist. However, this may be the exception in most practices, especially those in which ideal treatment is recommended for people whose financial resources do not permit them to readily complete such treatment. As we noted before, the alternative may be to do treatment in phases over a drawn out period of time — perhaps even years.

> After disease is under control, you can proceed at a deliberate pace in accordance with the patient's resources to pay for treatment or with the patient's readiness to accept treatment.

When the initial phase of treatment is complete, schedule the post-treatment conference. As for the completed patient, the history of treatment to that point should be reviewed — etiology, rationale, and limitations. Control of the dental disease must be accomplished in the initial phase — called by some dentists "the control phase."

After the disease is under control, you can proceed at a deliberate pace in accordance with the patient's resources to pay for treatment or with the patient's readiness to accept treatment. If you have a large number of patients, you may suggest this yourself, in order to accomplish treatment for more patients. This method permits gradual intake of procedures, so as to even the work load between periods of peak demand and those of low demand. Thus, there are many advantages of phasing treatment.

A *written plan* is advantageous for the purpose of scheduling treatment in phases. You may want to write one for the patient in plain language and one for yourself in technical terms. Treatment should be divided logically into portions that can be done independently of each other. In rare instances and always for edentulous people it may be impossible to do treatment in phases. Otherwise, you can complete restoration of the teeth in segments.

At the post-treatment conference the patient needs to know how much of the plan has been accomplished, what remains to be done, and what segment will be treated next. If the patient desires any particular order of treatment, that should be accommodated unless there are professional reasons for following a different order. Agreement should be reached based on trade-offs between patient desires and clinical problems. A patient's autonomy always deserves respect.

> Patients, not dentists, are responsible for their dental health.

Planning

The purposes of planning further activity are several. Most obvious is the preservation, and maybe the improvement, of the patient's dental health. Dentists are surely interested in progressing toward a higher trust/lower fear relationship with the patient. Many dentists have begun to look beyond the patient's dental health to a total view of health, often referred to as the holistic approach.

If dentists are to be helpers, as described in Chpater 11, they need to relinquish control to patients. Patients, not dentists, are responsible for their dental health. And so, patients must participate in planning future activities relative to their dental health.

As far as recall appointments go, we suggest that patients be given as much choice as possible. If we dentists believe (as Combs says helpers do) that people are able to manage their own problems better than anyone else can, we must operate our recall system for *their* convenience, rather than our own. It should support them in their quest for dental health, but not force them to do certain things. The system should provide choices for patients.

The first choice is whether they want to be reminded in any way of when they should return for preventive purposes. In the nonthreatening atmosphere of the helping dental office, they can surely choose to be responsible for making an appointment when they believe that they need it.

The dentist or hygienist can best determine the appropriate interval before the next visit and should recommend accordingly. If the patient chooses to vary somewhat from this, he has that right. Acknowledgment of this right would allay suspicion that the recall system serves the dentist's purposes, rather than the patient's. As it is, most dentists probably give patients the choice of the day of the week and the time of day for the appointment.

The patient can and should be given a choice as to how he will be notified of the appointment. That could vary: an advance appointment made at the last visit with no notification, a written notice of an appointment, a written notice to call for an appointment, a telephone call asking him to make an appointment. You probably have a favorite system. It may not be the favorite with all of your patients. Consider giving each patient a choice and manage the variations within the office. It may be well worth it in increased effectiveness.

Other Considerations

Who should conduct the post-treatment conference? As for the treatment planning conference, whoever has the skills and the knowledge could conduct the conference. You, the dentist, may prefer to do it, or you may delegate it to a qualified auxiliary. It could be a joint effort involving two or more team members. The treatment coordinator or patient communicator who is employed on some larger staffs is a natural for it. Regardless of who does it, the effectiveness of the process is crucial.

Another dental prophylaxis may be done when all other treatment is completed. Many dentists include this in their overall treatment fee, so that for financial reasons few patients would be reluctant to have it done. In fact, some dentists include the first recall preventive visit in their service fee. If a prophylaxis is not necessary, it makes more sense to compliment the patient for his effective home care and not do the prophylaxis.

The interdependence of the relationship should be reinforced at this time. If you have expressed appreciation to the patient for the opportunity to do his dentistry, if you have asked the patient for referral of friends, if you have stressed the importance of preventive maintenance, including appropriate services in the dental office, you have reinforced your mutual interests and concerns, and your interdependence. The patient continues to need your support, and you surely need each patient's support.

RECALL SYSTEM

Every individual patient should be aware of some particular reason why he should return on a periodic basis.

From a marketing perspective this time-honored term leaves something to be desired. "Recall" appears to be more for the benefit of the dentist than for that of the patient. "Prevention," "maintenance," "health promotion" are more attractive terms from the patient's vantage point. Although you may prefer to think of it as "the recall system," some other term such as preventive maintenance is more patient oriented. A positive term such as "promotion" is advantageous over a negative term such as "prevention." One can easily become finicky about semantics. Give it some thought and refer to the system appropriately. Even though "recall system" lacks market appeal, we shall use that term to avoid confusion.

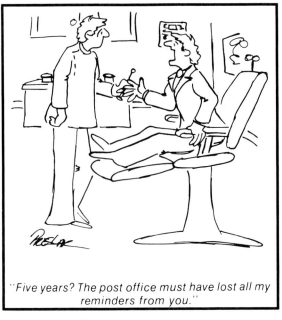

"Five years? The post office must have lost all my reminders from you."

Courtesy of *Cal* magazine.

Personalization

Every individual patient should be aware of some particular reason why he should return on a periodic basis. You can record potential problems to be evaluated at the next recall visit on the recall record card or dental chart. In the absence of perfect dental health, there are always restorative or periodontal problems, which need to be watched. Even in the perfectly healthy mouth the dental hygiene may be less than perfect. If you and the patient are striving for perfection in this regard, you (or your hygienist) may note the problem areas and assist the patient to accomplish his goal. A word of caution: Be sure the patient is actually committed to perfection (and few of us are). Otherwise, you will be nagging — not the way to make friends. If you have to try hard to find a problem that needs this kind of attention, you are providing a personalized and excellent service to your patients. They will feel that you are treating them as individuals.

As you do the treatment procedures, you can begin to build your case. Conditions that require a significant length of time for improvement especially need to be pointed out. You can stress early and regular care from the beginning as a means of treating dental disease that the patient cannot prevent.

Purposes

The recall system serves a variety of purposes. Among other things the system: (1) supports the patient; (2) re-establishes the relationship; (3) informs the patient of the dental health status; (4) updates the health history; (5) reinforces the feeling that we care; and (6) creates ambassadors of good dental health.

A goal to which the patient is not committed is no goal at all.

As helpers our first concern should be to support the patient. To do this we must update ourselves on the patient's goals. If we personalize our approach, we will be prepared to proceed on previously agreed-upon goals. We can challenge the patient to accept more ambitious goals, but we must respect his or her autonomy in choosing goals. A goal to which the patient is not committed is no goal at all.

As you and the patient update goals, you will be re-establishing the relationship. Also during this process it is natural to inform the patient of his dental health status. If the process is managed well, the patient will be impressed again that you care. And in accordance with their personalities, patients will be your goodwill ambassadors. All of this depends upon your responsiveness to their needs.

You will need to update the health history for medico-legal purposes as well as for the purpose of enabling you to better serve patients. An easy way to do this is to add to the history form more "yes/no" columns which will be dated when they are filled out. Elderly patients need close attention, because their health states change more than do those of young people.

Kinds of Systems

There are three basic systems: (1) advance appointment; (2) notification by mail; (3) notification by telephone.

Scheduling an advance appointment when the patient is in for his last visit is perhaps the simplest method. But it involves problems, both for patients and for the dental team. Patients may forget or schedule something that will conflict, such as a vacation. Some of the dental team may be out for continuing education, professional meetings, and even vacation. As noted previously, patients should be given a choice of whether they want to be notified and if so, how. You might be reluctant to honor a request not to notify. These are likely to be very rare, and if they occur, those patients are likely to show. We suggest that you give patients this choice and allow them to be responsible if they choose. Most will say "Please notify me." This can be done by mail, by telephone, or by both.

In the notify-by-mail system two basic variations are possible: (1) notification of an appointment time, (2) notification to call for an appointment. Some dentists give a discount on the recall fee (as an incentive to call) to those patients who call within a designated period of time such as a week, or maybe even a month, of the time of notification by mail. You can follow up by telephone a week or two after the notice is sent to "be sure the patient received it." In this way the appointment time can be confirmed or arranged. In many offices patients are asked at their last visit to address the post card or envelope in their own handwriting. The theory is that most people will readily open and read mail which they have addressed to themselves. Also the wording "As you requested" can remind them of the agreed-upon arrangement. Many dentists prefer envelopes with an enclosed note rather than a plain post card because it provides more privacy and projects a more professional image. An eye-catching color, such as azure, may be preferred for its attention-getting power.

Most people will readily open and read mail which they have addressed to themselves.

Notification by telephone requires more staff time, but those who use this system think it is more effective. Arrange making calls when you are most likely to reach the patient. It is a good idea to establish with the patients what will be the best times to reach them, and whether to call them at work or at home. Otherwise, you and your staff can end up wasting a lot of time. The calls for the month can be spread over the entire month so as to even the load rather than attempting to call at the first of the month for everyone in that month's file.

When you do contact the individual patient, your approach should be persuasive but not pushy. If your relationship with the patient has been perceived by the patient as being primarily for his or her benefit, there should be no problem in your arranging a previously agreed-upon visit. Being pushy on the telephone is likely to be ineffective. Personal situations do change, and each individual who is capable of dealing with his own problems can best determine what action is appropriate.

Being pushy on the telephone is likely to be ineffective.

Your appointment system should be flexible enough to satisfy the preferences of each patient within reasonable limits. The patient who wants to make an advance appointment and not be notified should be accommodated. So should the patient who wants a written notification with or without telephone followup. Also the patient who desires to be called by telephone to arrange an appointment. Most dentists have developed a recall system that seems most effective with their individual patients or easiest for the staff. We are arguing that the most effective (from the marketing standpoint) system is one that is flexible enough to accommodate the preferences of *all* of your patients.

Incomplete Treatment

For those patients whose planned treatment is not complete, you need a way of keeping track. A computer provides a very easy means. Otherwise, you can list the incomplete phases of treatment on the recall file card and check them off as they are completed, or you can check them off the written plan as they are done. Many dentists have developed forms for this specific purpose. You may choose to keep this information in a loose-leaf notebook with a page for each patient. The point is that the dentist who is really taking care of his or her patients needs a way of keeping track of their needs. How else can the dentist satisfy those needs? As in all other situations, this should be done in a caring manner respectful of the patient's autonomy.

RETRIEVING PATIENTS

Value

Although "retrieval" may sound a bit manipulative, you do need some system (whatever you call it) for communicating with drop-out patients. For most dentists who have been in active practice more than just a few years, there is enough uncompleted treatment in their files to keep them busy for a long time. Of course, even with followup it will never all be completed, and certainly without followup most of it will never be completed. With a good system of followup or retrieval for those patients who have dropped out of (or were never included in) the recall system, much of this uncompleted treatment can and will be accomplished.

Methods

For most dentists who have been in active practice more than just a few years, there is enough uncompleted treatment in their files to keep them busy for a long time.

How can you retrieve lost patients? By "lost patients" we mean those who are not expected to return to your office under active treatment or on recall. Most dentists prefer to review the recall system for persons who do not respond. In many instances, after a year, or whenever the patient would be due for the next recall visit after the missed one, a form letter is sent to the patient which says in essence, "We will no longer notify you about the need for a followup visit, but we will be happy to see you if you need us." Such a letter stimulates some patients to resume preventive visits. You may even choose to be more persuasive, especially with patients more susceptible to dental disease.

Color coding the patient records by the year last seen would enable your staff to sort out quickly the records of those patients who have not been seen for more than a year. Similar color coding of file cards in either a rotary file or drawer could also be done.

Computers can be used for this same purpose. In fact the computer with a word processor can generate letters for each patient being notified. It may even be possible to personalize the letter according to the patient's dental condition. Such personalization is more effective than a form letter.

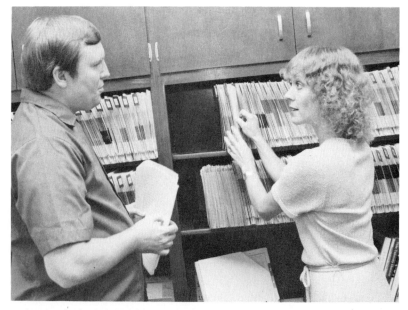

A receptionist briefs the dentist on her efforts to retrieve "lost patients" from the files.

Communication

Effective contact with the patient is your goal. As with the recall system, your communication should convey to the patient that you care about his health, not that you "need business." Wording should be carefully chosen for this purpose, whether your computer generates a letter, you develop a form letter, or you write a personal letter. If caringness is part of the office atmosphere and is portrayed in the letter, there is a good possibility that the patient will return. Of course, we all must recognize that patients' circumstances restrict what they can do. And we must face the fact that we cannot please everyone. It has been said that trying to please everyone pleases no one.

Correspondence should be followed up by telephone. If the patient fails to call within your prescribed period of a week to a month, your secretary can call "to be sure you received our letter," which makes sense in our highly mobile society. And to assure the patient that "we want to help in any way we can."

If caringness is part of the office atmosphere and is portrayed in the letter, there is a good possibility that the patient will return.

How can you follow up on the patient who has not responded since the treatment conference? You may feel that you have done all you can do and it would be unseemly to pursue the patient further. If you don't feel this way, your secretary can call the patient "just to check to see if there is any other way we can help you."

The "lost" patients may well be the "acre of diamonds" in your own backyard. Traditionally, more needed dentistry has been left undone than has been done for patients whose records fill our file cabinets. If you are marketing well, there will be fewer and fewer "lost ones" among your current patients. But look over the old records. They may prove valuable.

SUMMARY

Good marketing requires that the dentist understand and be responsive to the patients' needs. After treatment has been accomplished, the dentist should ascertain that the patient is fully satisfied. The patient should be informed as to the dentist's recommendations on how his dental health can be enhanced or, at least, maintained. Together, they should plan a continuing program. The dentist should support the patient in pursuit of his (the patient's) goals.

Further, the dentist should attempt to re-establish contact with patients who no longer seek regular attention. However, the control and autonomy of the patient must be recognized and respected. The marketing dentist always offers to help but never insists that the patient behave in a prescribed manner.

REFERENCES

Avila, D. L., Combs, P.: The Helping Relationship Sourcebook. Boston, Allyn & Bacon, Inc., 1973, pp. 300–412.

Brahe, N.: We Like These Ideas. Appleton, WI, Project D Publications, 1970, pp. 417–442.

Bregstein, S. J.: Interviewing, Counseling and Managing Dental Patients. Englewood Cliffs, NJ, Prentice-Hall, Inc., 1957, pp. 173–185.

Egan, G.: The Skillfull Helper. Monterey, CA, Brooks/Cole Pub. Co., 1975, pp. 182–232.

Hollander, L.: Modern Dental Practice. Philadelphia, W. B. Saunders Co., 1967, pp. 185–191.

Jacobi, H. P.: Dentists' Flight Manual to Success. Neenah, WI, Project P, 1967.

Levoy, R. P.: The Successful Dental Practice. Englewood Cliffs, NJ, Prentice-Hall, Inc., 1970, pp. 151–158.

16

Rewarding Patients, Staff, and Referral Sources

Dr. Jon Tillman leaned back in his chair after Joe Silverman had left his office. "I wonder," he mused, "if Mr. Silverman knows just how much I appreciate him as a patient?" Jon had been treating Mr. Silverman and his family for some years now. In addition to the income he had received from the treatment, the dentist was pleased with and felt a sense of pride in the improvements he had observed in the family's dental health. "I know Mr. Silverman is aware that I have said 'thank you' every time he or his family visits my office," Jon Tillman thought, "but perhaps I need to do something else, something more concrete to thank them."

WHY REWARD?

Many of us take for granted that our patients know we appreciate their patronage. And certainly, we realize that we have let them know of this by repeated "thank you's" and other remarks of appreciation. In this day of the marketing dentist, however, perhaps we could be more specific. And we shall see how in a moment.

By the same token, it is easy to assume that our employees, too, know how much we appreciate their efforts. We may not be able to increase their salaries as much as we would like (who *is* earning what he or she is worth, after all), but we do say thank you often enough, don't we? (Or do we?) In fact, we can't say thank you often enough and in enough different ways. This chapter is devoted to describing and discussing how we may show our appreciation to our patients, to

We can't say "thank you" to our patients and staff often enough and in enough different ways.

our employees, and to those people on whom we depend for patient referrals. By proper steps in this regard, we will be able to feel better about ourselves and our debts to the community, to increase or stabilize our practice incomes, and even to help people recognize the better dentistry we practice.

IMPORTANT FACTORS IN THE DENTAL PRACTICE

What factors in the dental practice are important to patients? Although the following report is from 1960, these factors are as important today as they were then (Stinaff, 1960, p. 201).

1. A clean, efficient office with adequate personnel.
2. Dentist's relations with patients — loyalty, interest, appreciation, compliments, respect, honesty, sincerity, kindness, and tact.
3. Ability of the dentist and durability and thoroughness of dental services.

Several comments about this list: First, the appearance of the office and treatment by auxiliaries are the most important factors for dental office patients. Second, the dentist's patient relations are next in importance in dental practice patronage. Words of interest, appreciation, praise, and kindness are used. Third, interestingly, the technical ability of the dentist comes last in importance. Apparently, patients do not discern major differences in ability among dentists, but they *do* notice personality and other personal differences. This is why we need to illustrate our personalities to patients and, in part, to reward our patients with thank you's, with followup notes, and with gifts.

COMMUNICATING WITH DIFFERENT TYPES OF PEOPLE

Marketing, as we have discussed earlier in this book, consists of understanding the needs of consumers and satisfying, or meeting, those needs in such a way as to earn a profit. In order to meet the needs of consumers, we need to be aware of two things: how people make purchasing decisions, and how to communicate with people.

Social Classes

Social class has a great influence on people's purchasing decisions.

Edwards (*Dental Economics,* June 1981) expresses the commonly used notion that social class has a great influence on people's purchasing decisions, and on the mechanisms by which we communicate with them. Edwards postulates three social classes: upper-middle, blue-collar, and white-collar — each subdivided by *age* into older and younger patients.

Older, Upper-Middle Class

This class consists of people thirty-five years and older, including professionals, managers, and heads of medium-sized corporations.

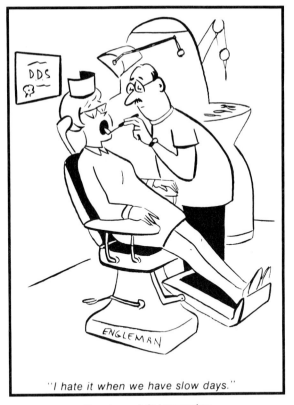

"I hate it when we have slow days."

Courtesy of *Cal* magazine

They have achieved most of their material goals and are concentrating on what has been called "self-actualizing" or self-fulfillment of the special potential of each person. They have come to a time when they want to develop themselves more, their minds and bodies, including their teeth. This is the largest market for esthetic dentistry. "Not the young and pretty, but the not so young who were never quite sure they were attractive or handsome," states Edwards.

What does this group "need" or want? They want an experienced dentist — this is the group most likely to read your diplomas on the wall. They want someone like themselves who has been "through the mill." Younger dentists should not be alarmed if they have fewer of this type of patient than do their older colleagues. Their time will come! These people also want recognition, even deference from you and your staff. Many of them are important and they want to be so regarded. This is the group which, most often, should be addressed as "Sir" and "Mrs. Jones."

Your office attire is important for the older, upper-middle class. Good taste, simple style, and lots of white might be the key words for describing the dress of you and your staff. Sport shirts are best left for sports occasions, not for as serious an occasion as a visit to the dentist, members of this group would usually believe. Your office location and its furnishings should reflect a similar, professional atmosphere.

Members of this older upper-middle class are best reached by verbal communications. They need to be thanked in person and, in

Your older, upper middle class patients may be your practice's best advertising medium.

some cases, followed up by telephone. This group probably is the least receptive to media advertising. They may notice your advertising, but they will not be as influenced by it as will other social classes. This group will be influenced by word-of-mouth, however. In fact, your older, upper-middle class patients may be your practice's best advertising medium.

Young, Upper-Middle Class

This class, usually under twenty-five years of age, acts or tries to act like the class above them. Because they do not have the esteem of their elders, they long for it, and anything you can do to help build their esteem will help not only them but also you. Give them the attention they want, all the while reminding them of who you are. You are not as important to them as they are to you. This is where the crucial skill of learning to really listen to people comes into play.

This group, with their children, may provide the largest numbers of patients for your practice. You may be able to keep them on a six-month check-up schedule. And usually they will accept your suggestions for dental care. Although they have other financial demands, these will usually not supercede their purchasing of at least adequate dentistry.

White-Collar Class

This is the traditional, older, lower-middle class group. Edwards calls them the "great imitators of the world." They tend to follow the leads of others. If you acquire as patients a few people from this category in a neighborhood, you will tend to get more of them. This group talks a great deal, and their conversation will often turn naturally to dentistry — and to you, *their* dentist.

The white-collar patient will not always be easy to work with. His or her complaints will tend to discourage you, but you must accept these and continue to recognize this person as an individual. Most importantly, you must be certain he or she is satisfied. Your auxiliaries should be aware of this need as well.

Blue-Collar Class

These people are frightened of cost and pain. They need great reassurance on both counts. They want relief from the anxieties which plague them. Your name will not be a household word, so you need to keep reinforcing your name and image with them. Frequent notes and cards will help; they get relatively less mail than do the middle-class people. Media advertising can help, too. The advertising you do, however, should not be subtle. It should be direct, pictorial, hard-hitting.

Blue collar people are frightened of cost and pain. They need great reassurance on both counts.

This group is used to taking orders from superiors and middle management people. Your being somewhat directive in the office not only will not turn them off, it will make them feel at home. Don't be surprised if this group of patients shows more gratitude to you than your others patients do. At times they will even thank you with gifts.

Summary

The middle classes need oral communication from the *dentist.* You will spend more of your personal time talking with them and reassuring them that they are, in fact, individuals and they are important and that you recognize them as such. The lower classes need written communications. Most of this work can be done by your auxiliaries, after you have set up a system. Letters, notes, and cards should be used after virtually every office contact with the white- and blue-collar groups. These written communications should reinforce the dental hygiene practices you have suggested, should promote regular dental care, and should thank them for their recent visit.

MOTIVATED BEHAVIOR

In most jobs, the best worker produces at a rate far exceeding the average worker's production rate. One of the major reasons for this higher-than-average production is *motivation.* Sometimes this is the most important reason for superior performance. Although psychologists do not agree on a definition of motivation, most experts would say at least that motivated behavior is goal directed. One important aspect of goal direction — the setting of those goals — is covered in Chapter Five.

Motivation in Organizations

The following characteristics have been cited as important to the consideration of motivation in organizations (Lawler, 1973, pp. 6–7):

1. *Money* plays an important role. Important to many people, money obviously can influence motivation. Thus, any discussion of motivation in work organization must consider how the way an organization handles its money influences the motivation of its employees.

2. Some type of *hierarchy* exists. Most organizations, including dental offices, of course, give more status and power to some people than to others. The possibility of promotion within an organization, or the unavailability of promotion, is often important to people and influences motivation.

Money plays an important role in the motivation of employees. However, people enjoy their jobs when they feel they are appreciated, when they are told "thank you."

3. People are given *assigned tasks* to perform. Research has shown that the way tasks are grouped to form jobs has a substantial influence on motivation.

In general, as the above list suggests, theorists do not include "thank you's" as a major determinant in employee behavior. We believe, however, that thanking employees is vital to the success of the dental practice. Salary levels for dental auxiliaries are not likely to be higher than for other, similarly trained individuals. In some areas they may not be as high. To stay in a dental auxiliary job for a long time, then, requires that a person enjoy his or her job. On one level, people enjoy their jobs when they feel they are appreciated, in short, when they are told "thank you." For this reason, we should take time to thank our employees often and in a variety of ways.

Are Your Employees Satisfied?

An interesting sidelight: apparently most dental office employees are happy with their work. In a survey done by *Dental Economics* in 1980, about 90 percent of all responding auxiliaries reported that they were very or somewhat satisfied. Figure 16–1 gives the survey statistics. Remember, however, that *any* dissatisfaction of employees detracts from marketing effectiveness.

WHAT IS A REWARD?

Most dictionaries will define reward as "something given (or received) in recompense for some worthy behavior." This is the sense in which we use the word. Positive reinforcement of desired behavior as an effective means of encouraging such behavior is a well-accepted principle. What are the things we can do, the rewards we can give, to reward and to promote behavior we wish to see in our patients and in our employees? The following are some of the "behaviors" many of us desire.

1. Regular patient visits
2. Patient referrals of other patients
3. Referrals from other dentists
4. Referrals from other professionals, civic leaders, businesspeople, friends
5. Referrals from auxiliaries
6. Pleasant, efficient, and correct office procedures by auxiliaries
7. Long and loyal service by auxiliaries

Rewarding Staff for New Patients

A staff that satisfies your current patients and brings in new patients is the most valuable resource of your dental practice. Keeping your staff in a marketing frame of mind at all times is very difficult, however. It requires constant attention and reinforcement.

To ensure attention to the things we are discussing, including the sending of birthday and graduation cards or gifts, following up of

	Hygenists	Chairsides	Receptionists
Very Satisfied	50%	53%	55%
Somewhat Satisfied	40	35	37
Somewhat Dissatisfied	9	10	4
Very Dissatisfied	1	2	4
Total	100%	100%	100%

Figure 16–1. Employee satisfaction. (Adapted from Dental Economics, September 1980, p. 52.)

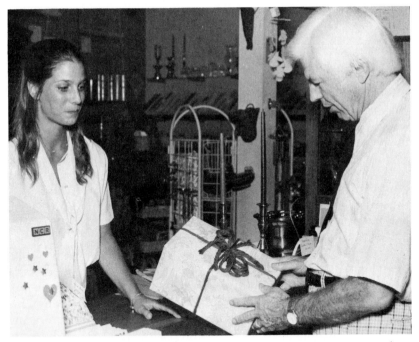

Rewarding employee performance that you'd like to see continue — such as referring patients — can be done with gifts for specific accomplishments.

patients' achievements with cards, and other clerical details, you will need to pay your staff well. It will also help for you to further reward your staff on frequent occasions.

What rule of thumb might you use for such rewards? You could set aside an amount, perhaps three to five dollars for each new patient who enters the practice, regardless of whether it is for a simple prophylaxis or for more complex and expensive work. At the end of each month, you can add up the new patients and divide by the number of hours worked by each staff member. This amount per hour worked can be paid to each person as a bonus. This bonus will make all staff members more cognizant of the value of bringing in new patients, and will cut down staff turnover and absenteeism. Only those hours that a staff member works during the month will be rewarded.

One variation would be to subtract from the bonus pool the same amount for each patient who has left the practice. This way, not only will staff members be interested in getting new patients, they will be interested as well in retaining current patients.

Most bonuses, however, should not be on a regular basis. If they are too regular, auxiliaries tend to build them in to their salary expectations, hence cancelling the bonuses' effectiveness as a special reward.

We think it is better to reward auxiliaries directly for patient referrals. You could offer a standard $5 for each referral or devise some other reward, perhaps in proportion to the amount of dental work each referral produces.

A staff that satisfies your current patients and that brings in new patients is the most valuable resource of your dental practice.

Rewarding for Correct Behavior

You may decide to reward auxiliaries directly for patient referrals.

Numerous examples exist of employee reward systems which reward one behavior while hoping for another. Universities have been used as an example of this phenomenon. Most universities reward professors based on publications, and hope that they teach well. Few examples exist of teachers being punished for bad teaching or rewarded (other than in a modest, short-term way) for good teaching. At the same time, universities hope that students will acquire knowledge, judgment, and maturity. However, these same institutions award admittance to dental and other professional and graduate schools on the basis of grades, apparently not considering that grades often are not a direct indication of knowledge, judgment, and maturity. We could find such examples in business, government, and other organizations.

In order to avoid creating a misplaced reward system in the dental office, we need to determine just what behavior is being rewarded. Do we give raises based on an auxiliary's smile or voice, or even looks? Do we reward auxiliaries who bring in additional patients and who help retain patients? Do we make a point of telling auxiliaries which of their activities and duties are most important to us, and which of them will be rewarded? (Kerr, 1978, pp. 307–321).

WRITING LETTERS AND NOTES

It may be too strong to say that your written communications make you or break you, but they are very important in creating your professional image, and in communicating with your patients and potential patients. According to Bregstein (1953, pp. 299–317), several rules will help you write interesting, effective, and professional communications:

1. Use the proper salutation. If you are on a first-name basis with the person to whom you are writing, use the first name in the letter as well.

Write all letters as though you were talking to people in person.

2. Get down to the facts early. People would like to get your message quickly. Give it to them as quickly and efficiently as you can.

3. Avoid repetitious use of "I" and "We" wherever possible.

4. Never use trite phrases such as, "We received your letter of the twelfth this instant." Instead, start with "It was nice to hear from you again," or "Thanks for choosing me as your dentist."

5. Eliminate participial beginnings, "Complying with your letter. . . ." It is more interesting to read, "Your dental appointment has been arranged for. . . ."

6. Don't antagonize the reader with expressions such as, "You have ignored our last statement . . ." unless it is your deliberate intention to indicate the exhaustion of your patience. Friendly, personal notes with openings such as, "Will you please let us know . . ." are preferable.

7. Eliminate such letter endings as: "Thanking you for past

courtesies. . . ." Better is a closing such as "Please use the enclosed reply envelope. . . ."

8. All letters going out from your office should be courteous. Never write in anger. You are more likely to win over the person with a friendly note.

9. Write all letters as though you were talking to people in person. Your letters using a simple, conversational style will be much more interesting and effective than those using stilted, "business-like" words and phrases.

10. A form letter telling a person that, in justice to himself and the dental services rendered, he ought to visit you after a stated period, is not an effective one.

Ehrlich and Ehrlich (1969, pp. 68–69) give other hints which will improve your written communications.

1. Every letter should be attractive in its layout and margins. The overall visual effect of the letter is important. Strikeovers, erasures, uneven type, and ink-clogged letters are all symbols of carelessness and reveal a lack of pride and competence.

2. The name, title, and address of the recipient must be clear and correct. A person's name is his most important possession and should be treated as such.

3. All words used in the letter should be spelled correctly. Misspelling diverts attention and damages your prestige.

4. The choice of words should be constructive, so that the tone of the letter will be friendly and positive. The letter should be correct, clear, concise, courteous, and considerate.

One last point about notes and letters. Many dentists prefer that most notes and some short letters be written by hand. An orthodontist friend of ours remarked recently, "I know how I feel when I receive what is obviously a form letter, so I don't want to do the same thing. If I'm going to thank someone, then I'm going to do it personally." Not everything from your office can be a personal message, but that is a goal for which we all might strive, especially for referrals.

REWARDING WITH GIFTS

How many times have you been given something you did not expect, such as a ticket to a basketball game, a piece of pottery made by a local artisan, or a set of monogrammed handkerchiefs? Do you remember how happy that simple gift made you feel? Well, you can generate that same kind of feeling in your patients, employees, and referral sources. We will now discuss a number of possible gifts for these people. You will not choose, nor will you always be able to afford, all of them. Not all of them would provide a suitable return on your "investment." Some gifts will meet all of these requirements, however. We suggest that you consider the following suggestions carefully and systematize your gift giving.

Gifts to Employees

When an employee is doing an exceptional job, being unusually productive for the practice, sometimes it is not possible or appropriate to reward him or her with a higher salary or promotion in job title or position. In these cases, and they are frequent in most active practices, it may be best to reward the employee with a gift. These gifts should be substantial, something the employee would not buy, and something that says, "I really appreciate your effort." You probably will wish to purchase these gifts yourself and have them gift wrapped. Clothing, household decorations, kitchen items, and sports equipment will usually be well received.

It is important that the other practice employees not be miffed or "turned off" by a gift to another staff member. That is to say, make certain that you are rewarding individuals for something done by themselves, not with the help of other people. If other people have been involved, be sure that they receive gifts as well.

Flowers to III Patients and Staff

Something as simple as a bouquet of carnations or a potted ivy can enhance one's outlook on life and put a smile on our faces.

Almost everybody likes flowers. Something as simple as a bouquet of carnations or a potted ivy can enhance one's outlook on life and put smiles on our faces. So it is with patients and staff. When they are ill at home or in the hospital, a gift of flowers can raise their spirits and bring you closer to them. We suggest you consider having your receptionist carefully read all newspapers carrying news of local citizens for items about your patients. When she comes across a notice that one of them is ill, you should consider sending flowers or a plant.

Ideally, you should have preselected a florist or plant store and

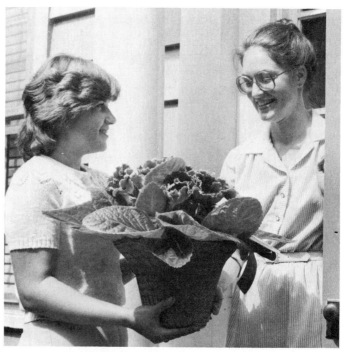

Flowers from the dentist can pleasantly surprise a patient and brighten the day.

made arrangements with them for delivery. If you send flowers or plants on a regular basis, the chances are great that one or more florist or plant stores in your area will be willing to grant you a modest discount, perhaps 10 or 15 percent. You are still going to spend a considerable amount of money, but it certainly will be worth it in terms of patient goodwill and practice revenues.

Gifts for Graduations and Weddings

Throughout this book, we have suggested that you attempt to differentiate your practice from other practices in your area. What better way can you think of than to follow your patients' lives closely enough to know when they or their children are graduating from some educational program or when they or their children are being married? Marking these events with modest gifts from you would make a great hit with most patients. We suggest again that you consider having your receptionist check all local newspapers, inquire from the patients themselves, and keep track of such events from patient records. It will be easy to know from these records when birthdays are coming up and even, roughly, when graduations from high school and college may be impending, which you can pin down with a phone call.

In most cases, you should be able to find and buy appropriate, modestly priced gifts in advance of the event, such as a pen and pencil set for graduations, or a pen and ink print, or a salt and pepper set for weddings. Such gifts may be wrapped at the store or in your office and sent out with a stylish card. In short, we are suggesting a procedure which you set up in advance and which is triggered by the awareness of someone on your staff that a meaningful event is about to happen in a patient's life.

Gifts will help increase activity in your office and eventually will increase practice revenues.

To be sure, the procedures we are suggesting will cost you and your practice some money. We believe the relationships that these gifts help develop, and the patient referrals they generate, will, however, pay for themselves many times over.

Free First Exams for Young Children

How many of your young patients do not see a dentist early enough in their lives, and how can you get people to bring their children in earlier? One way is to give a free first examination and to present the free examination as a "gift" to parents. A nicely printed, professional looking card or announcement could be used to award the gift. The exam can usually be scheduled for them when the office is not busy anyway. Such a gift will help increase activity in your office and, eventually, will increase practice revenues.

Rewarding of Referral Sources

You appreciate it when people refer patients to you. We all do. Why not tell them so, at least sometimes by a gift? We believe that dentists should, as a matter of course, send a thank-you note to anyone who has referred a patient. For people who seldom refer patients, a standard note, typed by your secretary or receptionist and signed by you, is fine. For those people who often refer patients, a note at least slightly different from previous notes should be sent. A note ought to be sent for each referral, in any event.

Further, for those people who often refer patients, an occasional gift is in order. The gift may be a standard one, perhaps something you also would send graduates or those getting married. Or, it may be an item reserved for referrals. If your town or state has a particularly popular artist who has issued a series of prints, it may be an excellent idea to buy a supply of these and send one, on occasion, to people who refer patients to you. It is necessary to keep a record of which print has gone to which person, of course. After all, you do not want to undo all of your good marketing efforts by sending the same print to the same person twice.

We believe that dentists should, as a matter of course, send a thank you note to anyone who has referred a patient.

Rewards to Staff for Long Service

When one or more members of your staff have served for a relatively long time, say five or ten years, you may wish to reward them and their spouses with a trip to a nearby beach or resort. One way to do this and ensure that there will be no tax problems for them or you is to send them to conventions at attractive places. The trip will then qualify as a business expense for you.

STAFF PARTIES

On occasion, it is advisable to get the staff, with spouses, together for an informal social event. This helps relieve some of the pressure in the office. It also helps the staff realize that while the dentist may be something of a martinet during office hours — because of technical demands — he is a relaxed human being during his leisure hours.

The dinner or party should sometimes be scheduled at a nearby restaurant or club and paid for entirely by the practice. On occasion, however, a pot-luck picnic or dinner is great for everybody. Most auxiliaries don't mind spending a little time preparing a special dish, and some will welcome the chance to show off their culinary abilities.

SUMMARY

Throughout this chapter we have suggested that you consider ways to make your employees, patients, and referral sources more aware of how much you appreciate them and what they do. Not all of our suggestions will work with all dentists. Further, not all dentists will feel comfortable with some of the suggested approaches to showing appreciation. We are simply suggesting that you explicitly recognize what people have done and what people mean to you and tell them about it in concrete ways. Nothing we have suggested is unprofessional. Done in a tactful and tasteful way, the gifts and notes we have discussed are all professional *and* productive.

REFERENCES

Blass, J. L., and Tulkin, I.: Successful Dental Practice. Philadelphia, J. B. Lippincott Company, 1947, pp. 207–10.

Bregstein, S. J.: The Successful Practice of Dentistry. Englewood Cliffs, N.J., Prentice-Hall, Inc., 1953, Chapter 15.

Communication with patients is key to dental marketing. Marketing News, 29 May 1981, p. 5.

Edwards, F. G.: How to communicate with your patients. Dental Economics, June 1981, pp. 56–70.

Ehrlich, A. B., and Ehrlich, S. F.: Dental Practice Management. Philadelphia, W. B. Saunders Company, 1969, Chapters 7 and 9.

Heiser, R. A., Hess, K. M., and Stallard, R. E.: Marketing Dental Services Professionally. Institute for Marketing Professional Services, Inc., 1981, Chapter 9.

Howard, W. W.: Dental Practice Planning. St. Louis, The C. V. Mosby Co., 1975, Chapter 13.

Kerr, S.: On the folly of rewarding A, while hoping for B. Academy of Management Journals, December 1975, pp. 769–83. Also *In* Frost, P. J., Mitchell, V. F., and Nord, W. R. (eds.): Organizational Reality, Santa Monica, California, Goodyear Publishing Company, Inc., 1978, pp. 307–21.

Lawler, E. E. III: Motivation in Work Organizations. Monterey, California, Brooks/Cole Publishing Company, 1973.

Lorsch, J. W., and Lawrence, P. R. (eds): Managing Group and Intergroup Relations. Homewood, Illinois, Richard D. Irwin, Inc., 1972.

Peterson, R. B., Tracy, L., and Cabelly, A.: Readings in Systematic Management of Human Resources. Reading, Massachusetts, Addison-Wesley Publishing Company, 1979.

Stinaff, R. K.: Dental Practice Administration, St. Louis, C. V. Mosby Co., 1960, Chapter 14.

17

Marketing Through Insurance

Faye Willingham had just hung up the phone when Mary Ledford came into the office. Mary wanted to talk about the dental insurance coverage for her proposed treatment.

"I got this note from my insurance company yesterday," Mary said, "after waiting for weeks and weeks. And look at this! Why aren't they paying more? It says here they're only paying $425. The bill is $750!"

"Let's review your chart, Mary, so we can find out more about this," Faye answered. "Oh, yes, on the day you came in for your examination, I talked with you about the total cost and estimated that your company would pay around $450," Faye replied.

"Well, I sure don't remember that!" Mary responded. "They told me at the plant that my work would be covered by insurance. And by the way, why am I just now finding this out? It's been two months since my exam and I told Dr. Green how anxious I was to have this done right away."

"I'm sorry it has taken so long, Mary. But you know we have a lot of paperwork here. Sometimes Dr. Green is so busy with patients that he just doesn't get around to signing the forms. *Now I remember* — the company sent the predetermination form back because they said two of the teeth involved didn't look like they needed crowns — so Dr. Green had to write back and tell them that two of the cusps were fractured and that that hadn't shown up on the x-rays."

Has an incident like this occurred in your office, or in the office of one of your friends? Obviously, we see here some form of communication breakdown. How can a dialogue like the above be averted? How can you and your team process insurance more efficiently — and please your patients more?

DENTAL INSURANCE

Growth

In less than two decades the growth of dental insurance programs has been nothing less than phenomenal. The number of persons covered by some form of dental insurance has increased dramatically since 1970. At that time there were an estimated four million persons enrolled in such programs. By 1975 that number had jumped to 42 million, then to almost double that — 74 million — in 1980. The number of Americans who will be covered by some type of dental insurance in 1985 is projected to be about 99 million!

As shown in Figure 17–1 (from *Delta Dental Update*, Summer/Fall, 79), the growth of dental insurance has been similar to that of major medical insurance with a ten-year lag. Apparently buyers of dental prepayment plans view them in much the same way they do major medical plans. If this trend continues, growth will level off in 1985 at about 42 percent of the population.

The attitudes of dental teams toward dental insurance have also changed. Initially insurance was perceived as a problem: interference in dentist/patient relationship, additional paperwork, and failure of patients to understand their insurance. Consequently, many dental teams did not welcome dentally insured patients with open arms. As the supply of dentists has increased, more and more dentists have recognized that dental insurance creates a new market, which enables the increased number of dentists to thrive. In a 1981 survey of *Dental Economics*, 86 percent of the responding dentists agreed that their current economic situations would be worse without dental insurance.

> In 1970 an estimated four million persons were enrolled in insurance programs. By 1975 that number had jumped to 42 million, then to almost double that — 74 million — in 1980.

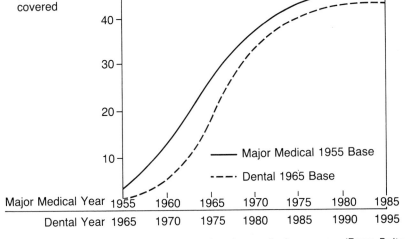

Figure 17–1. Dental prepayment and major medical coverage. (From *Delta Dental Update*, Summer-Fall, 1979, p. 3.)

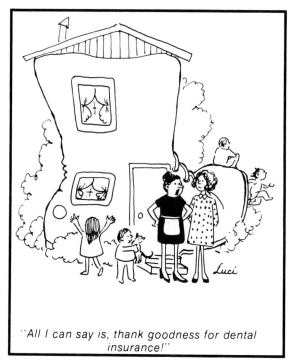

"All I can say is, thank goodness for dental insurance!"

Courtesy of *Cal* magazine.

Advantages

There are various advantages of dental insurance to patients and dentists: less direct cost to the patient, incentive for persons who have not done so to utilize dental services, more services purchased by patients, increased financial stability of dental practices, and enhancement of dentists' credibility.

Patients with insurance coverage can obtain dental service with less out-of-pocket cost.

Most of these advantages relate to the fact that the patient can obtain dental service with less out-of-pocket cost. This encourages people to seek care. Otherwise many of them would feel that they could not afford dentistry in the face of all their other needs. People who could only purchase basic dental care without insurance can now purchase more sophisticated services, such as endodontics and fixed bridgework.

These advantages to patients create more demand for dentistry, thus increasing the income of dentists. Also, stability of income may be achieved through insurance because many plans pay 100 percent for preventive services. A larger percentage of patients (especially children) will return for scheduled recall appointments because of the 100 percent coverage.

The dentist's credibility may also improve. Patients usually have no unbiased support in their decision to pursue a certain course of treatment. The approval of the treatment plan submitted for predetermination of benefits is endorsement of the dentist's recommendations by a third party. Credibility is especially enhanced if a dental consultant has given approval and the patient is so informed.

Problems

To list the advantages of dental insurance and ignore the problems would tell only half the story. So let us take a look at some of the problems. First, dental insurance creates *additional paperwork* for the office staff (and salary expense for the dentist) and secondly, *adds to the time* the office personnel must allot explaining pertinent information on coverage to patients and aiding them in filling out the insured's portion of the forms properly. These increased administrative costs can usually be readily absorbed, however, because of the gain in gross income that results from an increase in patients.

There can be a communication breakdown with patients regarding their financial responsibility.

Another problem is the involvement of a *third party,* the insurer, in the situation. Because of the coverage offered by the individual plan, the insurer can influence the treatment that the patient will accept. Insurance companies are not trying to dictate treatment, but they do reflect administrative cost controls for employers by suggesting an alternate mode of treatment, termed "adequate functional care." If the dentist includes a written explanation to justify more sophisticated treatment, it will often be allowed by the company. For example, the policy may offer more coverage for partials than for bridgework. In some cases the company may pay the entire fee for a partial, but not for a fixed bridge. In other cases the company will allow the fee for the partial to be applied toward the bridge fee, with the patient paying the difference. Naturally, some patients will be influenced by the amount they have to pay in deciding on the treatment they prefer.

There can also be a communication breakdown with patients regarding their *financial responsibility.* Some patients perceive dental insurance as an earned benefit of their employment, and occasionally may express feelings that the insurer should have paid a higher percentage. Therefore, it is important to inform patients early as to how their policies work and have them agree to pay any portion not covered by insurance. Financial arrangements for the portion of the fee to be paid by the patient must be firm.

The ability to communicate with patients regarding insurance is critical to the marketing of a practice. It is true that the dentist has the right to expect payment for services rendered. Even though insurance benefits upgrade the economic ability of patients, at the same time various methods should be available for patients to pay their portion of the fee.

Even though the majority of insurance dealings can be handled smoothly and with relatively little fuss, at times lack of communication between and among the parties can occur. However, any potential misunderstandings can be reduced if you can make it clear to the patient that there are two types of contracts involved when a patient has dental benefits: (1) the contract between the employer and the company providing dental benefits for employees, and (2) the contract between the dentist and the patient. You must explain that dentists have no formal relationship with third party insurance companies, but that you will do everything possible at no charge to ensure that each patient derives as much benefit as possible. If patients understand that, a relaxed and workable relationship between patient and dentist is likely.

Information File

An insurance notebook for quick and informative reference when conferring with patients can be invaluable. The notebook should contain booklets and information regarding benefits of the various plans in the community. As the receptionist (or the insurance clerk) becomes familiar with the information, explanations become much easier and require less time.

The information file should always be kept up-to-date, as benefits do change from time to time. For the past few years, the tendency has been for many businesses to improve dental benefits from year to year. Although this is continuing in some areas, the cost escalation of health care has forced some companies to re-evaluate their programs. In some instances there has been a decrease in monies allocated to health care when inflation factors have been considered.

It is a good idea, also, to request a supply of blank insurance forms from the local firms and industries that offer dental insurance coverage. Keep these forms on hand for those all-too-frequent occasions when patients forget to bring their own. This will enable you to get the patient's portion completed so the form can be mailed immediately for the predetermination of benefits.

KEEPING TRACK OF INSURANCE

There are several benefits to be gained by proper handling of insurance transactions. First, the practice gains from improved cash flow if forms are filed promptly. Second, the practice enjoys excellent relationships with satisfied patients, and third, the staff is gratified that they have done a good job.

To be efficient with insurance paperwork, a specific system is needed for filing forms for prior determination or payment, for recording payments received, and so on. The system should be designed so that (1) it does not lose track of patients, (2) paperwork is done immediately (within a few work days), and (3) payments are received promptly. A very helpful tool is an insurance log or an insurance summary record (see Fig. 17–2). This form contains data such as filing date, carrier's coverage estimate, dates of payments received, amount to be paid by the patient, and financial arrangements worked out in advance with the patient. Without some kind of system, it is very easy for some insurance paperwork to become lost in the shuffle, and to lose track of patients who have not returned for treatment.

Another method that might be considered is a ring binder or file folder to keep the claim forms in, categorized by (1) authorization pending, (2) authorized/under treatment, and (3) payment pending. The authorization pending category would include all forms submitted for predetermination before treatment is begun. The authorized/under treatment category includes authorized papers on patients who are under active treatment. The payment pending file contains forms that have been submitted for payment to the insurance carrier. When a payment is received, the form is removed

A helpful tool is an insurance log or an insurance summary record.

PATIENTS NAME	CARRIER	AUTHORIZATION REQUIRED		REQUEST FOR AUTHORIZATION MAILED		AUTHORIZATION RECEIVED			CLAIM FORM MAILED		AMOUNT RECEIVED FROM INSURANCE		AMOUNT PATIENT TO PAY	ARRANGEMENTS FOR PAYING BALANCE
		YES	NO	DATE	AMOUNT	DATE	AMOUNT	CLAIM NO.	DATE	AMOUNT	DATE	AMOUNT		

Figure 17–2.   Insurance summary record. (Courtesy of SYCOM.)

Form No. 274   Professional Budget Plan, Madison, Wisconsin, Printed in U.S.A.

from the folder and placed in the patient's folder. Regardless of the system you choose, keep copies of all insurance forms mailed.

The system you develop will begin to work to the benefit of the pratice immediately if insurance forms are properly filled out and mailed promptly. Followup on insurance claims should be stressed as one of the *most important duties* of the staff member who has been assigned the task of handling insurance. The summary record or file system should be thoroughly reviewed on a two-week to one-month basis to be sure all action is current. Without systematic followup, foul-ups will occur and cash flow will suffer. For example, forms of patients who do not return for treatment should be mailed to the carrier for payment if efforts to contact those patients prove fruitless. New forms can be filled out if and when the patient returns for resumption of treatment. If you have no way of checking on these patients, you may forget they never came back and fail to file for treatment that has already been completed.

Another helpful tool in keeping up with insurance is a code for use on charts and ledgers. The code can be as simple or complex as the dentist wishes to make it. A simple, very useful code, is to place an "I" in the upper right corner of ledgers and charts. This "I" can be used to identify charts of patients who are covered by insurance. The "I" code on ledger cards is useful in tabulating the percentage of each month's accounts receivable that involves insurance (Figure 17–3).

In order for any system of handling insurance paperwork to be effective, it should tie in to patient flow as shown on Figure 17–4.

> In order for any system of handling insurance paperwork to be effective, it should tie in to patient flow.

Coordination of Benefits

One should explain coordination of benefits when both husband and wife are employed and covered by dental insurance programs.

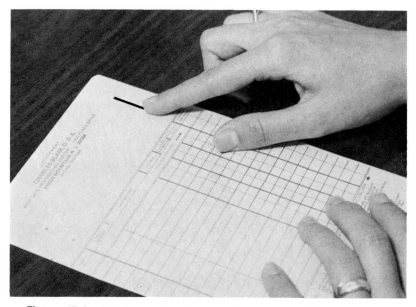

Figure 17–3. Keeping track of your insurance patients. An insurance sticker — "I" — on records helps to keep track of insurance patients.

Patient calls for exam appointment	Ask if insured. (If yes, ask to bring forms and booklet to exam).
Patient examination	Patient signs forms. Give patient written policy on insurance. Explain how policy works. Mail for predetermination and payment of exam fee.
Patient consultation	Give insurance benefit estimate. Make financial arrangements with patient for balance.
Predetermination received	Call patient and review: (1) Exact payment of benefit. (2) Exact liability of patient. (3) Payment arrangements. Schedule treatment appointment.
Treatment visit(s)	Can file for payment each time or wait until all treatment is completed. Collect patient's portion of balance.
Final treatment visit	File for payment. Collect final balance due from patient.
Insurance payment received	Record payment and file form in patient chart. Call patient if any additional balance is due.
Patient balance received	Record payment. Clear account balance.

Figure 17–4. Patient–insurance flow.

Tell them that in most cases the husband's policy provides primary coverage for him and the children and that the wife's policy is primary for her and secondary for her husband and children. At the same time spell out your office policy on accepting assignment when there are two companies involved — and further, the responsibility of the patient for payment.

You will find that it is next to impossible to accurately compute the amount the secondary carrier will pay because there are so many variations in the methods of determining liability among companies. Some secondary carriers will pay the difference between the primary coverage and the dentist's fee; others will pay the difference between the primary coverage and the maximum their own coverage allows. Still other companies will cover only a percentage of the remainder. Because of the delays in receiving prompt payment on coordination of benefits between two carriers, many dentists prefer that the patient pay the difference between the primary company's estimate and the total cost. In these cases, the secondary company makes payment directly to the patient.

Accidental Injuries

The treatment of the victim (as well as the finances) of a dental accident can be one of the most difficult areas the dentist must face. Some generalities will be made here, but because accidents can be covered by many different kinds of policies, there is great variance. For example, a patient may have accident coverage through a homeowner's policy, an automobile liability policy, a school accident policy, a business premises liability policy, Workmen's Compensation, and so on. You will find that each case must be dealt with on an individual basis and sometimes must be negotiated through a claims adjuster. Some types of policies (such as Workmen's Compensation) vary in their coverage from state to state.

The marketing dentist will do everything possible to secure additional benefits for his patients when he deems some future treatment necessary for the insured condition.

Generally speaking, accidents involving patients of record can be handled with very little difficulty, although at times it will be necessary to generate additional correspondence concerning the need for the proposed treatment. In the case of accidental injury to a child patient, the dentist often must explain that not only is the present treatment necessary, but future replacement will be needed as the child matures. The marketing dentist will make it his business to do everything possible to secure additional benefits for his patients when he deems some future treatment necessary.

Words of caution must be·said regarding patients who come to your office only as the result of an accident. Since accidents to teeth usually require some type of emergency treatment, many dentists find that if the patient is not known to the practice, it is best to perform the absolute minimum treatment and receive cash at the time of the visit. Of course, like any new patient, the accident victim presents a marketing opportunity. Since accidents will often result in the need for root canal treatment, full crown coverage, partials, or fixed bridges, which are high-cost procedures, predetermination of benefits should *always* be sought before any such extensive treatment is completed.

If the accident occurred on a neighbor's property, the neighbor may feel responsible for the accident and tell the patient to inform the dentist that his or her insurance will cover it. As in all accidents covered by insurance, the insurance company must acknowledge liability, not the neighbor. You need information on the insurance company and the accident so that you can file a claim. After the insurance company accepts your claim, you can proceed with confidence. Until then you must be responsive to the patient's needs, but consider that the patient alone is responsible for all charges.

The key in accident cases is to be responsive to the immediate pain and/or esthetic damage the patient has suffered, but avoid becoming a "victim" of the accident by ensuring that insurance benefits and payment arrangements are firm before you proceed with extensive treatment.

COMMUNICATION WITH PATIENTS

An understanding with patients relative to their dental insurance coverage is crucial to satisfying their needs. Most of the problems re-

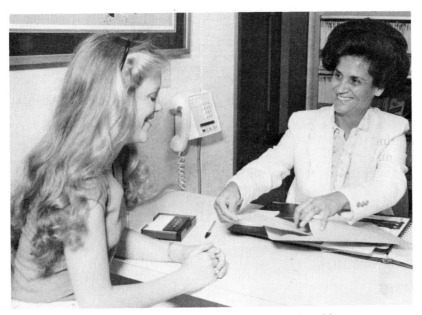

Receptionist is key in informing patient about her dental insurance.

late to the amount of coverage, annual limits, deductibles, copayments, and restrictions relating to time. Your staff should determine over the telephone at the time the examination appointment is made whether a new patient has insurance coverage, and request that the patient bring claim forms. If the insurer is a company unfamiliar to your practice, ask the patient to provide you with a copy of the company's insurance booklet to be added to your insurance notebook.

Terminology and Limitation of Coverage

Some of the terminology used by insurance companies can be confusing to patients and even to dentists. A dental practice with good marketing techniques will see the advantage in helping all patients remove the mystery surrounding their coverage. In simple language explain what is meant by individual and family deductibles, copayments, predetermination of benefits, and insurance limits. It is probably best to talk about these in terms of how they affect the patient and not try to explain how insurance works and the cost-control measures insurance firms employ. Remember, the patient is the important person here, and the focus should be on helping that patient.

An area of particular concern is the annual insurance limit, which can vary, typically from $500 to $1,500. Potential problems could arise in this area unless you determine whether part of this limit has already been used. For example, if the patient has been to another dentist or a specialist for treatment which was paid by the insurance carrier during the current annual limit period, the limit will be decreased or, in some cases, depleted. Simply ask the patient if any

Explain what is meant by deductibles, copayments, predetermination of benefits, and insurance limits.

dental treatment has already been provided this year, then contact the insurance company to verify the amount already paid and schedule treatment based on the balance. If the patient needs extensive treatment, you may mutually decide to take care of the most pressing problem areas first, then postpone the remaining treatment until a new plan year starts. The patient who desires more rapid completion of the treatment may sometimes be willing to make the payments personally rather than wait for the benefits.

Responsibility for Payment

Patients need to be made aware that there is a time lapse between filing for predetermination of benefits and beginning of treatment. If they are told approximately how long it will take, they should be notified if for some reason there is a longer delay. Some offices routinely schedule patients for the next appointment before forms are mailed, allowing a reasonable interval for predetermination to be returned from the insurance company. Others feel that it is better to telephone each patient as soon as the preauthorization arrives so that in addition to setting up an appointment, the exact treatment estimate and patient portion, with payment arrangements, can be reviewed before treatment begins.

As dentists, we understand that dental insurance supplements but does not completely cover dental fees. Our patients, however, often have a different view. In fact, a 1981 *Dental Economics* survey of dentists conluded that many patients think their insurance will pay the full fee and over half the dentists feel they have to justify their fees due to carrier actions. This makes it imperative that the staff seize the first opportunity to communicate effectively regarding the responsibility for payment. It is critical in the marketing effort to deal with this issue convincingly and tactfully.

Some dental insurance plans will pay 100 percent of the cost for checkups, but others will not. Although a few companies may provide 100 percent coverage for treatment, the vast majority require some copayment. Oftentimes, patients have mistaken impressions as to the degree of their coverage. They should be informed that coverage is determined by the plan bought by their employer — the higher the premium paid, the greater the benefits of the program.

It should also be clearly explained that the dentist does not determine patient benefits and that fees are the same regardless of insurance coverage. Of even greater importance is that patients understand their financial obligation. The dentist is happy to help the patient receive benefits by filing insurance forms, but any balance not covered must be paid directly by the patient. The receptionist should estimate the amount the insurance will pay and work out financial arrangements at the initial appointment or consultation. The most appropriate method of payment for the individual patient should be discussed with him or her.

When the insurance company's pretreatment estimate arrives, inform the patient by telephone and appoint him or her for treatment. At this time tell exactly how much the insurer will pay and review the payment schedule for the patient's share of the treatment cost. Since this was discussed previously, the patient will be expecting this confirmation call.

At times a procedure may need to be changed after the actual treatment is begun owing to unforeseen involvement. For example, a tooth that had been treatment-planned for an MOD amalgam may require full crown coverage if the tooth structure is weaker than could be determined through visual examination and radiographs. The dentist should fully explain that he or she is diagnosing the treatment to the best of his ability, but that the final procedure may vary and that the dentist will make every attempt to collect for the procedure from the company. However, the patient will be responsible for the actual treatment that takes place, over and above the benefits paid.

Some dentists, in these circumstances, work on the premise that no matter what treatment must be done, they will abide by the initial estimate. They also believe in reducing the patient's fee if the treatment proves less extensive than the diagnosis. Wouldn't your patients be grateful and tell their friends if you actually saved them money?

It is always to your benefit to determine the party responsible for finances prior to any treatment. Exercise caution in treating children of separated parents by determining which parent is financially responsible and by making payment arrangements *directly* with that person before any treatment is done. The natural father's insurance will usually provide the primary coverage for children and the natural mother's coverage will be secondary. In some cases, the stepfather (if the natural mother has remarried) will be the primary insurance source for the children. Taking the word of one party that a second party will be responsible is not wise — unless the first party agrees to pay for treatment should the second party fail to do so.

Exercise caution in treating children of separated parents by determining which parent is financially responsible.

Seeking additional information from certain patients can often facilitate insurance matters and avoid needless delays or nonpayment. For instance, when young adults come in, always find out their ages, whether or not they are students, and whether they are covered by their own insurance, their parents', both, or none. When any patient is unsure of coverage, this must be determined before treatment begins unless finances are no problem.

Scheduling Recall Appointments

The receptionist should schedule recall appointments at least six months after the last one unless the dentist and patient have planned for more frequent recall. This is a courtesy to patients because if an appointment is scheduled even one day before six months has passed, the insurance company will refuse to pay. This limitation of coverage on recall appointments to twice a year is one of the cost-control measures strictly adhered to by insurance companies.

When scheduling recall appointments, patients should routinely be asked if they are still employed by the company listed on the history forms, and still covered by dental insurance. If they have made a job change, they need to bring new insurance forms and a booklet from the present employer; if they are no longer entitled to dental benefits, you need to be aware of the situation so that personal financial arrangements for the entire balance can be made.

Assignment of Benefits

"I don't like dealing with insurance companies," said Joe Talant while lunching with his friend, Bob Broadwell. "I prefer to keep business strictly between me and the patient. After all, it's the patient's responsibility to pay for services."

"That's true," Bob replied. "And it works well when patients pay for services as quickly as insurance companies."

"Then you are in favor of accepting assignment of benefits?"

"Certainly. Let me give you an example. Recently I did $1,000 worth of treatment for a patient and insurance promptly paid $800. We made arrangements with her to pay the $200 balance during her four treatment visits, which extended over a period of six weeks. If she had been required to pay first and then be reimbursed by the insurance company, there would have been delay. Worse yet, she might have spent the money from the insurance company for some very urgent purpose, and I'd have been left holding the bag."

"I'd never really thought about it like that," said Bob. "Maybe it isn't such a bad deal after all!"

Accepting assignment of insurance benefits enables many patients to purchase your services who otherwise could not afford to.

While it is true that some dentists still resist accepting assignment, that number is decreasing steadily. A 1981 survey by *Dental Economics* revealed that 70 percent of the responding dentists are accepting assignment. Cash is the ideal method of payment, but if the patient does not have it readily available, the dentist must search for some alternative. By accepting assignment the dentist can receive the bulk of the treatment fee almost immediately (2 to 6 weeks). Prior to treatment, financial arrangements can be made with the patient to pay the balance before or during the treatment visits.

Remember that you are in business to serve patients, and accepting assignment of insurance benefits is a great marketing technique because it enables many patients to purchase your services who otherwise could not afford dental care. By refusing to accept assignment, the dentist will almost certainly fail to attract his share of the population.

Written Policy on Insurance

In addition to verbal explanations, it is advisable and very helpful to give the patient written information about how your office handles dental insurance. (Most people remember only a small part of what they hear.) This information should be presented in a positive tone. Insurance should be considered advantageous for both patient and dentist, not a problem. Remember, it is an aid to marketing. This can be included in the office handbook given to all patients and/or can be an additional single data sheet explaining pertinent insurance facts (see Figure 17–5).

TO OUR PATIENTS WITH DENTAL INSURANCE

We will be happy to help you file your insurance claim forms without additional charge and will do all we can to help you receive maximum benefits. Since many patients frequently have questions regarding their coverage, we have prepared this information to assist you in understanding more about dental insurance. If you have additional questions, please ask.

Determining Benefits

Your benefits are determined by your employer, not your dentist. These benefits are meant to aid you in paying for dental care, but most policies do *not* pay 100% of treatment costs.

Fees

Dentists charge the same fees to all their patients, regardless of insurance coverage. At times, the fee paid by the company may be lower than the fee charged by the dentist, depending upon the benefits allowed by the policy.

Responsibility for Payment

It will be your responsibility to pay any amount not covered by your benefits. We will be happy to arrange a payment plan for you to take care of this balance.

Deductibles

If your plan has a "deductible", this means that you will be required to pay a certain amount (usually $50 to $100) per year *before* the company will begin to pay. After these deductibles have been paid to the dentist by you, your company will begin to pay a portion of the fee for you.

Yearly Maximums

Most policies also have a limit that they will pay each year on each individual covered (usually from $500 to $1500).

Pre-Treatment Estimates

Most companies require that the dentist submit his treatment plan to them before treatment is started. We will contact you when the plan has been approved, and tell you the amount the insurance will pay, the amount you will owe, review your payment schedule, and schedule you for your next appointment.

Filing Claims

It is unlawful for us to submit any claim form for service not yet completed.

Figure 17–5. Sample data sheet explaining pertinent insurance facts.

COMMUNICATION WITH INSURANCE COMPANIES

Your office has a real marketing opportunity in communicating with insurance companies. Someone on your dental team (other than yourself, unless you are not very busy) should be responsible. This person can be a patient advocate with the insurance company, making sure that each patient receives all the benefits to which he is entitled. Such attention to patients' needs is effective marketing.

Contact Person

Your insurance personnel should become familiar with the contact person for each dental insurer your office deals with, along with that person's proper mailing address, title, and telephone number and even first name. Always ask if the company has a toll-free number. Courteous communication with the same person over a period of time is helpful in that the individual will tend to take more of a personal interest in seeing that your inquiries and problems are handled expeditiously. Always call the insurer when a problem arises regarding anything from predetermination to lost radiographs, and get it cleared up before treatment begins, if at all possible.

Always call the insurer when a problem arises, and get it cleared up before treatment begins, if at all possible.

Be especially prompt about contacting the insurer when a payment is late, because most companies are prompt in sending payment. Occasionally a company may erroneously issue a check to the patient when the form indicated it was to be paid to you. In such a case the company may issue a second check to you and deduct the amount of the payment made to the patient from his remaining benefit coverage for the year. If your paperwork was filled out correctly and the error was made by the company, insist that you receive the payment due you.

There is great variance in the format of insurance forms and it may be difficult to interpret each carrier's method. An easy way to standardize the "Dentist's Statement" portion is to attach a standard ADA claim form (with the dentist's portion filled out) to any nonstandard form. If a company still insists that you complete their form, write them a letter in which you state there is no charge for standard forms, but since theirs is not standard, you must add a clerical charge for adapting the information to their specialized form (see Fig. 17–6).

Some offices have found the "superbill," which is used with standard pegboard accounting systems, very helpful when they prefer to bill companies after each appointment. Other dentists who file for payment following every appointment use a copy of the predetermination form, with dates inserted as procedures are completed.

Timesaving Ideas

There are several other timesaving procedures that can be incorporated to expedite the mailing of claim forms. As stated in Chapter 10, insurance companies often request radiographs to assist them in determining coverage and confirming treatment. Instead of being placed in mounts, bitewing or periapical radiographs can be sent in a small envelope, stapled to the claim form; be sure to write the patient's name as well as your own name and address on this envelope. To facilitate prompt return of radiographs, stamp "PLEASE RETURN X-RAYS IMMEDIATELY" on the envelope. At times, insurance companies will send radiographs back separately from claim forms. If they are not identified by name, you will not know whose they are.

For routine visits such as examinations and recalls, you may wish to utilize a preprinted ADA standard form, which includes all information in the dentist's portion.

— Dentist's name, address, and identification number
— Individual ADA codes related to examination and recall visits

---

JAMES F. WHITE, DDS
3001 Remount Road
Escondido, California 92025

Dear Sir:

I have attached to your insurance claim form a standard ADA form with the "Dentist's Statement" portion
completed. Since the dentist's portion of your form
is nonstandard, I hope this attachment will be acceptable.

Our office charges a $5.00 clerical fee to transpose
information onto a nonstandard form if it should be
necessary. Thank you for your cooperation.

Sincerely,

James F. White, DDS

Figure 17–6. Sample letter to an insurance company concerning a nonstandard form.

— Fees for those visits

This procedure will save a great deal of work and effort on the part of the insurance clerk.

Permanent rubber stamps with the names and addresses of the insurance companies most used by your practice facilitate mailing. Stamps that include your name, address, and identification number are also helpful in filing for Medicaid and other federal and state programs.

Preprinted inquiries to be sent to insurance companies should also be considered. These forms may contain blanks to be checked (see Fig. 17–7).

Another preprinted form that can be very helpful allows explanations for unusual treatment. Rather than spend extra time composing explanations for the predetermination forms of each patient whose treatment must be verified, design a preprinted sheet. This should include the procedures that most often require additional interpretations in order for the insurance company to approve the treatment. As suggested by Ehrlich these should include items such as replacement of a full or partial denture or full crown coverage. Since every practice has different needs, each dentist can devise a form to fit his or her individual practice.

To:_____Insurance Company
From: Charles Letterman, DDS
      123 South Main Street
      Greenlawn, VA 11223

Patient_____ SS Number_____Date filed_____
—We have not received our x-rays. Please return immediately.
  Thank you.

—Predetermination has not been received. Please remit promptly. Thank
  you.

—We received your check for $_____. However, the predetermination
  stated we would receive $_____. Please advise or send additional
  check.

—We have not received payment. Did the payment go to the patient by mistake? Please investigate.

—It appears that the deductible amount of $_____ has been sub-
  tracted twice. Please check.

—It appears that the percentage of coverage has been calculated in error.
  Please refigure.

—We are forwarding your check for $_____ to Dr._____as
  we received it by mistake.

—We are returning your check for $_____ as it is a duplication and has
  already been paid.

Figure 17–7. Insurance inquiry form.

Any time-saving device that can be incorporated into insurance handling will make the job easier and less bothersome, and will also help trim salary overhead costs and facilitate receipt of benefit payments.

Local Clerks

It will also be beneficial for you and your insurance personnel to become acquainted with the insurance clerks of local industries. Again, personal contact and your willingness to deal with insurance may influence these individuals to refer patients to you who have become unhappy about treatment, inflexible financial arrangements, or inept management of forms in other dental offices. You may even want to consider extending professional courtesy to these local clerks.

It will help for you and your insurance personnel to become acquainted with the insurance clerks of local industries.

Always report poor cooperation on the part of the insurance carrier to the employer (local firm carrying dental insurance program) because the contract with the carrier must be renewed periodically, and a poor track record may influence the employer to seek another more helpful carrier.

Facilitating Cash Flow

Occasionally, one of the dentist's most difficult extractions can involve receiving prompt payment from insurance companies. Some dentists tend to blame poor cash flow on delayed insurance payments, but if filing is accurately completed on a regular basis, the mature practice will enjoy a steady income, even though several weeks go by between filing and payment.

New dentists will have a temporary cash-flow problem because of a lag in receiving insurance payments. But office overhead, filing forms, and delayed payments should be viewed as necessary costs of doing business. There are several steps you can take to speed up receiving payments.

1. Delegate insurance matters to an employee (you will not have time to handle them), but review forms before signing.

2. Complete forms at the office and mail them; don't rely on the patient to do it, especially if you are accepting assignment.

3. Have the patient sign for employed spouse.

4. Use a separate "Authorization to Pay Dentist," have the patient sign it, and staple it to the completed form.

5. Have the patient sign as many blank forms at the beginning of treatment as will be needed (with many companies it is possible to note "signature on file" in the signature section).

6. Request payment for the examination on predetermination form.

7. Complete forms accurately: patient name, address, birthdate, Social Security numbers, and so on; tooth numbers, ADA codes, and exact description of restoration (MOD amalgam, not just "amalgam" or the company may pay the least applicable benefit).

8. Make sure radiographs are of good quality and readable. For pretreatment estimates, send originals, but send copies after treatment has been initiated.

9. Describe unusual treatment (on preprinted check list) that cannot be detected on radiographs or the company will write for explanation (further delay). Study models (or duplicates) will also help in some instances. Note on claim form if models are being sent under separate cover. In most cases send models and claim form in the same container so they will not be separated.

10. File for payment promptly.

11. File for payment in phases during extended treatment periods (consider use of "superbill" for filing after each visit).

12. Call the patient immediately when preauthorization arrives, inform him of the exact benefits and payment arrangements, and set up the first treatment appointment.

13. Multi-doctor offices with large volumes of patients may want to consider a computer to generate claim forms and statements quickly and efficiently.

INSURANCE PLANS

Dental insurance is often referred to as prepaid dentistry because premiums are paid to insurance companies before dental services are provided. Most premiums are paid by employers as fringe benefits for employees. Individuals may buy dental insurance personally.

Of the current (1981) 74 million Americans who are covered by some form of dental insurance, the plans are underwritten by the following carriers, according to Elliott in *Dental Economics,* April 1981:

43 million — Commercial carriers (Connecticut General, Aetna, Prudential, etc.)

17 million — Delta Dental Plans

7 million — Blue Cross, Blue Shield

7 million — Other types, such as union funds, consumer cooperatives, employers, federal government

Methods of Payment

Commercial carriers compute payment for dental services in various ways. The *usual customary and reasonable* (UCR) method means that the carrier will pay your fee provided:

1. It is usual — the same fee is charged to insured and uninsured patients.

2. It is customary if other dentists in the area with similar experience and background charge similar fees. The company may decide that fees above a certain percentile are not customary.

3. It is reasonable if the first two criteria are met or if a peer review committee judges it as such.

In the *table of allowances* method, services are itemized, and a fee is set for each one. Because the carrier will pay only the maximum fee listed per service, the patient must be responsible for the difference.

In the *service plans,* fees are itemized for each service and the dentist agrees to accept the listed fees as *full* payment. Delta Dental is a service plan for participating dentists, but is a table of allowances for nonparticipating dentists. They are paid at usually the fifty-first percentile and can collect the difference from the patients.

Blue Cross, Blue Shield plans pay participating and nonparticipating dentists on the same basis, whichever amount is the *lowest:* (1) the dentist's prefiled fee, (2) charges as listed on the claim form, or (3) the maximum allowable by the company. If there is a patient copayment involved, a participating dentist can charge the patient only the difference between the maximum allowable by the company and the amount paid by insurance. The nonparticipating dentist can charge the *full* amount of the difference between his fee and what is paid.

Most of the other plans are service plans. *Caution:* it is fraudulent to collect from the patient the difference between the dentist's fee and the service fee.

Providers

The dentists (providers) may be in *open or closed panel.* Most current (1981) programs are open panel. Closed panel programs include health maintenance organizations (HMO), group practices, union clinics, industry-owned clinics, and participating dentists in a program that does not utilize nonparticipating dentists. In capitation programs, participating dentists (closed panel) agree to provide

Because the carrier will pay only the maximum fee listed per service, the patient must be responsible for the difference.

designated services to a certain population at a per capita charge. Methods of remuneration to the dentists vary from salary to entrepreneurial earnings in capitation programs.

Dentists may form an independent practice association (IPA). The IPA is a fiscal intermediary between the member dentists and employer or groups of employers who purchase dental services for their employees on a per capita basis. The IPA is a mechanism for providing dental services as a fringe benefit without the employer purchasing a plan from an insurance company. In fact the IPA is very much like an insurance company formed by dentists.

The IPA is a mechanism for providing dental services as a fringe benefit without the employer purchasing a plan from an insurance company.

Dentists may be subject to continuing pressure from insurance administrators. Certain ones have proposed to dentists that they agree to be "participating dentists." The agreement provides that the dentist will accept the insurance fee as full payment. It is implied that the dentist will attract additional business and consequently enjoy higher income.

Marketing Enhancement

Upgrading of benefits is a means of expanding the market for dentistry. A dentist may be influential in helping to improve dental benefits of local industries in several ways. The first is by direct contact with business management personnel. It is very possible that some of these individuals are patients within the practice. If so, it would be a very natural topic of conversation during a dental visit to discuss how upgrading dental insurance would be a very real fringe benefit leading to positive morale factors for employees. Another direct contact with management could occur at civic or business functions. In fact, the dentist could speak on the subject at club meetings around town.

An indirect approach, but probably a very strong one, is to talk to patients and encourage them to voice their wishes for increased benefits. If there is a union representative who is a patient, that person would be ideal for bringing the matter to the attention of management.

As a member of organized dentistry you may have countless opportunities to enhance third party programs. Committees and councils correspond with industries and attempt to convince them of the value of dental insurance as a fringe benefit. Certainly as more industries purchase more dental insurance, workers and dentists benefit. Your involvement in obtaining more benefits can be important in your community.

From the information covered in this chapter, it should be obvious that dentists in today's market and economy must cater to patients who have dental insurance. To increase patient load, you might consider the following ideas if you are not already incorporating them:

1. Participate in dental service programs offered in your area.
2. Join an Independent Practice Association.
3. Accept assignment of benefits, especially on large treatment plans.

4. Do not charge a fee for filing forms. Patients get the subtle message that you *could* be charging if you say "We will be happy to file these forms *without charge* to you."

5. Give a cash discount if payment in full is made at the beginning of treatment, and the insurance benefit is paid directly to the patient.

6. Always be cheerful and helpful in communicating with patients who have dental insurance.

7. Assist patients to get maximum benefits from their insurance.

SUMMARY

The present enormous volume of patients with dental insurance constitutes a vast, untapped market. It is certainly to the advantage of any dental practice to treat these individuals and to do so with very positive attitudes.

The dental team that is able to communicate effectively with the public and insurance carriers concerning insurance benefits will discover that it has a unique marketing advantage. Not only will the inclusion of these patients boost the gross income of the practice, but it will also be a most helpful marketing technique in encouraging other patients with dental insurance to seek quality dental services.

Any potential problems associated with the handling of insurance can be averted by proper planning and a systematic approach.

REFERENCES

Beacham, H., Kendall, M. B. A., Francis, S. R.: Capitation: some truths and myths. JADA, Vol. 103, July 1981, pp. 26–30.

Caffrey, R.: Delta Dental Update. Summer/Fall, 1979.

Description and Documentation of the Private Practice Dental Delivery System, Hyattsville, MD, U.S. Department of Health and Human Services, March. 1980.

Dewey, L. C.: Dental insurance: how to deal with it. Dental Economics, December 1977, pp. 55–59.

Elliott, P. S.: A disturbing look at today's problems with insurance. Dental Economics, March 1981, pp. 38–43.

Elliott, P. S.: Delta, blues most complex of all plans. Dental Economics, April 1981, pp. 68–78.

Ehrlich, A.: Pre-treatment estimates: key to faster insurance processing. Dental Practice, April 1981, pp. 38–40.

Farlow, F. E.: Dental insurance: blessing or curse? Dental Economics, December 1977, pp. 51–53.

Farlow, F. E.: Dental insurance: what an insurance consultant expects of you. Dental Economics, December 1977, pp. 60–67.

Few surprises in dental insurance survey. Dental Economics, July 1981, pp. 32–36.

Paine, S. G.: Coordination of dental benefits explained. Dental Economics, March 1980, pp. 105–106.

Paine, S. G.: Dental insurance made easy - part 2. Dental Economics, July 1979, pp. 73–77.

Policies on Dental·Care Programs. Council on Dental Care Programs, ADA, Chicago, January 1981.

Practice Management. Dental Clinics of North America, Philadelphia, W. B. Saunders Co., April 1978, pp. 269–278.

Schmidt, D. A.: Riding the wave of dental insurance: cranking up the cashflow. Dental Management, November 1978, pp. 45–46.

Schmidt, D. A.: Riding the wave of dental insurance: your fees. Dental Management, September 1978, pp. 69–71.

Understanding Capitation Dentistry. ADA, Chicago, 1980.

18

Marketing with Staff

Steve Seldon was puzzled about the interview he had just conducted with a candidate for his chairside assistant position. Ann O'Keefe had left his office after handling herself very well in the interview, and Steve was considering offering her the job. He had conducted similar interviews before and they had seemed equally good, but later, the person he had hired had proven disappointing. "How," Steve found himself musing, "do I find someone who will help build this practice? I want to be a marketing dentist. Therefore, the people I hire should be marketing oriented as well. Only how do I find them?"

THE TEAM CONCEPT

Why bother with trying to develop a *team* in the dental office? Wouldn't it be just as good for each person in the practice to do his or her best to please patients? No, it would not. Team action may be likened to football. An outstanding individual player cannot succeed by himself. Only with concerted effort of all team members can the team accomplish its goals — that of winning the game. In order to win the game, each team member must know and perform his or her task in synchronization with the performance of others.

To win the game, each team member must know and perform his or her task in synchronization with the performance of others.

Douglas McGregor suggested characteristics of an effective work team, a summary of which follows:

1. The group atmosphere tends to be informal, comfortable, and relaxed.

2. People talk to one another, and, for the most part, the talk concerns the job to be done.

3. The task or the objective of the group is well understood and accepted by the members.

4. Group members listen to each other, and people are not afraid to express their ideas and opinions. Disagreements are exam-

ined and the group seeks to resolve them rather than to dominate the dissenter. The group finds it possible to accept basic disagreements that cannot be resolved.

5. Most decisions are reached by a consensus, even though not all group members agree with all points.

6. Criticism is frequent, frank, and relatively comfortable. People are free in expressing their feelings.

7. When action is taken, clear assignments are made and accepted. The group frequently will stop to examine how well it is accomplishing its task.

8. The leader or chairman of the group does not dominate it; in fact leadership shifts from person to person.

Life in a close organization, such as dental practice, can become tense. It is common for staff members to get on each other's nerves, and for the dentist and staff members to become irritable with each other. These are normal reactions and occurrences, but we need to keep them from getting out of hand. In order to guard against frictions among the dentist or dentists and auxiliaries, frequent office staff meetings are helpful. These will be discussed in some detail later in this chapter.

JOB DESCRIPTIONS

Consider having each person draft his or her own job description, while you draft a description for each job as well.

Every job in the dental office should have an up-to-date description written for it. In writing each job description, you should consider at least four questions:

1. What is the purpose of the job in the office?
2. What specific duties are involved in getting the job done?
3. What education and experience are required?
4. What mental and physical skills are required for the job?

Obviously, there will be differences of opinion among the den-

Job Title	Receptionist
Job Summary	Receives patients and visitors, answers telephone, schedules dentist(s), hygienists, and dental assistants.
Major Job Duties	Schedules all office appointments. Welcomes patients and visitors. Makes contacts with patients by telephone or mail regarding appointments, followup visits, pretreatment conferences, and so on.
Job Qualifications	Education: high school graduate, some college or business courses and CDA preferred. Experience: typing, office work, or work with public preferred. Personal requirements: pleasant personality and telephone voice required.

Figure 18–1. Sample job description.

Classification: Secretarial assistant to be responsible for the smooth functioning of the business office.

Areas of Responsibility

1. Greeting and seating patients
2. Answering the telephone
3. Typing and filing
4. Handling patient records
5. Making and confirming appointments
6. Handling financial arrangements, records, and collections
7. Conducting patient education program, including the preventive recall system
8. Maintaining inventory control and purchasing
9. Maintaining office neatness
10. Substituting for other staff members if needed

Desired Characteristics and Skills

1. Pleasant personality and interest in people
2. Maturity
3. Pleasant voice
4. Ability to work well with others
5. Enthusiasm
6. Health
7. Intelligence
8. Adaptability
9. Basic secretarial skills
10. Ability to organize work

Figure 18–2. Sample job description for a secretarial assistant. (From Ehrlich and Ehrlich, 1969, p. 137.)

tists in the office, as well as among the staff members, as to the correct description. As a result, extensive and frequent discussion and negotiation are called for. You might consider having each person draft his or her own job description, while you draft a description for each as well. Comparing these two descriptions will indicate immediately where potential problems lie. When you have fully considered the suggestions of the people holding the various jobs, you could write the final descriptions and tell each auxiliary why you have decided what you have.

Remember that jobs in the dental office may change over time. Just because a particular duty was right when the description was written does not mean that it will always be so. You and your staff should review jobs periodically, perhaps annually, and make sure the job descriptions still fit. Another item to remember is that the description should not be written for a person, but instead for the work. In writing this description, try to remove the person or persons currently occupying the position or positions from consideration. Write the description as much as possible so that it will hold no matter who occupies the position. Figure 18–1 is a sample job description for a receptionist position. Figure 18–2 is a sample description for a secretarial assistant (from Ehrlich and Ehrlich, 1969, p. 137). There are many different suitable job descriptive forms; just make certain that the format chosen satisfies the dental team.

STRUCTURE JOBS FOR MARKETING EFFECTIVENESS

It is essential that the receptionist know what to say and how to handle all persons visiting the office.

Throughout your dental office, there will be duties that need to be structured and handled from a marketing standpoint. Your job descriptions, your training of employees, and your reward system must be structured to produce the best marketing job your office can perform. Following are some of the duties in most dental offices that we believe require generous marketing inputs. Without doubt, a serious consideration of the operation of your office will reveal others with which you should deal.

1. *Prompt and correct answering of the telephone.* The telephone is the first contact made with your office by patients and others. The telephone answering system during and after business hours may be the most important marketing tool you develop. Chapter 9 details the many considerations for the dental office telephone system.

2. *Prompt and correct greeting and handling of the reception desk.* The next most prevalent first contact for most patients (the first for some, of course) is the reception desk. It is essential that the receptionist know what to say and how to handle all persons visiting the office. Chapters 12, 13, 14, and 15 deal with patient visits to your office.

3. *Dental insurance.* This is a very common and timely subject with which you and your staff must be familiar. Chapter 17 treats this subject.

4. *Appointment system and practice bookkeeping.* In order to build your practice over time, and even the most experienced dentist needs to do this, you need appropriate and up-to-date techniques for scheduling appointments. A number of chapters in this book touch upon scheduling. On the subject of practice bookkeeping, Chapter 19, "Evaluating Marketing Effectiveness," and Chapter 20, "Improving Business Systems," detail some steps you should consider to determine which of your services and which of your technical and marketing practices are most cost/marketing effective.

As with telephone calls and reception desk visits, your practice's image and effectiveness will be judged by the look and content of your letters, notes, cards, and so on.

5. *Response through correspondence.* Chapter 10 takes you through the types of office correspondence you are likely to send and receive and how such correspondence should be handled. As with telephone calls and reception desk visits, your practice's image and effectiveness will be judged by the look and content of your letters, notes, cards, and so on.

6. *Efficient and unhurried responses to patients.* It is essential that your patients realize that you are interested in them as people, not just as technical problems. This requires listening to them, *real listening,* including observations of their nonverbal messages, sometimes called "body language." After you have listened to their questions and have "read between the lines," so to speak, you should give them a thorough, unhurried answer, attempting to deal with underlying as well as expressed concerns and needs.

7. *Public Speaking.* Both you and your staff are potential speakers to schools, civic groups, and other groups on the subjects of dental hygiene, advancements in dentistry, and so on. These efforts, if done well, can provide a distinct marketing advantage for your practice. However, you must be trained yourself and must provide rather ex-

tensive training for your staff. If you or a member of your staff goes out to speak before a group and does not come across with an interesting, effective talk or presentation, you can damage your practice and its image. One way to develop speaking ability for yourself and staff members is through participation in the local Toastmaster's Club. Most such clubs have breakfast, luncheon, or dinner meetings during which you can receive extensive practice in public speaking and constructive criticism on your speaking techniques and the content and effectiveness of your presentations on dental hygiene or whatever other topics you choose to speak about. In any event, you and your staff should develop written presentations, at least in outline form, and practice them on each other and on your families prior to appearing before groups.

SELECTING EMPLOYEES

The interview is one of the most commonly used means of selecting employees. However, it has been shown to be faulty, to the point that many mistakes in hiring are made because of unasked questions or misperceptions during the pre-employment interview. This section of the chapter will help you better conduct the interview

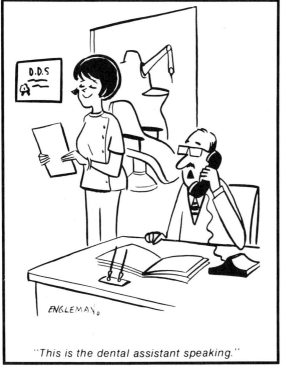

"This is the dental assistant speaking."

Courtesy of *Cal* magazine.

and determine how well a prospective employee will suit your office. Peterson, Tracy, and Cabelly (1979) have been used as our principal source here.

Candidate Sources

When you decide you need to hire a new employee, you should use the sources that have proven profitable in the past. Many dentists find newspaper classified ads helpful. In major metropolitan areas, local or regional daily or weekly newspapers should be considered, along with the metro dailies. It has been shown that housewives re-entering the job market tend to use these sources for employment possibilities. Others find that notices given to local schools and colleges are productive. Sometimes the local Employment Security Commission has appropriate job candidates. Your own office staff and personnel of other dental offices are excellent sources of new employees. You should ask all candidates to supply a personal data sheet or letter detailing their education and work experience. Be certain to ask for references on those candidates you believe are possible employees.

If your office is short-handed, your tendency will be to hire someone you may later be sorry you hired.

How Urgent the Hiring Need?

If your office is short-handed and you feel the need to get some immediate help, you are inclined to overlook potential problems with the person you are interviewing. Your tendency will be to hire someone you should not hire. Later, you will be sorry for your haste. One way to overcome this problem is to develop a standardized interview procedure and to hire a temporary person while you are sifting through your permanent candidates.

Structured Versus Unstructured Interviews

Should you have a set procedure for the interview or should you follow the interviewee's lead in discussion topics? Research has shown that structured interviews work best. (At least they should be structured in the dentist's mind.) All points must be covered, but the order of coverage is not important. Under a structured interview condition, the interviewer knows what to ask and what to do with the information. The interviewer can and does apply the same frame of reference to each interviewee. It has been shown that even with much experience in interviewing, one does not do a good enough job of interviewing without a structure.

Your interview with potential auxiliaries should cover the same topics for each person. Figure 18–3 is an interview record, to be filled out immediately after each interview and filed for future reference. The form was inspired by an article on office staffing in *Dental Economics,* December 1980.

INTERVIEW RECORD

Name of applicant _____

Address _____

Telephone __(___)_____   Date of Interview _____

	Excellent	Average	Needs Improvement
GENERAL APPEARANCE			
Facial expression	_____	_____	_____
Neatness of dress	_____	_____	_____
Smiles easily	_____	_____	_____
PERSONALITY			
Friendly manner	_____	_____	_____
Talks easily	_____	_____	_____
Seems alert	_____	_____	_____
Appears intelligent	_____	_____	_____
Has a sense of humor	_____	_____	_____
Appears mature	_____	_____	_____
Appears stable	_____	_____	_____
SPEECH			
Voice	_____	_____	_____
Diction	_____	_____	_____
Uses tact	_____	_____	_____
Enthusiastic	_____	_____	_____
BACKGROUND			
Education	_____	_____	_____
Dental skills	_____	_____	_____
Job experience	_____	_____	_____
Goal-oriented	_____	_____	_____

ADDITIONAL COMMENTS _____

_____

_____

Figure 18–3. Sample interview record.

Comparison Standards

By using the methods outlined in this chapter, you will improve your chances of selecting people who work out well.

The persons interviewed before a particular interview takes place can influence evaluation of a current interviewee. If you interview three or four poor candidates, and then interview a reasonably good one, you will be inclined to rate the last one higher than if you had not interviewed the poor ones first. Therefore, you should consider seriously the context within which you have conducted a particular interview and make allowances for particularly good or bad previous candidates.

Obviously, the purpose of the pre-employment interview is to predict which candidate will do the best job of assisting in the dental office and satisfying patients. What is the probability that you will be accurate in your predictions about interviewed auxiliaries? Research has shown that you will be able to record the facts about a job candidate rather accurately, but that you will evaluate those facts less accurately. That is, your record in predicting just how well a job candidate will perform in an auxiliary job will be less accurate. By using the methods outlined in this chapter, you will improve your chances of selecting people who work out well.

SELECTING NEW EMPLOYEES

After you have interviewed candidates, how do you decide which one or ones to choose? The appropriate people seem to have two attributes: (1) They will be able to work in a highly-structured, obsessive, compulsive kind of office where one must be in attendance and on time, must be detail-oriented, and must follow a rather tight schedule, and, (2) they will be able to fit in with the rest of the staff, will be friendly, patient-oriented, and sensitive to the needs of both patients and coworkers.

A procedure suggested in *Dental Economics* (September 1979, pp. 44–47) will help you find that special person who is "just right" for your marketing dental office:

1. Never select a new auxiliary in a hurry just because you have to fill a vacant position. Always take enough time to select the correct person. To paraphrase an "old saw," your acting in haste may allow you to repent at your leisure.

2. If you need a person to fill in until you can select the right permanent employee, do just that. Call one or more of your colleagues or a temporary employment service and find a person who will work on a temporary basis until you can find your choice of an auxiliary. In general, the person you use on a temporary basis should be a person not eligible for the long-term position. It will be harder for you to be objective about the qualifications of temporaries if they are in the office all day. And, their actions and attitudes will be colored by their wish to retain the job permanently.

3. If a job candidate is in an extreme hurry and not willing to wait the ten days to two weeks necessary for you to find the right person, perhaps you should not consider such an applicant. A person in a hurry may well be a person who invests little in finding the right

A person in a hurry to be hired may well be a person who invests little in finding the right position in the right dental office.

position in the right dental office, and may well be lured away with a few extra dollars per week from another office.

4. Use an interview form, such as the one suggested in this chapter. It will allow you to be much more systematic in your approach to evaluating potential auxiliaries.

5. Be sure to follow up on references from former employers. Most former employers will be candid with you and will tell you how the candidate is likely to fit in with other staff members, how good attendance and on-time records were, and so on. If a person gives only vague references or refers you to ministers, try to get a reference or two from some work experience, even if it is volunteer work with a charitable organization.

6. When you have narrowed the list of candidates to two or three, ask each of them to "work" in your office for a few days, observing you, the other staff, and, if possible, the person to be replaced. In order to get just the right person, you can afford to pay a total of a week or two of salary to these potential long-term employees. You should observe which one catches on the most quickly, relates the best to patients and other staff members, is the most energetic, enthusiastic, and eager to learn. And see also which trial employee improves the most as the days go by.

7. Your staff members may be qualified to interview job candidates and provide guidance to you. They, after all, must work with the new staff member. Perhaps the staff "interview" can consist of a group luncheon, paid for by the practice.

8. Whatever happens, do not make a quick decision about a matter as important as hiring a new staff member. Given the investment you have made in your education, in your office and equipment, in your other staff members, and in your patients, you certainly should be careful about whom you add to your practice.

Just what kind of person makes the best marketing dental auxiliary? Richard D. Hark in *Dental Economics,* September 1979, p. 47, has an answer for this:

> My own experience has shown this person to be very outgoing, can organize and direct others, can take added responsibility with enthusiasm and is the type of individual who truly enjoys working with people and developing harmonious human contacts. She has a great deal of energy, cannot stand to be idle and will look for work, asking other staff members if she can help to avoid being bored. She is a very feeling person, needs to be complimented and recognized for her good work, and is very sensitive to criticism. She is not going to be assertive and will often not tell you when things are bothering her until she explodes or cries. She likes order, likes to finish tasks and borders on being almost compulsive about details.

Marketing Through Applicants Not Hired

If you are doing the thorough job of interviewing we suggest here, there will be a number of people to whom you will have to say "no." Saying no correctly is an art, one which you will profit from learning well. During the course of the interviews, and in some cases, trial work periods, you will become well-acquainted with potential employees. The more you become acquainted with them, the harder

Be sure to follow up on references from former employers.

it will be to say no, but, of course, you must. You cannot hire everybody.

It is helpful to look upon the necessity of saying "no" also as an opportunity to recruit a new patient, or at least to encourage job candidates to refer patients to you. You should carefully explain to the candidates to whom you have said "no" that it was a very difficult decision for you, that you wish you could have hired more than one person, and that if the need for hiring arises later, and the candidates happen to be looking for a job, you would certainly like to consider hiring them at that time. You may also mention the possibility of suggesting the candidate to another dentist. Being refused a job is a bitter pill to swallow, but, using the "cushions" we have just described will mollify most people you must turn down.

Many job candidates whom you interview will be new arrivals in town. If the candidate does not currently have a dentist, you might close the last interview with the statement that you believe you practice good dentistry and would welcome her or him, this candidate's family, and any friends as patients. Done professionally, this will not "turn off" most refused candidates and might well result in new patients.

EMPLOYEE COMMUNICATIONS

Training in the Dental Office

It is assumed that the person you hire will be technically trained, or that you will be willing to undergo the training time and expense to bring that person up to the level you require. Even given previous academic or experiential education and training on the applicant's part, you will need a considerable reservoir of patience. Simply remember that people do not learn as quickly as we all believe they should, and that it takes time to indoctrinate them into the intricacies of a dental office operation.

The specifics of a training program for a new dental auxiliary will vary depending upon the job for which a person is hired, the age, education, and experience of the person and the number of people currently in the office who can serve as "models." Bregstein (1953) has suggested a number of steps in the basic training for a new secretary-nurse. The following training suggestions are inspired by Bregstein's list:

1. Conduct your new employee on a general inspection tour, pointing out the need for cleanliness, order, and accuracy. If you have had this person observe the office operation previously, this step may be shortened somewhat. The same may be true of other steps, but do not use this as an excuse for not conducting a thorough training program.

2. Throughout the office tour, emphasize the need for patients, and hence the need for patient satisfaction. If the employee has come from an office where patients were considered a "necessary evil," you may wish to have her read some recent issues of *Dental Economics* or

Look upon the necessity of saying "no" also as an opportunity to recruit a new patient, or at least to encourage job candidates to refer patients to you.

one of the other dental magazines that recognize the need for a marketing approach to dentistry.

3. Show the new employee where your printed forms, stationery, and sample forms are kept and how they are used.

4. Explain your recall system and its operation.

5. Explain your filing system. After the explanation, assign the new employee several items to find in the system.

6. Describe the telephone procedure used in the office. After the description, have the new auxiliary take several telephone calls, and monitor them for correctness.

7. Briefly describe your office meeting schedule and procedures. Encourage active participation in the meetings and suggestions for practice and office improvement.

8. If appropriate, brief the new employee on dental nomenclature.

9. If appropriate, indicate the names and uses of instruments and equipment.

10. Review again the hours of employment, vacation schedule procedure, holiday schedule, and other details of the office operation.

11. Review again the salary arrangements agreed to previously and review the promotion possibilities, if such exist within your practice.

Performance Reviews

You should conduct a performance review every six months for most employees, and certainly every year for long-term employees. For new employees, a performance review may be timely at the end of

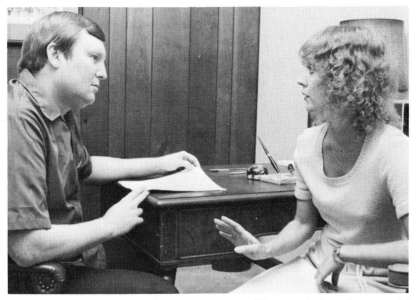

It is important for the dentist and for the auxiliary to sit down for a candid performance review every six months or so.

PERFORMANCE REVIEW

Name_____ Date_____

	Excellent	Acceptable	Needs Improvement
Cooperation with dentist(s)	_____	_____	_____
Cooperation with co-workers	_____	_____	_____
Working with/marketing to patients	_____	_____	_____
Follow through on assignments	_____	_____	_____
Optimistic attitude	_____	_____	_____
Personal cleanliness/attire	_____	_____	_____
Productivity in work	_____	_____	_____
Cleanliness in work	_____	_____	_____
Attendance/missing days	_____	_____	_____
Punctuality	_____	_____	_____
Patient referral	_____	_____	_____
_____ (other)	_____	_____	_____
_____ (other)	_____	_____	_____

Growth in above factors since last review

1._____

2._____

3._____

Goals for above factors for next month

1._____

2._____

3._____

Goals for above factors for next six months

1._____

2._____

3._____

Comments on strong and weak points_____

_____

_____

_____

Figure 18–4. Sample performance review form.

each of the first three months. Whatever the time schedule you choose for your office, the reviews should take place regularly. Nothing should cause you to put off scheduled reviews for more than a week or so.

Prior to the review, both the dentist and the employee should fill out the same form detailing the job the person has done for the period since the last review. You may then compare the forms prior to and during the review for differences of opinion between the dentist and the employee. All differences should be discussed and the reasons for the differences brought out. If you and your staff are to work as a team, you have to have mutual trust and belief in each other.

A performance review form is included as Figure 18–4. As with all of the forms suggested in this book, this should be adapted for your practice. You may wish to eliminate some of these items and add others.

> You should conduct a performance review every six months for most employees, and certainly every year for long-term employees. *

Exit Interviews

No matter how well your office is functioning, no matter how good an employer you are, some of your employees will leave occasionally. An exit interview can benefit your practice. You may determine if your exiting employee is likely to be a booster of your office in the future. If so, you may suggest to her that you would like to provide dental care to her friends. Remembering ex-employee birthdays, births, graduations, and so on will go a long way toward making them continuing boosters of you and your practice.

> Remembering ex-employee birthdays, births, graduations, and so on will go a long way toward making them continuing boosters of you and your practice.

COMMUNICATIONS IN THE OFFICE

Steve Seldon believes he is in close contact with his staff. He is with them at least thirty-six hours a week, after all. Now and then he sits down with whatever auxiliary is taking a break and has a cup of coffee. How could there not be good communication within the office? Steve might be surprised if he really knew how his employees felt. They happen not to feel that he understands their problems very well. Steve needs a feedback tool.

Figure 18–5 is a survey suggested by Robert Levoy in *Dental Economics,* November 1978. This can be used to determine just what your employees think of your office and how to run it. This survey may be used immediately and then periodically, as your staff turns over and you believe a recheck is necessary.

Staff Meetings

One of the very important means of communicating the "patient satisfaction" message to your staff is through regularly scheduled staff meetings. Some offices hold such meetings monthly, others find that a twice-monthly or weekly meeting is required. Whatever the

EMPLOYEE ATTITUDE SURVEY

	Strongly Agree	Agree	Disagree	Strongly Disagree
The doctor is fair with me.	_____	_____	_____	_____
I know well what is expected of me on the job.	_____	_____	_____	_____
I understand the reasons for changes in policies or procedures.	_____	_____	_____	_____
On-going training in this office is not satisfactory.	_____	_____	_____	_____
The doctor and staff appreciate my efforts to do a good job.	_____	_____	_____	_____
Development in job capabilities is encouraged here.	_____	_____	_____	_____
When I started in this office I was given adequate training.	_____	_____	_____	_____
This office has too much pressure on employees.	_____	_____	_____	_____
The office employees cooperate and help each other out when needed.	_____	_____	_____	_____
This job is adequately challenging.	_____	_____	_____	_____
The pay of employees is fair.	_____	_____	_____	_____
We should have more frequent staff meetings.	_____	_____	_____	_____
Office policies have been clearly communicated to me.	_____	_____	_____	_____
I was not told correctly what this job would be like.	_____	_____	_____	_____
I am paid fairly compared with other employees.	_____	_____	_____	_____
I like the working hours in the office.	_____	_____	_____	_____
Staff meetings are not helpful to employees.	_____	_____	_____	_____
If I have a complaint, I know how to get it resolved.	_____	_____	_____	_____
There is a satisfactory performance review system in the office.	_____	_____	_____	_____
This is a good place to work.	_____	_____	_____	_____
The doctor is truly interested in my ideas.	_____	_____	_____	_____
Some things that go on in this office are annoying.	_____	_____	_____	_____
The doctor and staff are friendly to me.	_____	_____	_____	_____
Some things in this office could be improved.	_____	_____	_____	_____
The doctor and staff give me the support I need.	_____	_____	_____	_____

Additional comments on any question or subject.

_____

_____

_____

_____

Figure 18–5. Sample attitude survey for employees.

schedule you decide upon, just make sure meetings are held regularly. If you indicate by frequent putting off of staff meetings that you do not consider them important, you can be certain your staff will soon agree.

Meetings should be held at a time when you and the staff are fresh and enthusiastic. This rules out most afternoons. Early or late morning are found to be best by most dentists. Mornings are good from another standpoint as well. If some criticism of a person or office technique is made during the meeting, there will be time to observe a criticized procedure, to institute and observe a new procedure, and generally to iron out any difficulties or bad feelings that might have been generated by the morning meeting. The bad feelings should not persist past the end of the day. Last, many practices tend to get busier as the day progresses, so time is usually more available in the morning.

Every staff meeting should include a discussion of marketing, what it is and how it pertains to your dental office. Auxiliaries should be reminded periodically that they are rewarded, in part, based on their marketing expertise.

> Every staff meeting should include a discussion of marketing, what it is and how it pertains to your dental office.

SUMMARY

Steve Seldon now is not so puzzled about his recent interview with a potential new auxiliary. It was comforting to Steve to learn that he is not alone in being unable to predict accurately which of the people he interviews will make good auxiliaries for his dental office. He now has job descriptions written for each of the jobs in his office; he interviews job candidates according to a standard procedure; and he is as objective as possible in evaluating them. His training of new

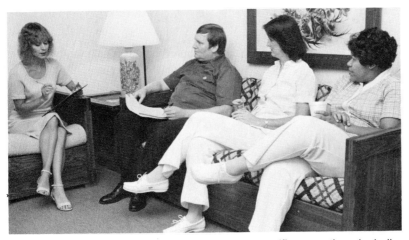

Regular meetings help you get staff input into your office operations, including all marketing programs.

employees is thorough, including a discussion of the previously untouched subjects of marketing and patient satisfaction. He reviews the performance of each of his employees regularly, holds productive staff meetings on a scheduled basis, and has a good idea of how well his auxiliaries like their jobs and his office's operations. "I don't have all the answers," Steve says, "but I feel more confident that I know what questions to ask and that my communication with my office staff has greatly improved."

REFERENCES

Bregstein, S. J.: The Successful Practice of Dentistry, New York, Prentice-Hall, Inc., 1953, Chapter 13.

Domer, L. R., Snyder, T. L., and Heid, D. W.: Dental Practice Management. St. Louis, The C. V. Mosby Company, 1980, Chapters 12 and 13.

Dyer, W. G.: Team Building: Issues and Alternatives. Reading, Massachusetts, Addison-Wesley Publishing Company, 1977.

Ehrlich, A. B., and Ehrlich, S. F.: Dental Practice Management. Philadelphia, W. B. Saunders Company, 1969, Chapters 15, 16, and 17.

Glueck, W. F.: Personnel. Dallas, Texas, Business Publications, Inc., 1979.

Hark, R. D.: What a psychologist can tell you about your staff. Dental Economics, September 1979, pp. 44–47.

Howard, W. W.: Dental Practice Planning. St. Louis, C. V. Mosby Company, 1975, Chapters 12 and 16.

Reap, C. A., Jr.: Complete Dental Assistant's, Secretary's, and Hygienist's Handbook. West Nyack, NY, Parker Publishing Company, Inc., 1973, Chapters 9 and 16.

Rowland, K. M., et al.: Current Issues in Personnel Management. Boston, Allyn and Bacon, Inc., 1980.

Peterson, R. B., Tracy, L., and Cabelly, A.: Readings in Systematic Management of Human Resources. Reading, Massachusetts, Addison-Wesley Publishing Company, 1979.

Stinaff, R. K.: Dental Practice Administration. St. Louis, C. V. Mosby Company, 1960, Chapter 8.

19

Evaluating Marketing Effectiveness

You have learned, by this point, a fair amount about the science, or art, of marketing professional services. We hope you have begun to apply some of the material you have absorbed. It is time now to assess how well you are doing with your marketing techniques. What works well for you? What doesn't? How can you tell for sure? What "fine tuning" needs to be done to sharpen the effectiveness of your marketing programs?

GRAPHING REVENUES AND PATIENT COUNTS

In order to evaluate our marketing programs, we have several possible courses of action; we should take all of them. First, we should look at the gross revenues of the practice. Often this is best done by graphing revenues by week or month. Those of us who have been in practice for some years should graph revenues by week for at least two years back. We can determine which weeks' revenues are lower than others and perhaps learn why. We might be able to decide *why* receipts are down simply by knowing *when* they are down. If weeks vary in length in your practice, and they do in most, you may wish to calculate an average daily revenue for each day you are open. If your days vary in length, you may wish to calculate an average hourly revenue per day and per week.

Second, we should do the same thing with patient counts, perhaps by week, but perhaps also by day or half-day. We can then see where our practice's "weak spots" fall, and make changes.

Variability of production during the year is natural. Typically, patients will defer treatment (because much of it is elective) from Thanksgiving to February. They will likewise put it off during the

Those in practice for some years should graph revenues by week for at least two years back.

297

week containing July 4, if many mills and factories close down for vacations. August is normally a busy dental treatment time for children, to get ready to return to school.

The next internal analysis procedure we should undertake is an analysis of our financial statements, including budget, income statement (profit and loss statement), and balance sheet. Many dentists concern themselves primarily with the income statement. We believe that dentists should be concerned equally with developing and using a budget and with their balance sheets. We hope what we are about to discuss will help. We shall be drawing here on Domer, Snyder, and Heid, *Dental Practice Management*. Remember that the real purpose of the financial analysis is to determine the effectiveness of your marketing program.

FINANCIAL ANALYSIS

Budget

Periodic budget analysis will assist you in keeping expenses under control.

The budget is a formal presentation of your spending plans for a forthcoming time period. Most dentists use a yearly budget, but it may be necessary for you, at least at times, to prepare a budget for a shorter time period, perhaps quarterly. Your budget development, of course, must be coordinated with the goals you have set, as described in Chapter 5. The budget forces you to think ahead about what revenues will be and what expenditures ought to be. The budget contains a list of expenses you expect to incur, including salaries, taxes, rent or mortgage payment, utilities, supplies, and so on. It may be developed on the basis of past expenditures or, if you are just starting, on the basis of your best estimates. Periodic budget analysis will assist you in keeping expenses under control.

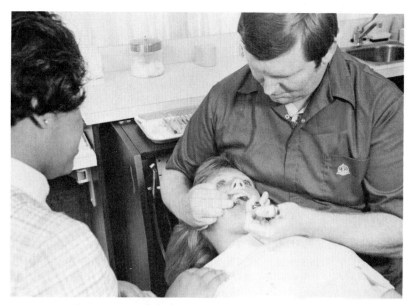

Painless injections are tremendous practice builders.

Income Statement

The income statement, sometimes referred to as the profit and loss statement or the operating statement, lists revenues, expenses, and, as a result of these, net income over a period of time. Figure 19–1 is a hypothetical income statement. The practice billed patients $100,000 and collected $90,000, a low average for marketing practices. Collection procedures are dealt with further in Chapter 20.

In Figure 19–1 it is shown that the dentist earned a total net income for 1982 of $40,500, which was 45 percent of the practice's revenues.

Using the percentage columns to the left, one can learn not only that expenses consumed 55 percent of the practice's revenues, but also what portion of revenues was taken by each of the expense categories. Incidentally, some accountants may suggest that you include an expense category called "bad debts," and include in this any accounts you decide are uncollectible in any given year. Others may simply suggest that you reflect uncollectibles in your revenue figures, as we have done in Figure 19–1.

By itself, a one-year income statement is very revealing. However, its real worth lies in analyzing the trends or growth of the practice. If, as your marketing improves and your practice fees increase, all of your expenses increase by the same amount, your net income will not increase. Tracking annually, and perhaps more often than that, just which expenses are increasing and then taking steps to hold down the increases will help to ward off this problem.

JANUARY 1–DECEMBER 31, 198–

PRACTICE BILLING (fees)		$100,000	
Collected Revenue		90,000	100.0%
Expenses			
Wages and Salaries	18,800		20.9
Laboratory fees	11,000		12.2
Rent or mortgage payment	6,900		7.7
Supplies	2,300		2.6
Office utilities	2,000		2.2
Payroll and other taxes	1,900		2.1
Telephone	1,400		1.5
Professional development	1,400		1.6
Accounting expenses	1,200		1.3
Postage	1,200		1.3
Insurance policies	900		1.0
Miscellaneous	500		.6
Total Expenses		49,500	55.0%
Net Income		40,500	45.0%

Figure 19–1. Sample yearly income statement.

Balance Sheet

The balance sheet shows the apparent wealth of the practice, its assets and liabilities. Assets less liabilities equals the owner's net worth or equity in the practice. Figure 19–2 illustrates a hypothetical balance sheet for a dental practice. Unlike the income statement, which was for a period *of* time, the balance sheet is for a period *in* time, in this case, December 31, 198–.

What can a balance sheet tell us? Among other items, it can tell us whether or not we are keeping too large a cash balance on hand. In Figure 19–2, a cash balance of $8,000 probably is too high given accounts payable and taxes payable accounts of $4,700 and $3,300 respectively. Probably some of the cash should be invested in a money market certificate or fund, or in a savings account, depending upon their respective interest rates. In some cases, depending upon the interest rate of the long-term liability, it may be to your advantage to pay off some of this liability.

Again, a one-time balance sheet is revealing in and of itself. The

DECEMBER 31, 198–

ASSETS

Current Assets		
Cash	$ 8,000	
Accounts receivable	12,500	
Supplies	8,500	
Total current assets		$29,000
Fixed Assets		
Furniture	$ 8,500	
Equipment	26,800	
Total fixed assets	35,300	
Less accumulated depreciation	12,100	
Net fixed assets		23,200
Other assets		
Deferred expenses		1,800
Total Assets		54,000

LIABILITIES

Current liabilities		
Accounts payable	$ 4,700	
Taxes payable	3,300	
Total current liabilities		$ 8,000
Long-term liabilities		
Notes payable	$26,000	26,000
Total liabilities		34,000
Owner's equity		20,000
Total liabilities and owner's equity		$54,000

Figure 19–2. Sample balance sheet.

most profitable use of the balance sheet, however, is in making comparisons over the years, in determining what progress is being made by the practice.

Productivity Analysis

Production refers to the total amount of dental services rendered. *Productivity* refers to the amount of dental services rendered per hour or per auxiliary. This is done by simply dividing the number of hours the practice was operating each month (or week, if you wish) into the total practice revenues. For example, if you were "open" for 140 hours in a month and had $9,800 in fees for that month, your productivity was $70.00 per hour. If you have the same $9,800 revenue and employed the equivalent of three auxiliaries, your productivity per auxiliary was $3,267.

By being aware of your productivity, per hour and per auxiliary, you can have a better idea of where you stand, what improvements you must make, what goals to set. By comparing your productivity over time, perhaps weekly, certainly monthly, you will be able to track your practice growth.

By being aware of your productivity, per hour and per auxiliary, you can have a better idea of where you stand.

SURVEYS

After you have completed analyses of your revenues and expenses and your practice productivity, it is time to consider the most important people in your practice — your patients. Most of us also need to think about those people who are not our patients and determine how we might attract them to our practice.

This basic tool for finding out about our patients and those who are not our patients is the survey. We will first discuss the types of survey's in general; then we shall offer some hints on how to conduct them.

There are three basic ways to conduct surveys, whether of current patients, former patients, potential patients, or the community in general. These are personal interviews, telephone surveys, and mail surveys. Let's look at each in turn.

Personal Interviews

Personal interviews, as the name implies, consist of the dentist or some other person sitting down with a person and asking questions. This is the best way to get to the heart of the matter. It is easiest with personal interviews to ask the followup questions necessary to probe a respondent's initial answers. For example, when a patient states, "I don't feel very comfortable in the dental office," and seems content to leave his answer at that, the interviewer can ask: "Why is that?", or "What do you mean by that?" Face-to-face, with a skilled interviewer, people will answer questions more frankly and thoroughly than they will by any other means.

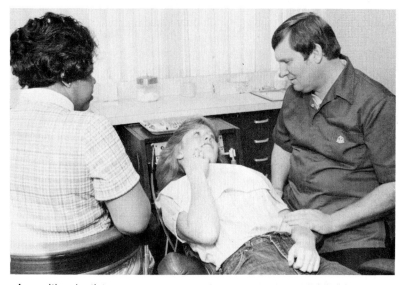

A sensitive dentist encourages teen patient to check her jaw after injection.

The major drawback with personal interviews is that they take considerable time and money. Most dental office surveys will take at least fifteen minutes of time from one of your auxiliaries. Further, the dental office may not be the place to conduct surveys. Privacy must be provided for such interviews, just as for the initial interview. When treatment is completed, an interview such as that described in Chapter 15 can provide very helpful information.

It is possible to have personal interviews done for you by someone else, but the cost is probably going to be in the range of $15 to $20 per interview. One way to get around the high cost of personal interviews is by means of a relatively new technique called *focus group interviews*. Focus groups, as the name implies, consist of bringing together 8 to 14 people and interviewing them as a group. A skilled interviewer can introduce the subjects of dental care, dental offices, dentists' techniques, and so on, and can allow the group to interact and discuss the subjects, always bringing the discussion into "focus" on the desired topic. This technique is certainly beyond the skill level of most dentists and dental auxiliaries. Thus you would need to contract with a marketing or public relations agency, or with a skilled individual — unless you happen to possess such skills yourself.

Focus groups consist of bringing together 8 to 14 people and interviewing them as a group.

Mail Surveys

Mail is probably the most common and popular method of conducting surveys. Many people will take the time to complete a mail questionnaire. The anonymity promised will encourage candid responses. And the results can be tabulated in the dentist's or the auxiliaries' spare time. Thus, many dental offices will find mail surveys the most suitable type.

Mail surveys, however, do present some problems. Because

response is at the option of the person to whom the questionnaire is sent, it is difficult to know if you have an adequate, representative sample. Also, mail surveys require considerably more clerical work than do the other types of surveys. In assuring anonymity, you are "encouraging" the recipient to throw the mailing away and not respond.

Further, with the continuing rise in postage costs, it is becoming more difficult to justify mail surveys economically. Most dental offices will find it suitable to send surveys first class. Thus, a survey of 500 patients will cost about $200 (or more, as costs continue to inflate), plus the cost of paper, envelopes, printing, stuffing, and salaries. Mail surveys, however, are the easiest type of survey to administer. The work can be done by your auxiliaries in their spare time and, perhaps, by you and your family in the evening at home.

Many dental offices will find mail surveys the most suitable type.

Assuming a mail-out of 500 questionnaires, a one-third return, and a total cost of a mail survey at $300, the cost per completed questionnaire for the survey will be approximately $1.80. If your return is less than one-third, which is often the case, your unit cost will be proportionately higher.

Telephone Surveys

Perhaps the best survey method for many dental offices is the telephone. People are used to talking on the telephone and will answer freely. You can be certain that you have a sufficient number of completed interviews, and, if it seems called for, the interviewer can probe for additional answers.

Most telephone companies have what are called Reverse Telephone Directories, which are telephone books arranged by street

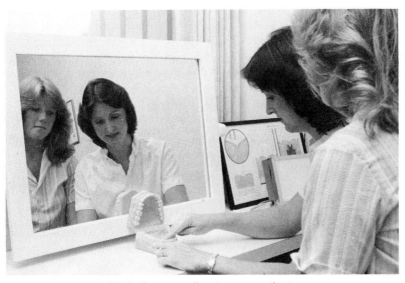

Hygienist counseling teenage patient.

address. Medium- to large-size cities also will have "City Directories," which provide the same information. (Check with your Chamber of Commerce.) In this method, you may determine who the people are on the streets you wish to have surveyed: these people and these people only may be surveyed. Further, you can go through the list and eliminate other dentists or other people whom you do not, for whatever reason, wish to survey. Telephone surveys, depending upon how and by whom they are done, will cost from about $3.00 to $5.00 per completed interview.

Who Is To Do The Surveys?

By now you will have realized that surveys are complicated, technical, and somewhat difficult to do. Usually, such surveys will be beyond the scope of people in your office. Many dentists turn to consultants or other types of people to do their surveys. Your telephone directory will list possible survey sources under "Market Research and Analysis," "Management Consultants," "Research Consultants," "Research Service," or perhaps some other listing. Other possible sources include contacting nearby colleges or universities for marketing, management, or, sometimes, economics, journalism, or sociology professors who do survey work in their spare time. In a few instances, it might be possible to employ a high school teacher to do such work. It is important that the person you choose be experienced in interviewing and work in a highly structured manner.

Sometimes it will be possible to have such surveys done internally, especially if your auxiliaries have spare time to devote to it, and you can locate a professional marketing person willing to train and supervise them.

If it is possible to have the survey done by your auxiliaries in their spare time, the out-of-pocket cost to you is small. You are utilizing people already on the payroll, from an office for which you are already paying, and on your office telephones. If this is not possible, you may be able to hire experienced part-time people to conduct the telephone interviews from their homes in the evening. It is necessary that a knowledgeable person train them in how to interview and supervise their work, however. Without an adequate job of interviewing, the results you receive will be worthless, even misleading.

Many dentists turn to consultants or other types of people to do their surveys.

SURVEYS OF ACTIVE PATIENTS

The first type of survey you do probably should be a "Patient Information Form." Much of this information can be gathered from your current records. You are interested in such information as age, sex, education, occupation, address, number of children, and so on. You are, of course, interested in income, but it probably is better not to ask income for fear of "turning off" the patient. A suggested patient information form is included as Figure 19–3.

If any of the information on the patient information form is not currently in your files, your receptionist can start collecting it as

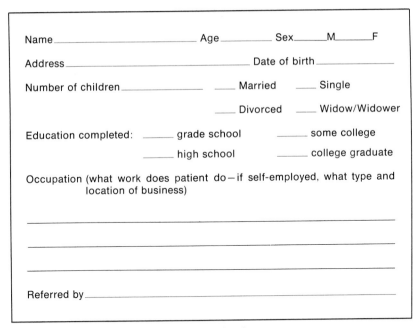

Name_____ Age_____ Sex____M____F

Address_____ Date of birth_____

Number of children_____ ____ Married ____ Single

____ Divorced ____ Widow/Widower

Education completed: _____ grade school _____ some college

_____ high school _____ college graduate

Occupation (what work does patient do—if self-employed, what type and
location of business)

_____

_____

_____

Referred by_____

Figure 19–3. Sample patient information form.

patients come in for service. In six months to a year, you will have the
information on current patients up to date.

After information on current patients is collected, you can start
your analysis. This consists of counting those items that can be
counted, such as age, sex, marital status, and so on and analyzing the
rest. The count should be made a permanent part of your records, so
that you can trace these counts over time and can tell if your practice
is handling more young people, more older people, more higher
educated people, and so on.

The two major analysis items are address and occupation. Addresses should be displayed on a map, usually with pins, but marks by
colored pens may be used as well. This should give you an accurate
idea of the geographic area from which you draw your various types
of patients. Undoubtedly, you will find some areas underrepresented,
even unrepresented. These areas are the ones in which you especially
need to do some development work, such as arranging to hold
examination clinics in the schools.

The second analysis question is that of occupation, and from
occupation, income. Many dentists will find a standard occupation list
helpful, such as the following:

Executives and proprietors of large concerns and major professionals.

Managers and proprietors of medium concerns, lesser professionals, and minor officials.

Administrative personnel of large concerns, owners of small
independent businesses, and semiprofessionals.

Owners of small businesses, clerical and sales workers, and technicians.

*The two major analysis items
are address and occupation.*

Skilled workers.

Semiskilled workers.

Unskilled workers.

Retirees unless assigned to one of the above.

Military unless assigned to one of the above.

Students.

With a little study, and perhaps with the help of the local Chamber of Commerce, you should be able to determine an average income for each occupation. Even if your patient's income is different from the average, it will still be within the range; hence, you can have an idea of what income classes your patients are in. In order to make the occupation-income analysis, you will want to get as complete a description as possible of the patient's work. An answer such as "Republic Steel" or "work for the county" is not satisfactory. Some description of the type of work is required.

How may you use this information? First, you may use it for deciding upon your level of fees for each specific service. Second, you may use the information in communicating with patients. As discussed in Chapter 16, people with different occupations have different needs and respond positively to different types of communication. Last, as an overall statement, the more you know about your patients, who they are as personalities, and what they do in work and in leisure, the better you will be able to handle your practice.

> The more you know about your patients, who they are as personalities and what they do in work and in leisure, the better you will be able to handle your practice.

SERVICES USED

Your patient records may already be in a form that will enable you to analyze services used by each type of patient. If so, then it will simply be a matter of transferring the services used from the patient record to the Patient Information Form. Some dentists utilize a service code such as the following:

Code	Service Provided
1	Crowns and bridges
2	Dentures
3	Endodontic treatments
4	Examination and x-rays
5	Fillings and inlays
6	Oral surgery/extractions
7	Orthodontic treatments
8	Periodontic treatments
9	Prophylaxis
10	Other (specify) _____

You could use the second and third digits of the ADA procedure code.

This information on the Patient Information Form will enable you to know exactly which of your services are being used most, and which least. Further, it will let you see what type, age, sex, and so on of patient utilizes which of the services you offer. If you observe that a certain service is underutilized by certain types of patients, that will be a clue for you to mention the service to and discuss it with particular patients who you believe need the service. Such information will also stimulate you to increase chairside, newsletter, brochure, and other types of patient education regarding certain underutilized but key dental services, such as fixed prosthodontics.

If your patient records are not in a form suitable for transfer to the Patient Information Form, have your receptionist start keeping a 5 × 7 inch card file on all patients coming in for treatment. Most questions can be answered when the patient arrives at the office: the treatment information can be transferred to the Patient Information Form after treatment. In a few months, and certainly within a year, you will have an up-to-date card file on all your active patients.

PATIENT SATISFACTION

In addition to the relatively easy-to-obtain patient information we discussed earlier, it will help your practice greatly to know how well patients are satisfied with your current services and whether you need to add new services. Some dentists may believe that if patients were dissatisfied, they (the dentist) would know it, or if new services were needed, patients would ask for them. This is not necessarily the case. People are often reticent to voice to a professional their dissatisfaction with current services or their desire for new services. In fact, many people do not realize that they are unhappy until they have left the office after treatment and experience nagging pain. Some do not realize it until after they have received their statement.

People are often reticent to voice to a professional their dissatisfaction with current services or their desire for new services.

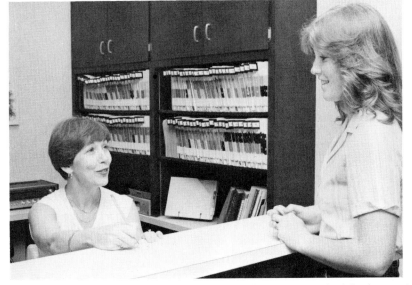

The young patient, already gaining a sense of autonomy, schedules her next appointment.

All of this means you need to conduct a survey of current patients at least every two years. Some dentists find that they need to conduct such a survey every year. The survey can be done in the office, while patients are awaiting treatment or after they have received treatment. A suggested survey form is included as Figure 19–4. The post-treatment questionnaire (Chapter 15) can be used for the same purpose.

You will find it productive to think through what items are important to you and your patients and construct the categories or questions accordingly.

NON–PATIENT SURVEYS

So much for surveys of your current patients. Now let us deal briefly with surveys of people who are not your patients. First, you must decide what kinds of things you would like to know about these individuals. Some suggestions are:

— What kinds of people in your community are without dental care?

— What is the image that the public holds of your practice and of the practices of other dentists?

PATIENT SURVEY

We need your help in order to improve our services.
Please complete the following questionnaire and return it to the receptionist in the envelope provided. Do not sign your name.

PLEASE RATE EACH OF THE FOLLOWING

	Excellent 4	Good 3	Fair 2	Poor 1	No opinion 0
Capabilities of dentist(s)	_____	_____	_____	_____	_____
Capabilities of assistants	_____	_____	_____	_____	_____
Capabilities of hygienist	_____	_____	_____	_____	_____
Capabilities of receptionist	_____	_____	_____	_____	_____
Personal treatment by staff	_____	_____	_____	_____	_____
Level of fees charged	_____	_____	_____	_____	_____
Payment plan	_____	_____	_____	_____	_____
Convenience of location	_____	_____	_____	_____	_____
Convenience of hours	_____	_____	_____	_____	_____
Length of wait for appointment	_____	_____	_____	_____	_____
Length of wait for treatment	_____	_____	_____	_____	_____
Other (specify)_____	_____	_____	_____	_____	_____

Figure 19–4. Sample patient survey.

— How do people in your community choose a dentist?

— How important is location in choosing a dentist?

— How attractive is your location to people who may be choosing a dentist?

— How does the public view dentists who advertise?

—What kinds of advertising, if any, would be viewed positively?

—What dental habits do people have?

— How do these habits differ by age?

— What dental knowledge does the public possess?

Decide what information you want to collect on the basis of what you want to do with it. If you will not wish to, of if you will not be able to, make changes based on what you learn from your survey, then do not bother to ask for the information. You will just be wasting time and money as well as others' time.

One inexpensive and easy survey method would be to distribute questionnaires to people examined in schools or other places where you do examinations. Keep the questions simple so that it takes a person no more than five minutes to complete the survey. Do not ask for names and addresses. Make it clear that you are not soliciting business (although perhaps you can ask for each respondent's section of town). And, as with all of the survey work you do, make sure it is consistent with the professional image you wish to maintain and the professional work you wish to do.

Another possibility is a telephone survey of people with names drawn at random from the telephone directory. With proper training and experience, your auxiliaries and/or family members could carry out such a project in the evening using home telephones. You may also be able to hire college students or housewives.

The opening words of the survey script should state simply that dental care data is being collected in your city, guarantee anonymity, and emphasize that all answers are voluntary. An introductory statement might contain the following:

> "Your participation in this interview is completely voluntary. If you want to stop the questioning at any time, please feel free to tell me and we will stop. Nobody will know who you are because we are not interested in individual answers, but rather in how this community feels in general about dental care."

In no event should the telephone interviewer reveal the name of the dentist or dentists sponsoring the survey. If the respondent will not supply answers without knowing the name of the sponsor, then the interviewer should politely terminate the conversation, perhaps by saying: "Thank you for your time but I regret that for professional reasons, the survey sponsor may not be disclosed. Good-bye and thanks very much."

All the questionnaires should be tested before a final questionnaire is decided upon. This means calling ten to twenty people and using the draft questionnaire and then making the revisions that seem to be indicated. If many revisions are necessary, it may be best to test the revision before a final questionnaire is accepted.

The survey script should state that dental care data is being collected, guarantee anonymity, and emphasize that all answers are voluntary.

REFERRAL ANALYSES

Referrals to Your Practice

All of us get referrals of patients from dental colleagues, suppliers, staff members, other patients, and other sources. How many of us do regular analyses of who provides the referrals? We suggest you develop statistics in two forms. First, Figure 19–5 is a Referral Source Analysis. Ask this question of each new patient: "Can you tell us who referred you to this office or how you happened to come here?" Then keep a monthly tally of *types* of persons or organizations referring patients to you. By checking this tally from month to month, you can determine where the bulk of your referrals are coming from. Then you can concentrate on developing these sources further. By the same token, you can determine where you are *not* receiving referrals and can work on developing these potential sources.

On a separate list, we suggest you keep the actual names of each person or organization supplying a referral. This can be done on a simple notebook page with room for names, and with a place at the end of the name to mark duplicate referrals. Among other uses, this notebook can serve as a notice to you of when you should reward your referral sources, which is discussed in Chapter 16.

REFERRAL SOURCE ANALYSIS

MONTH OF _____, 19_____

Referral Source	Tally
Drop-in	
Yellow Pages	
Patients	
General dentists	
Dental specialists	
Other professionals	
Staff	
Former staff	
Suppliers (labs, etc.)	
Organizations	
Other	

Figure 19–5. Sample referral source analysis form.

Listed below are services and names to suggest to patients:

SERVICE	NAME	ADDRESS	TELEPHONE
Physician			
Ob-Gyn			
Eye specialist			
Orthodontist			
Psychologist			
Veterinarian			
Hairdresser			
Attorney			
Real estate agency			
Funeral home			

Figure 19–6. Referral suggestions.

Referrals to Other Professionals and Businesses

From time to time, you will be called on to refer patients to other professionals and businesses. It will be helpful to your receptionist to have a list of suggested names. Figure 19–6 is such a list. You may wish to expand the list to include several physicians, orthodontists, and so on, or you may simply change the list from time to time.

SUMMARY

Evaluation of a dental practice comes from both within and outside the practice. Within the practice evaluation consists of analyzing financial statements for each accounting period and, over time, trying to spot trends in revenues and expenses. The income statement, the balance sheet, and productivity analyses are three types of internal analyses.

External analyses consist of surveys of patients and the community. These may be carried out in person, by mail, or by telephone. In many practices, professional help is necessary for surveys. The Patient Information Form may be used by all practices to gather readily available data from active patients. Some of these data will already exist on patient records. Other data may be obtained as patients visit your office.

REFERENCES

Blackstrom, C. H., and Hursh, G. D.: Survey Research. Evanston Illinois, Northwestern University Press, 1963.
Churchill, G. A., Jr.: Marketing Research. Hinsdale, Illinois, The Dryden Press, 1976.

Co-op to market traditional dentistry, motivate consumers, combat rival "cut-rate" franchises. Marketing News, May 29, 1981, pp. 5–6.

Domer, L. R., Snyder, T. L., Heid, D. W.: Dental Practice Management. St. Louis, C. V. Mosby Company, 1980, Chapter 19.

Kinnear, T. C., and Taylor, J. R.: Marketing Research. New York, McGraw-Hill Book Company, 1979.

Levoy, R. P.: The Successful Professional Practice. Englewood Cliffs, NJ, Prentice-Hall, Inc., 1970, pp. 159–71.

Morabito, P. A.: What do your patients think of you? Just ask them! Dental Economics, April 1976, pp. 37–41.

Sowter, J. B. (ed): Dental Laboratory Technology. Chapel Hill, North Carolina, The University of North Carolina, 1967.

20

Improving Business Systems

Some dentists may bridle at having their practices referred to as "businesses." We have no quarrel with that; we believe that dentists and dentistry should operate as professionally as possible, and if that means removing the word "business" from your vocabulary, do it. Our main concerns are that society has the best possible dental care and that you make a good living providing it. There is, however, one aspect of your operation that certainly must be akin to a business — your business system, the business-like operation of your office procedures.

Let us look now at your practice's business systems, including your appointment and recall system, patient records, personnel records, and account collections. We will offer you some ways of determining the adequacy of your business systems and suggestions for improving any that you find inadequate.

THE STAFF MANUAL

An absolute essential for all dental offices is the *Staff Manual*. We all want our offices to run when we are not there; when we are there, we want not to be interrupted constantly to answer procedural questions. Therefore, a good idea is to develop a manual to which everyone concerned with the practice is privy and with which each person is familiar. Using such a manual, you do not have to *guess* how things are being handled in your office; you know how. Your employees know what is expected of them, and they know what to expect of you. You can use the established procedures set forth in the manual as a means of evaluating your employees. The manual may also be used if you should have to fire an auxiliary for dishonesty, poor performance, or gross misconduct.

The manual, we suggest, should be kept in two copies, one for your private office and one either near the reception desk or in the employees' lounge or coffee area. You may even wish to keep a third copy at home. Every new employee should be required to go through

Using a staff manual, you do not have to guess how things are being handled in your office; you know how.

313

the manual and ask questions about any portion of it. During each regular staff meeting, it would be productive to discuss at least one section of the manual, making certain auxiliaries understand the contents of the section, then inviting suggestions for changes. Auxiliaries may also suggest sections to be discussed at these weekly meetings. It probably would be most productive to prepare a simple staff meeting agenda in advance, so that auxiliaries can know what topics will come up.

What should you include in the staff manual? This depends upon what you consider important. However, among the topics we believe you ought to include are (1) Practice philosophy; (2) Job descriptions; (3) Rules of office conduct; (4) Personal hygiene; (5) Personnel policies; and (6) Appointment control.

Such a manual will not answer all the problems of your practice. But at least the routine concerns will be handled with dispatch. And you will have more time to deal personally with the important nonroutine questions.

Practice Philosophy

Your practice philosophy is your own and you must develop it. This does not mean that it may never change, however. As you acquire experience, you may find that what served you well previously has to be updated. In developing your practice philosophy, we suggest you remember some basic statistics.

1. Only 48 percent of the population receive *any* dental care.
2. Only 28 percent of the population receive *regular* dental care.
3. 46 percent of the children in the United States *never* see a dentist.
4. 75 percent of black children under seventeen years of age *never* see a dentist.

Not only is there a great untapped dental market out there, but there is also a great societal need for dental care. Your practice philosophy should perhaps take these statistics into consideration.

> Each person in your office, over time, should consider the descriptions of every job and be made to feel free to recommend changes.

Job Descriptions

As suggested in Chapter 18, job descriptions should be written for each job in the practice. Each person in your office, over time, should consider the descriptions of every job and be made to feel free to recommend changes. The mechanics of writing job descriptions and two sample descriptions can be found in Chapter 18.

Rules of Office Conduct

The *Staff Manual* is a good place to summarize just what you expect from your employees. McCure and Elliott, *Dental Economics,* Sep-

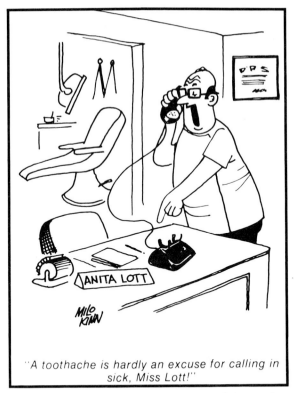

"A toothache is hardly an excuse for calling in sick, Miss Lott!"

Courtesy of *Cal* magazine.

tember 1979, suggest the following guidelines (slightly altered here). While some of these may be too strong or "military" for your taste, you may find others appropriate for your situation.

1. Employees are expected to perform their jobs as outlined in their job descriptions and to maintain all information related to patients in strict confidence. Employees are also expected to keep in confidence information concerning the doctor's financial position.

2. Actions that indicate subpar or negligent employee conduct include:

   —absence from work without permission.
   —leaving the work area without legitimate reason.
   —habitual tardiness.
   —improper care of or unauthorized use of practice property.
   —violation of safety rules.
   —faulty workmanship.
   —inattention to work.
   —vending, soliciting, or collecting contributions on doctor's premises without authorization.
   —poor attitude toward patients, showing lack of courtesy and respect.
   —use of the telephone for personal reasons beyond negotiated limits.
   —failure to cooperate with other staff members.
   —offensive language.

Orderly and courteous behavior should be the rule.

3. Orderly and courteous behavior should be the rule. Any time staff members behave otherwise, they will be informed of the problem created by their behavior. It is expected that everyone will be able to correct his or her own behavior with the aid of constructive feedback. Repeated problems could result in a written reprimand or lead to dismissal. In addition, your office manual should include "intolerable offenses," actions that are grounds for immediate dismissal, such as the following:

- —stealing property from the premises.
- —removing letterhead, prescription pads, and so on for improper use.
- —injecting, ingesting, or inhaling unprescribed drugs that are classified "dangerous" while on the premises.
- —falsifying records.
- —willfully obtaining or disclosing unauthorized confidential information.
- —willful damage or destruction of property of the dentist or the property of other employees.
- —vending or soliciting for any illegal purpose on doctor's premises.
- —willfully causing a physical disturbance or injury while on doctor's property or in the performance of a job assignment.

Dress and Personal Hygiene

Expectations should be clear in this area also. Staff members should realize that sloppy dress and careless hygiene are offensive to many patients, and for that reason cannot be tolerated. Some dentists have a list such as the following:

1. Cleanliness is a must. No body or mouth odors are permissible. Toothbrushes, toothpaste, mouth fresheners, and body deodorants are provided for your use in the office.

2. Cosmetics and hair style should be conservative and generally unobtrusive. Bouffant type or long, loose hairdos are discouraged. Very little perfume or cologne should be used. Use only clear or very light colored nail polish.

Staff members should realize that sloppy dress and careless hygiene are offensive to many patients.

3. Pantsuits or street-length style uniforms should be worn. Uniforms should be clean and pressed, reflecting the modern office decor. Shoes should be low-heeled, clean, and polished.

4. Chewing gum is not appropriate for a dental office.

5. Smoking by auxiliaries is discouraged, and permitted only in the rest room and employee lounge.

Personnel Policies

You will find, especially if you ask specifically at one of your regular staff meetings, that a number of concerns are on your employee's minds. A specific policy should be developed for each of these. Following are suggestions:

Office Hours

The office is open on the following schedule. You are expected to be present fifteen minutes before opening and you may leave fifteen minutes after closing, unless there are no more patients or other duties to attend to, in which case you may leave at closing time.

Monday	8 to 12 and 1 to 4
Tuesday	7 to 12 and 1 to 4
Wednesday	8 to 12 and 1 to 4
Thursday	1 to 5 and 6 to 9
Friday	8 to 12 and 1 to 4
Saturday	9 to 12

You will be scheduled for forty hours a week. In the unlikely event that you must work over forty hours in any week, you will be paid time and one-half for the overtime hours.

You will find, especially if you ask specifically, that a number of concerns are on your employees' minds.

Vacation and Holidays

One week of annual vacation is given after twelve months of employment, two weeks after three years, and three weeks after five years. Vacation will be scheduled in March, with the employee with the most seniority having the first choice, etc. No more than one person may be gone in a given week. (This statement may not be necessary if your office closes and all vacations are taken at the same time.)

Generally speaking, vacations must be taken in one-week or more increments. Vacation time not used or scheduled will be paid for at the end of the year at the salary rate in effect on December 31. Vacation time may not be carried over from year to year.

The office will be closed on the following dates to commemorate holidays: (these should be reviewed in the manual from year to year, and generally should follow local business and industry holidays). Employees are paid for these holidays.

Sick Leave

After three months' service, sick leave is earned at the rate of one-half day per month of service. The employee will not be paid sick leave in excess of that earned in any year. Employees are asked to take sick leave only when they or their families are actually sick. Sick leave should not be confused with vacation time or considered as extra vacation. Some offices pay unused sick leave as a bonus. This encourages employees not to take sick leave unless necessary.

Other Fringe Benefits

It is difficult for us to outline for any dentist just what his fringe benefits for employees should be. Generally, they should follow the policies of local business and industry, and other local general dentists and dental specialists. Included in the fringe benefit package might be some or all of the following, as well as other benefits: paid parking, hospital insurance (may be only partially paid), uniforms, or a

Your fringe benefit plan may become more extensive as an employee's service time increases. This should help reduce employee turnover.

uniform allowance, pension plan (may be only partially paid), group investment plan, profit sharing, continuing education courses (may be contingent upon satisfactory grade), professional organization membership dues, and so on. Your fringe benefit plan may become more extensive as an employee's service time increases. This should help reduce employee turnover. In addition, of course, most dental offices provide free dental care or discounts to employees, and in some cases, to their families, too.

Appointment Control

Appointment difficulties may be caused by a poor appointment control policy.

Appointments will not just take care of themselves. They must be controlled. In most dental practices, the appointment book is the control center of the practice. With good appointment control, the doctors, staff, and patients are scheduled efficiently and the patient load is seldom, if ever, over or under what it should be. It is critical, however, that appointment control be responsive not only to the needs of the dentist and the staff, but also to those of the patients and potential patients. Whether or not patients are satisfied by the appointment control process can be deduced from patient reaction. If patients often show a personal negative reaction to their appointment schedule or if many patients miss appointments time after time, it may not be the fault of the patients only. Such appointment difficulties may also have been caused by a poor appointment control policy.

RECALL SYSTEM

You are aware, from your experience and the material in this book, that new patients are very important to your practice. You are also aware that retention of your existing patients is equally vital to the life of your practice, or even more so. Your recall system should be examined frequently and improved when necessary.

Recall System Examined

To examine your recall system, determine the number of active patients in the practice and count the number of patient visits to your hygienist or hygienists during the past twelve months. What portion of your active patients are answering your recall notices? The recall percentage will never be, or perhaps never even approach, 100 percent. But if the number is smaller than you would like, perhaps some modification of your recall system is in order.

Are the telephone calls being made correctly, with the right frequency and followup for hard-to-contact patients? Do you need to follow recall telephone contacts with postcards, notes, or letters? Most importantly, are your patients happy with your recall system? The marketing dentist will have a system that is pleasing to and correct for the patient, yet efficient and effective for the practice.

You will also want to outline the recall system in your staff manual.

Recall Schedule

Many dentists have a set recall schedule, usually six months, because of the ease of administration. Some practices find it advantageous to employ a recall system tailored to the individual. In consultation with the patient, a recall schedule of four, five, six, or seven months can be established, based on the patient's dental needs, psychological needs, and wishes. The recall period chosen should be a joint decision, and explained to the patient so that it does not appear arbitrary on your part.

> The marketing dentist will have a recall system that is pleasing to and correct for the patient, yet efficient and effective for the practice.

FEES AND BILLING

Presumably, you have determined the general level of dental fees in your area and have developed an average fee for each service. Many dentists will then charge that average, slightly below the average, or sometimes slightly above it. This is not a correct method of setting fees. Your fees should be determined by considering the normal factors used by businesses to set prices.

Your Costs

Generally, these consist of time and materials. How much staff time does a procedure take, and how much of your personal time? What materials are used in the procedure? What is the cost of those materials? If you are able to treat more patients than you are treating, and want to increase your patient load, perhaps you should not worry much about the cost of your office overhead. Because overhead costs will basically be the same whether or not you perform a particular service, perhaps your price for this service may be lower than it would be if you were considering "full costs," including office overhead. Patients tend to compare standard procedures such as emergency extraction, examination, and recall. Many practices charge at least what Medicaid or welfare agencies would pay for such procedures.

Demand

If there is a great deal of consumer (patient) demand for a particular service, and therefore the service is less price-sensitive than others, then perhaps you are justified in setting a higher fee on the service than you might otherwise do. If there is little demand, one way to help build demand may be to set a slightly lower fee, at least until demand builds.

Your Fee Strategy

Basically, you have two alternative strategies in setting a fee. You may wish to appeal mainly to those people who are willing to pay the fee for the service even though it is rather high. In such a case, your patronage will be relatively low and your revenue per patient will be high. This has been termed "skimming the cream off the market."

The second alternative has been labelled "market penetration." This consists of setting a fee low enough to attract a great many patients for that service.

Do you want and need more patients? Or do you simply wish to raise the revenue per patient? The choice will also depend upon how much you wish to work. Obviously, setting a lower fee for a service, given that there is some price elasticity for your dental services, will bring in more business and will cause you to work harder. It may also cause your revenues to rise faster than your costs, thereby increasing your net income.

As an example of the use of this strategy, let us consider the case of a dentist whose patient load has fallen off drastically for reasons beyond his control or of a dentist who has simply never been able to build his patient load sufficiently to provide the level of income he wants and needs. One approach — some would say a theoretical approach — to using the fee level to increase patient load would be to offer a free examination to all new patients for a limited time. Such a dentist might also consider reducing the cost of prophylaxis to only slightly over direct costs during this time. This special "introductory" fee could be advertised in a professional manner. Again, given that there is some price elasticity or sensitivity in dentistry, the chances are that this dentist might gain new patients during the introductory period, enough to keep him busy and increase his income for a long period of time.

THE CORRECT TYPE OF BILLING SYSTEM

In 1978, *Dental Economics* conducted a survey of dentists. One of the topics on which information was requested was the billing system. The survey results were reported in March 1979. They are reproduced as Figure 20–1.

Eighty-one percent of the dentists responding reported using a manual system for billing. Thirteen and one-half percent reported using a computer service, 4 percent reported using microfilm, and only 1.5 percent reported using an in-house computer. The fact that more than four-fifths of the respondents reported manual billing indicates that most dentists have clung to traditional ways of billing patients, perhaps with good reason. With all its faults, cost, slowness, mistakes, and so on, manual billing at least allows you to keep a semblance of control over your monthly statements. However, if you are ready to consider other alternatives, we now offer you brief comments about each of them.

Computer Billing Services

Computer billing services will take the manual work out of your billing procedure. Your auxiliaries prepare the information for the computer and the service computes, prints, and mails patient state-

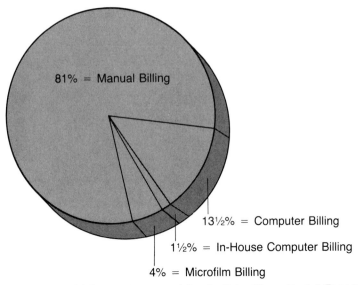

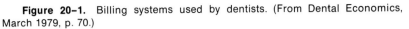

Figure 20-1. Billing systems used by dentists. (From Dental Economics, March 1979, p. 70.)

ments or insurance forms. Most such services will also provide you with nearly any other report you wish, including analyses and aging of accounts receivable, production reports for you and your auxiliaries and your laboratory, collection analyses, and almost any other analysis you are willing to pay for. The tendency may be to ask for too many reports, because they would be "interesting to see," but not to make use of all of them.

Computer billing services usually charge a minimum of $100 to $150 per month; many practices find such services run from one to three percent of gross billings. Your postage and envelopes, at least, are normally an additional cost.

Microfilm Billing

Otten reports that microfilm billing in the St. Louis area costs approximately fifteen cents per statement, in addition to postage. With this system, your ledger cards are microfilmed each month and then printed from the microfilm and mailed to patients. Essentially, you can retain your manual ledger card system, but someone else does the copying and mailing. In addition, there is an independent record of each month's statements kept in a separate place, the microfilm company's office.

In-House Computer

An in-house computer is a major step for a dentist to take. In general, unless you send more than 1200 statements per month, this step is not recommended. If you do decide to use a computer, it is advisable to become familiar with the computer's operation and programming. Even so-called "canned" programs might require some adaptation for your office.

In general, unless you send more than 1200 statements per month, an in-house computer is not recommended.

What do you get from the $10,000 or more you will invest in your own computer? First, you will get independence. No longer will you be completely at the mercy of your auxiliaries' sick leave or dependent upon the efficiency and timing of a computer service firm. However, in some cases, you will have transferred your dependence to the computer company! If your practice is large enough or active enough, buying your own computer may make sense. Go slowly, though, learn as much as possible about computers in general as you can, and visit several dental colleagues who have already installed computers. Do not do anything concerning computers in haste.

1. How much does the complete system cost?

2. Does this total include software as well as hardware?

3. What hardware components are included in this price?

4. What additional charges are there for delivery, installation, etc.?

5. What programming language is used?

6. Is this system designed specifically for use in a dental office?

7. Can the computer generate account status at the time of each visit?

8. How are treatment and fee information transmitted from the operatory to the computer?

9. Does the patient receive a computer-generated statement of receipt at the time of visit?

10. How are data entered into the computer?

11. How many active accounts can be stored in the computer's memory?

12. Can a daily journal page be generated? Does it show any transactions changed or deleted during the day?

13. How are errors corrected? How can I check for errors or omissions in accounts and other records?

14. What kind of paper forms will I need? Will they require special printing? How difficult is it to change from one form to another?

15. How are statements produced? How long will this take per 100 statements?

16. What is required to convert from my present system to the computer?

17. How much training is required for my office personnel? How much assistance can I expect from you during the conversion and start-up period?

18. Do you provide your own service for the hardware? How much does the service contract cost?

19. Can the software be updated as new programs are developed? Can it be modified to meet specialized needs of my practice? How is this handled?

20. How long has your company been in business?

21. Will you supply names of other dentists who are using your system?

Figure 20–2. Questions to ask computer vendors. (Derived from Ann Ehrlich, *The Role of Computers in Dental Practice Management.* Colwell Systems, Inc., Champaign, Illinois, 1981.)

Perhaps a suitable first step in acquiring an in-house computer facility would be an in-house terminal. Your patient billing data are entered in your office and transmitted to the computer elsewhere via the telephone. The total term cost of this type of system is considerably less than having your own computer, yet you are able to do many of the items you would like to do but could not do previously because of a manual system.

Ann Ehrlich in *The Role of Computers in Dental Practice Management* suggests a number of questions to be discussed with computer vendors. Answers to these questions will go a long way toward helping you make your buying decision. See Figure 20–2.

IMPROVING COLLECTIONS

The monthly requirement of having statements prepared and mailed, and following up on slow payers can usually justify some time and attention for most offices. The overall average of collections in the dental office is reported to be between 90 and 95 percent. You will not reach 100 percent collections, but you *can* improve your average considerably by choosing your patients well and by carefully considering your collection policies.

Note to Delinquent Accounts

Delinquent accounts are a problem for any office except those with a time-of-visit payment policy. Time-of-visit policy offices have their own problems, which we will discuss later. For the rest of us, *Dental Economics,* June 1978, offers a good suggestion. After one month of appending the note below to the statements of hard-to-collect accounts, the practice not only received back payments, but also received phone calls and notes of apology. Mrs. Ruth Maffett, Dr. Robert T. Clagett, Dr. William T. Clagett, and Dr. Dan Ray Clagett of Elizabethtown, Kentucky, are responsible for this suggestion.

An established policy of this office is that monthly payments are required. If this policy is not met in the future, then full payment will be required with each visit.

(doctor's signature)

This form may be too harsh for some tastes, but you may be able to develop acceptable alternative wording.

Time-of-Visit Payment

Will instituting a time-of-visit payment policy reduce your receivables? Most assuredly. Will such a policy also lose patients for you? Yes it will. Although all of us like the idea of reducing receivables, few

Would you rather have nearly 100 percent of $100,000 or 95 percent of $150,000?

of us have patients to spare. Time-of-visit payment policies will work for many practices, but they must be tempered with common sense. First, there are some instances where the fee is too high for most people to pay at one visit. For these situations, spreading the fee among three or more payments is a reasonable way to keep the patient, yet still collect your fee. Second, there are times when a patient forgets his or her wallet or checkbook and, after treatment, tells your receptionist. Of course, you then have no choice but to give a statement to the patient and hope that it is paid before the time comes to send a followup statement. In short, time-of-visit payment can work for some practices, but it can never be accomplished 100 percent of the time.

Would time-of-visit work for your practice? We can't answer for you. You yourself must determine this. We ask only that you go slowly, so as not to lose too many of your patients over an ill-considered new policy. Perhaps one way to look at this question is: Would you rather have nearly 100 percent of $100,000 or 95 percent of $150,000? The marketing advantage is with the dentist who is concerned with the needs of his patients, including their financial needs. Some flexibility and understanding go a long way.

OFFICE MANAGEMENT

Your office will not just operate; you have to manage it. It is clear that such management takes time. Much of that time will have to be your own. It is *your* office, after all. But the time you spend on improving your office can pay handsome rewards.

Work Simplification

One answer to improving office management is to simplify the office procedures. Work simplification consists of analyzing each of the office procedures to determine if they can be done faster, more easily, more efficiently, or less expensively. The dentist who does this can better meet the needs of his or her community. It is a means to an end — better service with lower fees — not an end in itself.

One approach to the problem of work simplification is time and motion studies. These consist of breaking office procedures down into *what* is done, *who* does it, *when* it is done, *where* it is done, and *how* it is done.

Under this approach, all members of the staff plus the dentists should ask themselves and offer for discussion such questions as the following:

— Can a different procedure be used? Can procedures be eliminated or combined?

— Can someone else perform a procedure, other than the person normally performing it?

— Can an office procedure be done at a different time? Or not done at all?

— Must a procedure be accomplished in the room or section of the office where it is normally accomplished? Can it be done more efficiently and effectively out of the office, or by an outside contractor?

— Are we certain that the way a procedure is performed is the correct way? Why have we come up with all of these answers? Are we satisfied with them?

Absences from the Office

While you are absent from your office, whether to dental meetings, on vacation, or simply taking an afternoon off, are your auxiliaries making the best use of their time? Or have you not made it clear what needs to be accomplished in your absence.

While you are absent from your office, are your auxiliaries making the best use of their time?

Although you may have a service that cleans your office regularly, your auxiliaries can help by cleaning those areas not normally covered by the service. Much dusting and time-consuming stain removal can be accomplished in the hours you are absent. Files can be reorganized and, perhaps, reviewed when you are gone; this type of work is difficult, if not impossible, in a busy office.

This time may be used for your auxiliaries to make calls on local businesses and industry; it may be an ideal time for them to conduct the surveys discussed in Chapter 19. These are your decisions; adequate consideration of them can improve your office's efficiency, even while you are gone.

Purchasing Policies

Rather than running out of supplies frequently and having the dentist make purchasing decisions several times a week, successful dentists will provide purchasing policies that will give auxiliaries the authority to purchase supplies when they are needed. Ehrlich and Ehrlich provide several factors to consider before setting the minimum inventory levels that trigger a purchase order.

1. The quantity used annually.
2. The shelf life.
3. The storage space required.
4. The possibility of a new product soon replacing this item.
5. Quantity purchase savings.
6. Investment required. (Does an expensive item, purchased in large quantity, represent a sufficient savings to justify the capital outlay?)

Succesful dentists will provide purchasing policies that will give auxiliaries the authority to purchase supplies when they are needed.

In consultation with your auxiliaries, perhaps at your regular staff meetings, these reorder inventory level points may be set, as well as the appropriate order quantity. You may find it beneficial to review these quantities quarterly or semiannually.

Purchasing decisions can be helped by the use of a computer. If you find a computer suited to your practice, you can use it for inventory control.

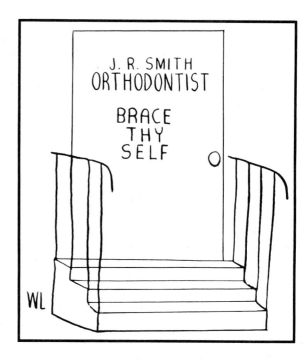

ANNUAL OFFICE CHECKUP

How do you know when your office is operating effectively and efficiently? None of us can be certain that all is well without a systematic procedure. Appendix B suggests a number of questions that will help us determine practice weaknesses and decide upon needed improvements. No such practice evaluation list can be all-inclusive. As with many of the topics covered thus far, there are questions on this list that will not apply to all dental offices. However, many of them will apply to any given office, and pave the way for improvements.

None of us can be certain that all is well in our office without a systematic procedure.

We suggest that you turn now (or at your convenience) to Appendix B and answer this list of questions.

How did you come out?

SUMMARY

Your office will not operate efficiently and provide the maximum income for you all by itself. You must make it happen. It will happen only if you consider all office procedures and question whether they are appropriate for your practice. The key to a successful office operation is the *Staff Manual*. It may take some time to prepare a manual that is right for your practice, but the time will have been well spent. You also need to think carefully about the billing and record-keeping process you use, along with the question of whether an in-office computer would serve you well or ill. Perhaps another key to a successful practice is a periodic office checkup; once a year is usually enough.

REFERENCES

Blass, J. L., and Tulkin, I.: Successful Dental Practice. Philadelphia, J. B. Lippincott Company, 1947, Chapters 9 and 13.

Bregstein, S. J.: The Successful Practice of Dentistry. New York, Prentice-Hall, Inc., 1953, Chapters 14 and 17.

Corby, C. S.: Are you ready for a computer? Dental Economics, August 1978, pp. 32–6.

Domer, L. R., Snyder, T. L., and Heid, D. W.: Dental Practice Management. St. Louis, The C. V. Mosby Company, 1980, Chapters 15, 16, 17, and 18.

Ehrlich, A.: Business Administration for the Dental Assistant. Champaign, Illinois, The Colwell Company, 1973.

Ehrlich, A.: The Role of Computers in Dental Practice Management. Champaign, Illinois, The Colwell Company, 1973.

Ehrlich, A. B., Ehrlich, S. F.: Dental Practice Management. Philadelphia, W. B. Saunders Company, 1969, Chapters 3, 12, and 18.

Frederick, P. M., and Towner, G.: The Office Assistant. Philadelphia, W. B. Saunders Company, 1956, Chapters 6, 7, 8, 11, and 13.

Howard, W. W.: Dental Practice Planning. St. Louis, C. V. Mosby Company, 1975, Chapters 10 and 15.

Marcotte, O. P.: My computer has been the best management tool I ever invested in. Dental Economics, September 1978, pp. 50–52.

Otten, W. L.: Here's an Alternative to Computerized Billing. Dental Economics, February 1978, p. 60.

Powell, B. J.: Your Office Needs a Yearly Checkup. Dental Economics, December 1979, pp. 51–55.

Reap, C. A., Jr.: Complete Dental Assistant's, Secretary's, and Hygienist's Handbook, West Nyack, NY, Parker Publishing Company, Inc., 1973, Chapters 6, 7, 14, and 18.

Stinaff, R. K.: Dental Practice Administration. St. Louis, The C. V. Mosby Company, 1960, pp. 192–95.

The best billing system. Dental Economics, March 1979, p. 70.

THE FIRST MARKETING OPPORTUNITY OCCURS FOR THE DENTIST ENTERING PRIVATE PRACTICE. ALSO, THE PRACTITIONER WHO MAKES A MAJOR CHANGE SUCH AS RELOCATION HAS THE OPPORTUNITY TO PLAN ACCORDING TO MARKETING PRINCIPLES. CHOOSING A LOCATION AND PLANNING AND STAFFING A FACILITY SHOULD ALL BE DONE ON THE BASIS OF THE COMMUNITY'S NEED FOR DENTAL SERVICE. NOW IS THE TIME TO PLAN FOR SERVICES NEEDED BY THE COMMUNITY, RATHER THAN TO PLAN SERVICES TO BE "SOLD" TO THE COMMUNITY.

21

Starting or Altering a Practice

Dwight Parrish, senior dental student, is in a quandary about his career plans. He has been so intent on finishing his requirements for graduation that he has given very little thought to what to do afterwards. In the school's Community Dentistry program he was exposed to a number of career options, such as public health, hospital dentistry, and the prison (corrections) system, as well as private practice — group and solo. Private practice had always been his first choice, but recently he has had second thoughts.

Even though solo private practice had been his first choice all along, he has begun to consider the problems of getting into practice. First of all, is he really cut out for it? He studied hard all the way through school and was not very socially inclined. Would he be able to promote or market himself as everyone now says a dentist has to in order to do well? Could he manage employees and relate to patients? Although he has a lot to learn, Dwight believes that he can develop the skills he will need for private practice.

A series of other questions now have to be answered. Where should he locate? Should he consider employment in a department store clinic in order to improve his financial situation more immediately? Should he try to find a practice for sale? Join a group? If he opens his own solo practice, should he incorporate? How should he design the office? Develop the business systems? Select equipment? Finance the office? Select and employ staff? So many decisions!

PRIVATE PRACTICE

Private solo practice requires a broad spectrum of management skills. The solo practitioner needs to be able to answer "YES" to the following questions:
— Do I possess leadership and initiative?

First of all, are you really cut out for private practice?

— Do I inspire confidence?
— Do I recognize and take advantage of opportunities?
— Do I act without direction?
— Do I seek responsibility?
— Do I make quick and accurate decisions?
— Are others pleased to do things for me?
— Am I an organizer?
— Am I industrious, friendly, flexible in my views?

A great many dentists have succeeded very well without being able to answer all or even most of these questions affirmatively. However, as we enter the marketing era, such qualities are more vital to one's success.

The absence of some of these qualities need not mean that Dwight Parrish could not do well in private practice. If he is merely friendly and pleasant so that others like to do things for him, and if he inspires confidence, he may succeed admirably in taking care of patients as a team member. He would do well to work as an employee or as a member of a group where the active leadership is supplied by others. Whatever his deficiencies, he should attempt to find a situation where others complement his skills. If the practice provides all the necessary management skills, any competent dentist who wants to treat people (not merely treat teeth) can do well.

LOCATION

Marketing begins with the selection of a community and then of a site within the community. It is at this time that you need to determine what group (segment of the market) you wish to target as your prospective patients. Initially you may choose to serve anyone who seeks your services. However, you must engage in a rather complex process in which you decide first on some general geographic areas where you would find the living agreeable and then determine

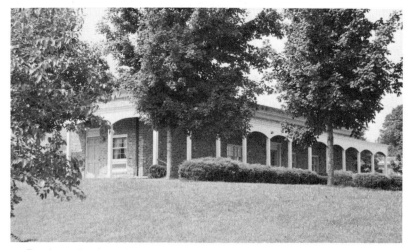

Dentists who have located in this attractive and accessible medical office building are doing well.

whether those areas offer the professional opportunity you seek. At any rate, keep in mind your total requirements: select an area and community that needs your services. In other words, market by providing services that are needed.

At one time dentists could locate wherever they wanted to live and achieve success. Every community needed more dentists. Even now that dentists are not in such short supply, you should strive to answer two questions in the affirmative:

— Will I (we) enjoy living here?
— Can I succeed in practice here?

To answer these questions, let us examine personal, professional and economic considerations.

Marketing begins with the selection of a community and then of a site within the community.

Personal Considerations

If you are married, you and your spouse have an interest in the following factors: geographic area, kind and size of community, schools, cultural activities, recreation, religion, and social life.

Your selection of the geographic area is largely personal, with the usual constraints of health problems, such as allergies. Moving to an unfamiliar area may create personal problems — distance from family and friends, for instance — and some professional problems — perhaps the lack of acquaintances who might refer patients to you, and the necessity of another licensure examination.

Selecting a community is based on its composite features. Large cities provide a variety of schools, cultural activities, recreational facilities, churches and synagogues, and opportunities for social life. They also may feature high noise levels, a hurried pace as well as congestion, pollution, and unsafe streets. The advantages of large cities are the disadvantages of small towns. And vice versa.

The advantages of large cities are the disadvantages of small towns. And vice versa.

Professional Considerations

These relate to both your satisfaction in practice and your economic success. The considerations, with their accompanying questions, follow:

— Satisfactory practice arrangement: Is there a practice opportunity of the type I am looking for?
— Adequate population: Are there enough people in this community to support me? Dentists may locate outside corporate limits at an easily accessible location and do very well, provided there is sufficient population within reasonable traveling distance.
— Need for dental services: A rhetorical question in most communities.
— Educational level: Is it high enough to cause people to value my services and keep me as busy as I want to be?
— Population per dentist: Is this so low as to indicate a saturation of dentists?
— Demand for dental services: Given the mix of educational

level, income, and population per dentist, is sufficient demand
for my services likely to develop?
— Dentist busyness: Are dentists busy enough that I can attract
an adequate number of patients? You can get a handle on this
by talking with community residents: dentists, physicians,
pharmacists, public health nurses, and consumers. Busyness
of dentists may be the most prognosticative indicator of
success for a new dentist.
— Availability of colleagues: Will I be able to interact with other
dentists enough to satisfy me?
— Availability of dental specialists: Will there be enough specialists to care for patients that I would refer?
— Availability of qualified auxiliaries: Will there be enough for
me to staff my practice?
— Availability of satisfactory continuing education: Will it be of a
high enough quality for me and my auxiliaries?
— Receptivity of community dentists: Will the dentists (especially
those in their prime) be receptive to me as a new dentist? As
you call on community dentists (which is good marketing), you
can assess how receptive to your coming each would be.
— Accessibility of service for dental equipment: Can I get my
equipment serviced without crippling delay?
— Access to commercial dental laboratory: Will the service available and the transportation arrangements be satisfactory?
— Access to dental supply house: Will the time required to
deliver orders suit me?
— Other professional activity: Are there good opportunities for
part-time employment, such as public health clinics or teaching programs?

Economic Considerations

Communities can be compared with each other and with the state
as a whole relative to: *per capita income, per capita retail sales, effective
buying income* (personal income less taxes and other payments to
government), *unemployment rate,* and *taxes.*

The ADA publication, Distribution of Dentists in the United
States by State, Region, District and County, provides information on
each of these except unemployment rate and taxes. Unemployment
rates can be obtained from the U.S. Job Service local office and you
can call local government offices for tax rates.

This information is significant for various purposes. High effective buying income indicates high potential for discretionary purchases, such as dental service. Per capita retail sales divided by per
capita income is a marketing index that indicates the strength of the
community as a market area. Third party funding upgrades economic potential.

Information on dental practice in the community is helpful: *fees,
business expenses, dentists' incomes* — gross and net. If such information
cannot be obtained directly from dentists, it can often be obtained
indirectly from bankers and dental dealers. The averages can be

compared with the current ADA Survey of Dental Practice. If the community dentists are doing well financially, you are likely to do well also.

Various other items of information deserve your attention. What is the *type of employment*? Is it balanced among industries? Single-industry communities are vulnerable to the swings in fortune for the industry. Educational institutions and government facilities tend to stabilize the local economy.

What is the growth potential of the community? Although chambers of commerce tend to be overly optimistic, they can provide helpful information. Also, city planners, utility companies, and banks project growth trends. Information from these sources can even be applied to neighborhoods when you are ready to decide where in the community to establish your practice.

Although chambers of commerce tend to be overly optimistic, they can provide helpful information.

Other financial information is of more personal interest. Is *financing* available and at what rate of interest? Does practice in this community entitle you to forgiveness of your educational loan? Later on, after you have accumulated some capital, what are the local opportunities for investment?

Summary

How completely should you evaluate the community? If you expect to remain during most of your foreseeable professional career, you should evaluate it fully and carefully. Economic factors relate closely to how well you can expect to do financially. Heavy financial commitment (e.g., beginning a solo practice) should be based on favorable economic evaluation. Personal and professional considerations relate to all other aspects of your practice and personal life. Only you (and your spouse) can weigh the various factors according to your own criteria and make a sound decision. There is — as you probably can feel already — a great deal riding on your decision. Make it thoughtfully. Appendix C should be helpful.

Site Selection

If you decide to start a solo practice in a sizable community, your next decision is precisely where in the community you should establish your practice. Again, if you are to serve the needs of your chosen community well, you must select your office location so as to ensure ready access for your patients.

To do this, consider the following questions:
— What segment (age group, socioeconomic group) do I wish to serve?
— Where do these people live?
— Where do they work? (go to school or otherwise spend the day?)
— Where are the growth areas for these people?
— Where are the dentists and physicians who currently serve these people?
— What locations are most accessible to these groups?

City planning departments can provide many of the answers. To locate dentists and physicians you may have to plot their offices on a city map using the telephone directory as a source. The most accessible locations can be determined by considering city transportation routes and vehicular traffic arteries.

Beyond accessibility you should consider the following:

— Adequacy of the lot or office suite for the planning period (usually 3 to 10 years).
— Parking (if it is provided) sufficient for you, your staff, and your patients.
— Zoning that permits you to practice dentistry in the location.
— Physical characteristics (such as character of the soil and ground elevation) of the lot, if you are building.
— Utilities available on lot.
— Prestige of the site. A prestigious site will attract people of high socioeconomic strata but may repel those of lower strata. A "low-brow" site may do the opposite.
— Cost, which is usually high in central and prestigious areas but may well be justified.

Prior to final selection, you should talk with other dentists, physicians, dental supply salespeople, and bankers. Architects are especially trained for determining feasibility and you should consult one, preferably one whom you may employ for the design phase. If you have not yet selected an attorney you should do so, and consult him or her regarding possible legal problems.

> Prior to final selection, you should talk with other dentists, physicians, dental supply salespeople, and bankers.

ASSOCIATESHIPS

The term associateship here describes any situation where the associate works in a practice without owning at least part of the practice. The associate may be an *employee* who is paid a salary, a salary plus a percentage of production, or a straight percentage of production. The employer is required to withhold income tax and Social Security taxes from the employee's compensation.

Or the associate may be an *independent contractor* who is affiliated with, but not employed by the practice. He or she pays personal income tax and Social Security taxes directly to the Internal Revenue Service. The independent contractor manages his or her own practice: collects fees, pays laboratory bills, generally employs and pays a dental assistant, owns or leases equipment (often from the practice), and pays rental for space to the practice. Although the independent contractor takes risks, the opportunity to develop an affiliated practice within an established practice may be far preferable to going it alone.

Associateships may well appeal to the new graduate. There are several possible advantages:

— Minimal or no capital required.
— Immediate patient load with consequent assured income.
— Limited commitment, which provides the associate flexibility

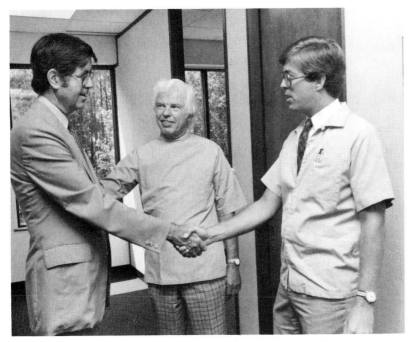

Senior dentist introduces patient to his new associate.

to later engage in advanced training, relocate, or go into another practice situation.
— Opportunity to practice and develop skills in clinical dentistry and in relating to patients.
— Camaraderie of and interaction with peers.
— Opportunity to buy into the practice.
— Limited responsibility in management.
— Opportunity to learn management skills.

The possible disadvantages, though fewer, could be troublesome.
— Personality conflicts and philosophical differences.
— Restricted variety of patients and procedures.
— Restricted income.
— Limited autonomy.

Bringing an associate into a practice has several possible advantages for the established dentist(s):
— Increased capacity to satisfy demand and thus enlarge the practice.
— More free time.
— Increased profits.
— Opportunity to select patients and procedures.
— Opportunity to learn from the associate.
— Transition into retirement.

A young dentist who is interested in an associateship should carefully study the practice and point out the advantages to the established dentist(s). It may be necessary to "sell" the practitioner on the idea.

Sufficient time to discuss important issues and to agree on them must be invested by the associate and by the established dentist. The

A young dentist who is interested in an associateship should carefully study the practice and point out the advantages to the established dentist(s).

agreement should be formalized in a written contract, which you should check out with your attorney. If the practice is incorporated, all dentists are employees of the corporation, but the terms of the employment agreement for associate dentists differ from those for owner dentists.

The contract should address the following issues:
— Employment: length of time of agreement.
— Termination: notice required (usually 30 to 90 days, should be the same for both).
— Other employment: whether prohibited or what (if any) is permitted.
— Duties: hours and days for working and general description of work to be done.
— Compensation: amount of salary, or percentage if on production, and expenses (if any) such as laboratory, charged against production, and when payment is due.
— Fringe benefits, such as insurance (especially professional liability), and retirement programs.
— Facilities and personnel available and assured to the associate.
— Compensated time (if any): vacation, meetings, and disability.
— Buy options (if any): corporate stock, partnership, or other sharing arrangement.
— Assignment of previous and new patients.
— Ownership of records.
— Contact with patients upon dissolution: prohibited or permitted.
— Covenant not to compete: customary and enforceable if reasonable as to time (approximately 2 years) and distance (depends on density of population).
— Amendment: procedure for.

BUYING A PRACTICE

An active practice for sale provides an excellent avenue into solo private practice. The interminable hours of planning for and setting up an office can be avoided, and time and energy can be spent in more productive activity, such as getting acquainted with patients. Access to an established panel of patients is invaluable to the new dentist. He or she, with orientation, can go right to work in the office with functional equipment, adequate systems, and auxiliaries who know the patients. A well-managed transition in most thriving practices will assure the buyer of a sufficient patient load. As the market for dentists becomes more saturated, the value of an active practice will increase.

A well-managed transition in most thriving practices will assure the buyer of a sufficient patient load.

Finding a Practice

There are several sources of information on practices for sale:
— Advertisements in dental journals.

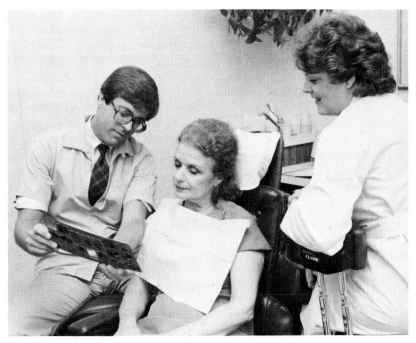

Associate gets into step with this marketing dental office by exploring treatment options with patient.

— National Health Professions Placement Network — computerized matching service.
— Dental schools.
— Word-of-mouth from dentists and dental supply representatives.
— Practice brokers who function as agents for the seller, much like real estate agents. Brokers advertise their services in the dental journals.

If you are fortunate enough to find more than one practice for sale in an area where you would like to live, you need to evaluate the alternatives.

Value of the Practice

In order to arrive at a value of the practice you need to examine several factors: (1) facility; (2) equipment and furnishings; (3) supplies; (4) management factors; and (5) goodwill.

If you purchase the land and building, the value is a matter of appraisal. If you do not purchase the *facility,* you will need to discuss the lease with the landlord and be assured that the terms are satisfactory to you, that the lease can be extended, and for how long. A value should be assigned to the lease-hold improvements, if the seller owns them. Evaluate the office floor plan for good traffic patterns. This can hardly be assigned a monetary value but should be considered. If the seller owns the facility and you prefer to lease, you can negotiate a lease separate from the purchase of the practice.

Equipment and furnishings should also be appraised, probably by a dental dealer. A rule of thumb for depreciating equipment for appraisal purposes is 20 to 30 percent the first year and 10 percent annually thereafter until it reaches a value of 10 percent, which it maintains during its useful life. The quality of maintenance and the way it has been used may modify this somewhat. You should make sure that seller's equity is as represented.

Supplies should be inventoried and appraised for tax purposes separately from equipment. They are immediately deductible to you as a business expense, whereas you must depreciate equipment over its useful life. If the inventory includes supplies that are of little value to you, you may use this fact as a negotiating point in arriving at a final price.

The *management factors* relate to the value of the practice, but they are difficult to evaluate. The fee schedule, if too low, could be negative. Other negatives are: (1) low gross and net incomes; (2) high overhead ratio; (3) low number of patient visits; (4) large proportion (over 20 percent) of accounts receivable over 60 days old; (5) accounts receivable in excess of two months gross; and (6) auxiliary salaries below average. Each of these except accounts receivable is included in the ADA Survey of Dental Practice. And you can compare the practice with national norms. Less tangible, but important, are the efficiency and effectiveness of operation. Even more important is the philosophy of patient care. It need not be in complete accord with yours, but you need to be aware of the differences and plan your approach to patients accordingly.

Transferability of patients determines the value of *goodwill* and is enhanced by:

1. the seller staying on and introducing you to the patients.

2. a letter from the seller to all patients of record endorsing you strongly.

3. the practice comprising patients who live and/or work in an area readily accessible to the office.

4. staff who relate well to patients and who will continue working for you.

You should ascertain that there is no significant ill will, such as a pending malpractice lawsuit or questionable reputation of the seller.

> It is reasonable to set the value of goodwill at whatever additional income you would earn over income from starting your own practice.

In the absence of ill will you need to compute the value of goodwill. It is reasonable to set the value of goodwill at whatever additional income you would earn over income from starting your own practice. The value may be very high in areas where it would be difficult to start a new practice. The rule of thumb has been 25 percent of the annual gross, but it could range up to one year's gross. Another method of determination is to pay a set percentage of production on all seller's patients for a prescribed period of time — perhaps 25 percent the first year, 15 percent the second, and 5 percent the third.

The sales agreement should list the various components of the price of the practice. Goodwill should be listed at a minimum because you cannot depreciate it for tax purposes. You can depreciate a covenant by the seller not to compete, which you should insist on. The proceeds of the sale attributable to the covenant are taxed as ordinary income to the seller. More attractive to the seller are proceeds attributable to the sale of patient records, because they are taxed as capital gains. The contract most favorable to you and to the seller will show a large portion of what you might think of as goodwill under the price of records. At least a token amount should be shown as goodwill, because the Internal Revenue Service recognizes that there is always value to goodwill. Since laws and court opinions change, you should confer with an attorney knowledgeable in taxes.

Sales Agreement

As for an associateship, you need a written sales agreement that not only describes the sales items and the price but also the conditions by which you both will abide. It is in your interest to have a definite understanding of the following:

— the date of your assuming ownership.
— the termination date for the seller working in the facility.
— seller's working arrangement if termination date is after you assume ownership.
— your working arrangement if you work before assuming ownership.

Furthermore, you need an understanding with the staff about their continued tenure in the office.

Buying an active practice is an excellent opportunity, but not risk free. It is an alternative along with associateship or starting your own practice. Carefully evaluate your available alternatives. Select the most feasible one for you and your needs.

Buying an active practice is an excellent opportunity, but not risk free.

	Buyer	Seller
Equipment	Depreciation	Ordinary in excess of book value
Supplies	Expense	Ordinary income
Covenant not to compete	Amortize over the period of covenant	Ordinary income
Patient records	*Amortize over 5–7 years	*Capital gain
Goodwill	Not depreciable— part of cost for computing sale later	Capital gain

In general, tax advantages beneficial to the buyer are detrimental to the seller and vice versa.

*Sale of patient records at the highest allowable price benefits both buyer and seller.

Figure 21–1. Tax implications in sale of practice.

PRACTICE ORGANIZATION

Practice organization includes the concepts of ownership and mode of practice.

Ownership

How are practices organized as legal entities? Just as ownership of other businesses varies, a dental practice can be owned by one person or by two or more persons. If it is owned by one dentist, it may be organized as a sole proprietorship or as a one-person corporation. A practice owned by two or more dentists can be either a partnership or a corporation.

Investor entrepreneurs will continue to exert political pressure to change dental practice acts to permit non-dentist ownership.

Further changes are quite likely in the traditional dentist ownership of dental practices. Although all the early department store clinics were owned by dentists, there is a trend toward non-dentist ownership. Avrom King and others say that investor entrepreneurs will continue to exert political pressure to change dental practice acts to permit non-dentist ownership.

Figure 21–2 shows the possible arrangements of ownership and mode of dental practice. Ownership is a legal entity and is regulated by state laws. Mode refers to whether you practice with others and by what arrangements.

Practicing Alone

There is a trend toward practicing with others, but most dentists still practice alone. Within the last couple of decades solo dentists have been permitted by law to incorporate their practices. Corporate practice enables the dentist, as an employee of his or her practice corporation, to set aside a higher proportion of pretax earnings for retirement purposes than is possible as a sole proprietor. There are certain other benefits for this "employee" dentist not available to a

MODE OF PRACTICE	OWNERSHIP		
	Sole Proprietorship	Partnership	Corporation
ALONE			
Solo	X		X
Expense Sharing	X		X
WITH OTHERS			
General Dentistry Group	X	X	X
Multi-Specialty Group	X	X	X
Single Specialty Group	X	X	X
Mixed Group	X	X	X

Figure 21–2. Possible arrangements of ownership and mode of dental practice. (Adapted from Domer et al, 1980.)

proprietor dentist, such as group life insurance, health and accident insurance, tax free death benefit, and an opportunity to accumulate capital with certain tax advantages. (For further information consult a tax attorney.)

Given the advantages, why shouldn't every dentist incorporate? Dentists who do not set aside a significant amount of pretax earnings for retirement may not find the other benefits of corporate practice sufficient to justify the problems. These include:

— Being salaried.

— Additional legal and accounting expense.

— Behaving like a corporation with minutes of meetings and employment agreements.

—Taxes on corporate profits.

Others view the discipline imposed by the corporation as facilitative toward their financial goals.

Expense sharing arrangements are quite varied. Some dentists share complete facilities and work different times. A common arrangement is for dentist A to work early hours one week and late hours in the alternate weeks with dentist B working the other hours. Ingenious scheduling may even accommodate dentist C.

Less complete sharing may include:

— Certain facilities such as reception room, laboratory, dark room, and possibly even a treatment room for emergencies.

— Personnel, especially receptionist and hygienist.

— Expensive equipment such as panoramic x-ray machine.

— Quantity purchasing at more competitive prices.

Another sharing arrangement is a group of dentists practicing together, but not organized as a group practice. Several dentists can share a common facility in which there is one reception area and each dentist occupies his or her individual treatment area. Personnel such as receptionist(s), hygienist(s), and laboratory technician(s) can be shared, but chairside dental assistants may be employed by their individual dentist. The dentists can be sole proprietors or individually incorporated with retirement plans designed for their individual needs.

> Without being organized as a group practice, several dentists can share a common facility in which there is one reception area and each dentist occupies his or her individual treatment area.

Practicing with Others

A practice of two or more dentists presents various possibilities for *ownership*. It can be owned by one dentist who may be organized either as a sole proprietor or as a professional corporation, and all other dentists are then employees. If the practice is owned by two or more dentists, it can be organized as a partnership or as a professional corporation and may employ other (nonowner) dentists. All dentists in the group may be owners and can be organized either as a partnership or as a professional corporation.

Prior to states authorizing professional corporations, dentists could share ownership only as partners. Personal liability for a partner's acts is a distinct disadvantage of partnerships. A partner's act resulting in a judgment from a malpractice lawsuit for which there is insufficient professional liability insurance creates a grim situation

> Personal liability for a partner's acts is a distinct disadvantage of partnerships.

for all. The answer is sufficient insurance of partners or the professional corporation. Only the assets of the corporation are at risk in a malpractice lawsuit, but of course they should be protected with adequate insurance also. Dentists sharing ownership are well advised to do so through the professional corporation rather than through partnership.

There are also various possible *modes* of practice for a group. A general group may comprise dentists who all do a broad spectrum of general dentistry. Such a group is much like the single specialty group in that they all do about the same things. Or they may "specialize," in which case they resemble the multi-specialty group and can probably provide a broader spectrum of care. The mixed group comprises generalists and specialists providing a broad spectrum of general and specialty care.

Marketing varies among the groups. The advantage to the public, and therefore to marketing, is with the groups providing the broadest spectrum of care. The generalists who specialize must coordinate their marketing activities. Effective marketing methods differ among the groups. The speciality groups have traditionally marketed primarily to general dentists, and the general dentists primarily to the public. The trend now is toward more marketing to the public by specialists.

OFFICE DESIGN

The relatively competitive market in dentistry results in few graduates designing their own facility before going into practice. For those who plan a complete new facility, we suggest you consult authors such as Domer (Chapter 7), Kilpatrick (Chapter 2), and Howard (Chapter 7). In this book we want to call your attention to a few major points in planning a facility.

As Winston Churchill said, "We shape our buildings, and afterwards our buildings shape us."

Marketing

At this time you need to continue your consideration of marketing which you began in selecting your location. The facility ought to be planned to satisfy the total needs of your patients. An acronym "erthn" (environment responsive to human needs), coined by Wilson Southam of Cox Systems, Stoney Creek, Ontario, Canada, speaks to the importance of considering human needs (patients and dental team) in design. As Winston Churchill said, "We shape our buildings, and afterwards our buildings shape us."

Architects and Designers

Should you hire an architect? If the law requires it, of course you should. Otherwise, you will need to decide whether to encumber yourself with the additional expense of an architect's fees. Architects are well qualified by professional training to deal with problems of site

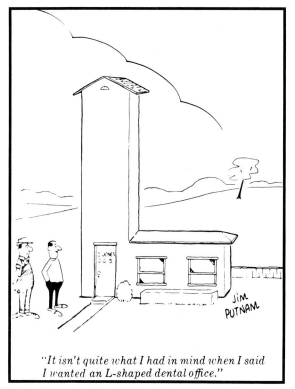

"It isn't quite what I had in mind when I said I wanted an L-shaped dental office."

From Gerald Epstein, *You Said A Mouthful,* New York, Dickerman Printing and Publishing Co., 1966.

selection, design, contracting, and construction. If you feel that you need assistance in these areas, you should engage an architect.

Ways of selecting an architect will be similar to those of selecting any other professional. You should first compile a list of architects from a variety of sources: bankers, builders, others who have recently completed a similar project, from the local chapter of the American Institute of Architects, and even from the telephone directory. You can contact the various architectural firms, ask for literature, ask if they are interested in doing your project, and ask about similar projects each firm may have recently completed. Finally, you will need to interview the candidates themselves and select one in whom you have confidence.

You may decide that you need a designer to work with the architect or in conjunction with a builder if you choose not to engage an architect. Designers, who may be available through your dental dealer, design floor plans and assist you in the selection of decor and furnishings.

General Considerations of Construction

E r t h n calls for attention to a variety of environmental factors: air conditioning, lighting, color, materials, privacy, and safety.

Heating, ventilating, and air conditioning should provide air that is clean and odor free, and at the proper temperature and humidity, with gentle air movement. Although expensive, charcoal or electrostatic air filters are most effective. Cold climates may require humidification of heated air. Balance of the system, and perhaps zone control, are necessary to ensure even temperature throughout.

Lighting ought to be of sufficient quantity and proper tone. The Illuminating Engineering Society has determined requirements for areas in the dental office as follows:

Area	Foot Candles
Reception room and general areas	0015
Reading areas	0030
Treatment room	0250
Operative light	1000
Laboratory	0100
Recovery room	0005
Business area	0100

The tone of light should be appropriate to the activity. The Valtronic Aurotron, Duro-test, or Auralux fluorescent tubes enable one to select correct tooth shades. Incandescent lighting provides a warm soft tone where such is desired, for example in the reception room and your private office.

Appropriate *color* interacts with lighting to achieve a pleasing esthetic effect, which minimizes eyestrain. In areas where critical seeing tasks are performed, such as in the laboratory or the treatment room, the recommended colors are those with high light reflectance (70 percent or more), meaning pastels with a high proportion of white. To avoid monotony, use a somewhat darker color on the wall opposite a window. In other areas a darker and richer wall treatment such as panelling or wallpaper will do well.

Beyond its interaction with lighting, color helps to determine the mood of the room. The problem in each area is to use a color that creates a desired mood. The reception room and treatment rooms (at least the portion the patient views) should be relaxing. Stimulation, if desired in areas such as preventive ones, can be achieved with warm bright colors. An interior designer with expertise in the communication of color can be of invaluable assistance in selection of colors.

Various *materials* can be used. The architect or engineer will select suitable structural materials. Others, such as ceilings, floors, partitions, doors and trim, permit choices. Acoustics and privacy need to be considered in these selections. A suspended acoustical tile ceiling provides access to space for tubing, wiring, and duct work. Carpet of wear resistant nylon, impregnated with a soil retardant and factory treated to be static-free, is an excellent floor covering. If you are concerned about mercury hygiene, seamless vinyl floor covering is also very good.

Privacy (tactile, olfactory, aural, and visual) is of concern in e r t h n, and relates to selection of materials. Because we dentists invade tactile privacy as a matter of course, we need to show as much respect for it as we can by providing enough space for people. Although the "dental office smell" is less a problem than it once was,

E r t h n calls for attention to a variety of environmental factors: air conditioning, lighting, color, materials, privacy, and safety.

we do need effective air filtration. The air turbine, our worst offender of aural privacy, needs good sound dampening provided by acoustical ceiling, wall, and floor coverings. Careful attention to lines of sight will provide visual privacy. Privacy, a form of autonomy, deserves respect.

Safety for the dental team and patients is essential. Radiation safety requires safe equipment (pretty well assured by regulations) and walls, floors, and ceilings that will block the transmission of x-rays. The Occupational Safety and Health Act (OSHA) of 1970 requires every employer to provide an environment free of hazards such as air contaminants, mercury, gases, and unsatisfactory safety exits.

Space Requirements

How much space do you need? To determine that, you must first decide how many treatment rooms you will have. You need as many treatment rooms as it takes for you and your staff to care for your patients. How many patients will you have? Now that is a question you would really like to know the answer to, isn't it? In spite of the fact that you cannot determine patient volume in advance, you should estimate as carefully as you can — perhaps partly on the basis of how many patients the other dentists treat.

The number of auxiliaries determines the number of treatment rooms.

The number of staff depends on the number of patients and your work patterns. The number of auxiliaries determines the number of treatment rooms. Suggested combinations are as follows:

Number of Auxiliaries	Number of Treatment Rooms
1–2	1
3	2
4 (1 Dental Hygienist)	3
5–6	4

Length of appointments may modify this. Very long appointments mean fewer treatment rooms (and probably fewer staff), and vice versa. If you begin practice with no patients, you need only one treatment room until you get busy enough that you need more staff. However, it makes sense to provide at least two treatment rooms, only one of which you may equip at first. Or, if your market research indicates that you will be quite busy within a year or two, you may prefer three or four treatment rooms (including one for the hygienist). The minimum size for a treatment room is 8' × 10' and you may prefer 10' × 10', 9' × 11', 10' × 14' or even larger. The cost and your feelings about space will determine what is best for your practice. The rule of thumb is that three treatment rooms require 1000 to 1500 square feet of total office space.

Other space requirements are the following:
— Reception room: 15 to 25 square feet for each occupant.
— Business office: about 70 square feet for each business auxiliary.

— Laboratory: 6 and preferably 10 linear feet of bench.
— Darkroom: at least 9 square feet and up to 25 square feet if you have an automatic processor.
— Staff room: 15 square feet per staff member.
— Private office/consultation room: 80 to 150 square feet.
— Lavatory: 15 to 40 square feet with $5' \times 5'$ clear area for a wheelchair.
— Panoramic x-ray: $5' \times 5'$ (some a bit less).
— X-ray room for chair and conventional machine: $6' \times 6'$.

In addition to deciding the number of treatment areas, you will need to decide what other areas you will have and how much space for each. Beyond essentials (treatment room, reception room, business office, dark room — unless you use a daylight loading automatic processor — laboratory, and lavatories — unless provided elsewhere), you will need to decide on what other areas to provide and how much space for each. Will you have a consultation room? Private office? (with lavatory?) Staff room? (with lavatory?) Separate sterilizing area? Separate x-ray area?

As we have mentioned, we believe you need a consultation room, which may double as a private office, or staff room or team room (for both dentists and auxiliaries). A private office and no staff room communicates to staff that they are less important. So does a private lavatory for the dentist, but none for staff. You may prefer a separate sterilizing area, rather than using a laboratory or treatment room. A separate x-ray area permits economy of equipment but means moving and possibly queuing patients.

A private office and no staff room communicates to staff that they are less important.

Floor Plan Design

Now the elements need to be arranged in the most useful design. Domer (pages 90–100) discusses this problem thoroughly. The problem is one of arranging the office so that it provides e r t h n for everyone. As C. M. Deasey says, the design exerts control on behavior, and the basis for design is to make human beings more effective in work and enjoyment.

Figure 21–3 illustrates a rational relationship of the elements. (It should be noted that "private office" refers to the consultation room as we have described it.) The solid line shows patient traffic and the broken line shows staff traffic. Additional suggestions are:

— Hygienist's operatory should be near the front to minimize traffic of hygiene patients into the dentist's treatment area.
— An operatory that is used primarily for emergencies should be similarly located for the same reason.
— Consultation room (private office) located adjacent to the business office can be used as an adjunct business office for private conferences and telephone calls by the receptionist.
— If you can afford it, you may include a private office which can be used as a retreat. Such an office should be in the back of the office suite — away from the traffic.
— Hallways should be wide (5 feet) unless there are separate halls for patient and staff traffic.

Hallways should be wide (5 feet) unless there are separate halls for patient and staff traffic.

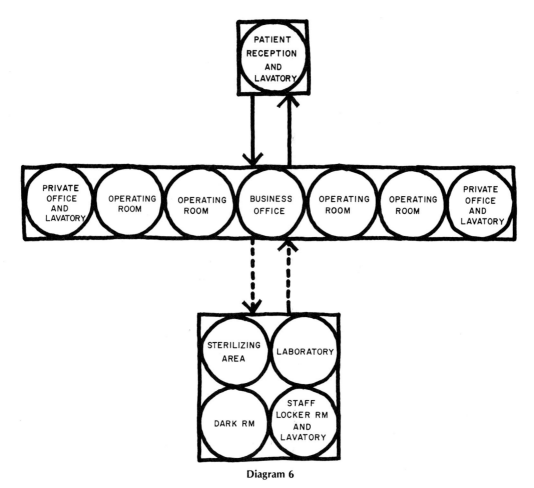

Figure 21–3. Traffic control within dental offices: fundamental principles. (From Kilpatrick, H. C., *Work Simplification in Dental Practice,* 1974, p. 47.)

— Open design with dividers permits ready visual communication among staff but limits aural privacy.

Remember that after you shape your building, it will shape you, your staff, and your patients. It will vitally affect your marketing.

EQUIPMENT

If you need to select equipment, remember that it is part of e r t h n — principally for the dental team. As Joe Dunlap says, patients do not pay very much attention to dental equipment — so long as it appears neat and works well. The selection of equipment should be on the basis of efficiency and effectiveness of the dental team. Your dental equipment should enable you to simplify your work. In the words of Harold Kilpatrick, "Work simplification is the right tool placed in the right position at the right time."

For a more comprehensive discussion we refer you to Kilpatrick, Chapter 4. We would like to direct your attention to some important considerations, however.

Kinesiology

The principles of mechanics and anatomy in relation to human movement should be considered in the design and placement of dental equipment. While working at the chair the dental team should observe the following principles:
— Torso and neck should be nearly vertical and not rotated.
— Upper arms and elbows should be in light contact with the rib cage.
— Hands should be at or slightly above the elbows.
— Sitting is preferable to standing, but occasional standing for short periods of time is healthful.
— In the sitting position the thighs should be nearly together and approximately parallel with the floor.
— The eyes should be naturally directed toward the work area.
You may choose to depart from these principles on occasion but should not be forced to do so by the dental equipment.

Asepsis

Features of the equipment that facilitate asepsis are the following:
— Autoclavable or disposable devices used intraorally or in contact with the patient's face or hands.
— Slick plastic hoses that do not retract.
— A mechanism in the water line to the handpieces to prevent aspiration of fluids from the mouth into the handpiece water line.
— Smooth surfaces without knurling on any equipment handled by either dentist or assistant.
— Foot controls for the patient chair and for height adjustment of the stools for dentist and assistant.
— Foot- or leg-activated controls for water and soap at sink.
— Disposable covers for chairs to be used for patients with hepatitis.

Dental Unit

Before selecting the unit, you need to answer a number of questions for yourself.
— Am I going to sit or stand most of the time while working?
— Am I going to work alone or with a dental assistant?
— If I work with an assistant, what tasks do I expect the assistant to do?
— What are the most convenient locations for the various dynamic instruments (handpieces, air and water syringes, and oral evacuator)?
— What particular dental unit or custom design provides the most convenient location for the dynamic instruments?
— What particular dental unit(s) are easily maintained?

Are you going to sit or stand most of the time while working?

— What particular dental unit is most favorably priced?
In addition to convenient positioning of the dynamic instruments, the
unit should not restrict the movement of the dental team, nor should
hoses and attachments invade the tactile privacy of the patient.

Dental Chair

Although its function is designated by the term patient position-
ing unit (PPU), it should by all means be comfortable for the patient.
Additionally it should:
— Be conveniently operable by both the dentist and the dental
    assistant.
— Have a thin, narrow back.
— Be capable of placing the patient's mouth at the operator's
    elbow level (seated or standing) in all operating positions.

Other Dental Equipment

Operating Stools

Operating stools should meet the following requirements:
— Be completely mobile with a broad stable base with five casters
    (and foot support for the assistant).
— Have large adequately and firmly padded seats.
— Be height adjustable by foot pressure (with range 14 to 21
    inches for dentist and 20 to 27 inches for the assistant).

Intra-Oral Light

Intra-oral light can be mounted on chair, wall, or ceiling. A
chair-mounted light remains directed in mouth as the chair is raised
or lowered but is less stable than a wall or ceiling mount. Ceiling
mounts are less restrictive than wall mounts. Intra-oral illumination of
1000 to 1200 foot candles should be provided by a long-lasting bulb
that can be readily changed by office personnel.

High Velocity Evacuation

High velocity evacuation (HVE) equipment should (according to
William R. Thompson, D.D.S.) meet the following requirements:
— Move 10 cubic feet of air at 150 miles per hour at negative
    pressure of 3 but no more than 5 inches of mercury through a
    10 mm orifice of all units that could be in use at any one
    time.
— Provide for separation of solids and drain water directly.
— Be operable by either the assistant or the dentist with variable
    suction control.
— Be activated when picked up.
— Not occupy useful floor space or evacuate air directly into the
    office suite or near the compressor.
— Be capable of providing continuous suction.

Air Compressor

The air compressor should provide dry filtered air at adequate volume pressure to operate all air-powered equipment that might be in use at any one time.

Radiographic Equipment

Radiographic equipment should be adequate for your practice. Do you need a panoramic x-ray machine? It may be too expensive, but it does have the following advantages:
— Much diagnostic information is provided that is not available in a periapical survey.
— Little time is required.
— Procedure for the patient and operator is facilitated.
— Radiation is minimal.
— Patients can understand the panoramic film better than the full mouth series.

How many conventional radiographic machines do you need? At least one. But you need no more than that until you have sufficient patient load. Where should you put it? This is largely a matter of personal choice. If you have a second room equipped for examination and emergencies, it makes sense to put it there.

Do you need an automatic processor? Again, this is largely a matter of personal choice. If you have daylight loading, you may choose to eliminate the dark room. However, it is better to have a dark room in case the processor fails. A dark room with developing tank is always reliable.

If you have daylight loading, you may choose to eliminate the dark room. However, it is better to have a dark room in case the processor fails.

A *radiograph duplicator* is essential for the production of copies when you want to (and should) retain the original in your files.

Laboratory Equipment

Laboratory equipment is another decision. The tendency is to buy more than you will use. You probably need a dental engine, vibrator, lathe, and model trimmer — possibly a glazing furnace. Be sure you will need it before you order anything else.

Sterilzing Equipment

Sterilization equipment should meet the following criteria:
—The equipment should be easily cleaned.
—The equipment should be easily filled with water or fluid (if required).
—It should have an automatic timer.
—It should operate quietly.
—It should accommodate a sufficient number of instruments.

Business Office Equipment

Business office equipment should not be an afterthought. Your business assistant needs serviceable equipment just as you do. At a minimum it should include the following:

— Electric typewriter.

— Electronic calculator with tape.

—Copy machine.

In order to save money, you may choose to shop for a used typewriter and used copy machine — in good condition.

Additional Considerations

Also consider the following when making decisions about equipment.

— Used equipment of the type you want in good condition may be hard to find but can minimize your investment.

—Backup is advantageous (especially if service is not readily available) in case of failure of such items as: twin motor or extra motor for compressor and HVE, handpieces, separate control panels for x-ray machines.

— Buy only equipment that you need. It makes little sense to pay finance charges on equipment that is not used.

The environment you create with dental equipment is also important to your dental team and to your patients. Choose carefully.

FINANCING

Money is the inescapable essential for your entry into solo practice. The feasibility of any project is based on its cost measured against its potential return. So you need to examine and evaluate the possible alternatives of financing. For a more complete discussion than is within the scope of this book, see Domer (Chapter 8) and Howard (Chapters 8 and 9).

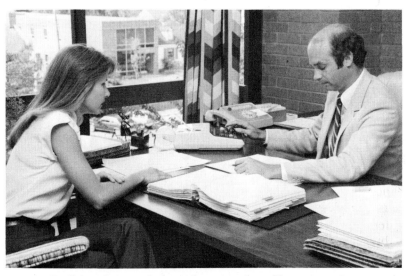

Dentist explores cost of opening a practice with an accountant.

Sources of Financing

The most usual source is banks. Savings and loan associations usually lend money for real estate purchases, whereas commercial banks lend for most other purposes, such as purchasing equipment. Large banks offer more services, but small banks in small communities may extend more credit if the officers feel that the project, such as the dental practice, is important to the quality of life in the community.

The Small Business Administration (SBA) is a possible source of a loan if you are unable to obtain one from the commercial banks. Actually the loan is through the commercial bank with a substantial portion (90 percent) guaranteed by SBA so that the bank is willing to make the loan. The bank may even be willing to assist you with the application, which is rather involved.

Do not overlook personal sources. If you own whole life insurance, the cash value can be borrowed at a favorable interest rate. Substantial equity in a home enables you to refinance or obtain a second mortgage. Relatives and friends who have the resources may lend you money or assist you to borrow. In order to substantiate your business deductions of interest payments, you should insist on a written note with a stated interest rate, which may well be less than that from the bank.

The Small Business Administration (SBA) is a possible source of a loan if you are unable to obtain one from the commercial banks.

Negotiation

You should expect to negotiate with a bank for a loan. Remember the banks want to lend money to people who can repay, and they want your business later when you are successful. So, you need not go with hat in hand. But you should go prepared with documentation (as discussed by Howard):

— Amount needed and for what (list of equipment and other items).
— Estimated business expenses.
— Estimated income.
— Personal budget.

Consult with more than one banker and let each know that you are shopping. You need to consider the following factors:

— The annual percentage rate (APR) of interest.
— The payback schedule.
— Penalties for prior payment, if any.
— Possible refinancing.
—Interest of and compatibility with the banker.

The most desirable answers include a payback schedule of 7 to 10 years with initial payment delayed six months, no penalties for prior payment, and possible refinancing if necessary.

Financing of real estate is inadvisable except in unusual circumstances. For those with financial resources, it is usually an excellent investment. In small communities, it may be necessary to build in order to obtain a satisfactory facility. Usually a local investor is willing to build for you. If not, you may need to develop your personal resources and finance the project yourself.

LEASING

In ordinary circumstances most financial consultants advise leasing real estate and purchasing equipment. As financing real estate may be justified, so may leasing equipment. If you are unable to obtain financing for dental equipment, you should consult further and re-examine your plan. The banker, especially in small communities, may not understand that the potential earnings of a dental practice justify lending with inadequate security. On the other hand, the banker may have carefully evaluated the potential of your dental practice and decided that your loan request was not feasible. In that case, you need to trim your sails—reduce your request, or perhaps even abandon your plan to enter practice on your own. If, however, the banker's decision does not seem reasonable, you may attempt to finance outside the community, or you may decide to lease.

Leasing is a business and must return a profit. The lessor finances equipment which he then leases. The gross profit is essentially the difference between lessor's finance charges and lease payments. In other words, it costs you more to lease than to buy equipment. It may still make sense (even if you could finance the purchase) for items that may become obsolete quickly or items you are not sure you want to keep.

> It may make sense to lease (even if you could finance the purchase) for items which may become obsolete quickly.

Leasing office space brings up a whole series of questions that you should take up with your attorney. Remember that standard leases are written by lawyers to protect landlords and lawyers. Also remember that any item in the lease is negotiable, and you should be satisfied.

STAFFING

Staffing is covered in considerable detail in Chapter 20. For the dentist organizing his or her practice a few additional comments are in order.

First you should decide what you need assistance for. If you enter as an associate into a practice with a heavy patient load, you need assistance in the production of dental services. However, if you begin a solo practice, you need marketing assistance.

The tendency for the new dentist is to feel that he or she wants chairside assistance to make the work easier. Then when the telephone rings, the assistant answers it, and she takes care of other business functions as she has time. The danger is that the personal contact at the desk and on the telephone, which is so essential to marketing, may be slighted. As a consequence, the practice may fail to develop as it should. So give serious thought to first hiring a desk person, and letting yourself do the dental treatment without assistance.

> Give serious thought to first hiring a desk person, and letting yourself do the dental treatment without assistance.

If this is unacceptable to you or if the demand for your services is quite high, you can hire a business assistant and a chairside assistant initially. By all means you need a business assistant who relates easily to people and makes them feel welcome in your practice. Your marketing station, the desk and telephone, should have someone present at all times.

SUMMARY

If you have made good decisions relative to location, your practice, office, financing, and staffing, you are on the road to success.

REFERENCES

Born, D. O.: Dental Manpower Planning and Distribution. A Survey of the Literature, ADA, 1975.

Diseker, R. A., Chappell, J.: Practice Location: A Rating System for Comparing Communities. Resident and Staff Physician, April 1977, pp. 161–167.

Domer, L. R., et al.: Dental Practice Management. St. Louis, C. V. Mosby Co., 1980.

Goldbert, M. J. (ed.): The Business Side of Dental Practice. Stamford, CT, Professional Publishing Company, 1969.

Howard, W. W.: Dental Practice Planning. St. Louis, C. V. Mosby Co., 1975.

Jergi, C. R., et al.: Group Practice and the Future of Dental Care. Philadelphia, Lea and Febiger, 1974, pp. 301–317.

Kilpatrick, H. C.: Work Simplification in Dental Practice. Philadelphia, W. B. Saunders Co., 1974.

Layman, G. A., Redmond, P.: As your practice grows. Dental Economics. Tulsa, PPC Books, 1977.

Medical Group Practice Management. Cambridge, MA, Ballinger Pub. Co., 1977.

Roach, J. M.: Simon says decision making is a satisficing experience. Management Review, Jan. 79, pp. 8–17.

Thompson, W. R.: The Dental Clinics of North America. Philadelphia, W. B. Saunders Co., July 1967.

Twelker, P. A., Smith, R.: Locating a Dental Practice. Washington, D.C., U.S. Public Health Service, 1972.

Afterword _____

Thank you for exploring with us the realm of marketing for your dental practice. We sincerely hope that our association over these approximately 400 pages has helped you launch, improve, or expand your practice as a professional marketing dentist.

We are certain that you have already found—or will shortly find—that patients appreciate your marketing consciousness. Such an approach is implicitly *more* professional, *more* dedicated, and *more* patient-oriented than traditional non-marketing approaches.

A few closing notes:

—*Marketing for the Dental Practice* does not pretend to be inclusive of every possible dental marketing idea or technique. You and your staff, possibly prompted by some of the points we've mentioned, will surely come up with new and perhaps even more workable marketing ideas. We'll be delighted if we have been a stimulus to your own brainstorming.

—Despite our perhaps too-frequent use of words such as "should," "need to," and similar imperatives, we hope you will not perceive us as having attempted to dictate to you how you can best manage your own practice. Chalk up a healthy percentage of those imperatives to the limits of the English language. Consider that most of what we've said was offered to you in the spirit of suggestion—though based on sound research and decades of experience in both dentistry and marketing.

—We welcome your criticisms and other thoughts and earnestly hope that you will take a few moments to send them to us by mail. This is, please be assured, much more than a perfunctory request. Please *do* write, to this address:

> Dr. Charles Milone
> School of Dentistry
> University of North Carolina
> Chapel Hill, NC 27514

Especially would we be grateful to you for letting us know how things work out as you implement some of the techniques we have discussed here. We would appreciate receiving any anecdotes you may want to share, as well as any data.

Our work of conceptualizing, researching, and writing this book was, we found, quite a challenge, at times intimidating or discouraging, at times exhilarating, but almost always rewarding. We think that your efforts to become a marketing dentist, with a marketing-oriented staff (or to improve upon a marketing approach) may provide a similar challenge. Inevitably, there will be "downs" and discouraging moments. But there will also be upbeat moments and exhilarating ones, too. Through it all, you will grow, personally as well as professionally, and both your staff and your patients will share in your gains.

Charles L. Nielsen

Charles Blair

James R. Littlefield

Appendix A

ADA Principles of Ethics and Code of Professional Conduct*

PRINCIPLE — SECTION I

Service to the Public and Quality of Care. The dentist's primary obligation of service to the public shall include the delivery of quality care, competently and timely, within the bounds of the clinical circumstances presented by the patient. Quality of care shall be a primary consideration of the dental practitioner.

CODE OF PROFESSIONAL CONDUCT

1-A Patient Selection

While dentists, in serving the public, may exercise reasonable discretion in selecting patients for their practices, dentists shall not refuse to accept patients into their practice or deny dental service to patients because of the patient's race, creed, color, sex or national origin.

1-B Patient Records

Dentists are obliged to safeguard the confidentiality of patient records. Dentists shall maintain patient records in a manner consistent with the protection of the welfare of the patient. Upon request of a patient or another dental practitioner, dentists shall provide any information that will be beneficial for the future treatment of that patient.

1-C Community Service

Since dentists have an obligation to use their skills, knowledge and experience for the improvement of the dental health of the public and are encouraged to be leaders in their community, dentists in such service shall conduct themselves in such a manner as to maintain or elevate the esteem of the profession.

1-D Emergency Service

Dentists shall be obliged to make reasonable arrangements for the emergency care of their patients of record.

Dentists shall be obliged when consulted in an emergency by patients not of record to make reasonable arrangements for emergency care. If treatment is provided, the dentist, upon completion of such treatment, is obliged to return the patient to his or her regular dentist unless the patient expressly reveals a different preference.

1-E Consultation and Referral

Dentists shall be obliged to seek consultation, if possible, whenever the welfare of patients will be safeguarded or advanced by utilizing those who have special skills, knowledge and experience. When patients visit or are referred to specialists or consulting dentists for consultation:

1. The specialists or consulting dentists upon completion of their care shall return the patient, unless the patient expressly reveals a different preference, to the referring dentist, or if none, to the dentist of record for future care.

2. The specialists shall be obliged when there is no referring dentist and upon a completion of their treatment to inform patients when there is a need for further dental care.

1-F Use of Auxiliary Personnel

Dentists shall be obliged to protect the health of their patient by only assigning to qualified auxiliaries those duties which can be legally delegated. Dentists shall be further obliged to prescribe and supervise the work of all auxiliary personnel working under their direction and control.

1-G Justifiable Criticism and Expert Testimony

Dentists shall be obliged to report to the appropriate reviewing agency instances of gross and/or continual faulty treatment by other dentists. If there is evidence of such treatment, the patient should be informed. Dentists shall be obliged to refrain from commenting disparagingly without justification about the services of other dentists. Dentists may provide expert testimony when that testimony is essential to a just and fair disposition of a judicial or administrative action.

1-H Rebate and Split Fees

Dentists shall not accept or tender "rebates" or "split fees."

PRINCIPLE — Section 2

Education. The privilege of dentists to be accorded professional status rests primarily in the knowledge, skill and experience with which they serve their

357

patients and society. All dentists, therefore, have the obligation of keeping their knowledge and skill current.

PRINCIPLE — Section 3

Government of a Profession. Every profession owes society the responsibility to regulate itself. Such regulation is achieved largely through the influence of the professional societies. All dentists, therefore, have the dual obligation of making themselves a part of a professional society and of observing its rules of ethics.

PRINCIPLE — Section 4

Research and Development. Dentists have the obligation of making the results and benefits of their investigative efforts available to all when they are useful in safeguarding or promoting the health of the public.

CODE OF PROFESSIONAL CONDUCT

4-A Devices and Therapeutic Methods

Except for formal investigative studies, dentists shall be obliged to prescribe, dispense or promote only those devices, drugs and other agents whose complete formulae are available to the dental profession. Dentists shall have the further obligation of not holding out as exclusive any device, agent, method or technique.

4-B Patents and Copyrights

Patents and copyrights may be secured by dentists provided that such patents and copyrights shall not be used to restrict research or practice.

PRINCIPLE — Section 5

Professional Announcement. In order to properly serve the public, dentists should represent themselves in a manner that contributes to the esteem of the profession. Dentists should not misrepresent their training and competence in any way that would be false or misleading in any material respect.*

CODE OF PROFESSIONAL CONDUCT

5-A Advertising

Although any dentist may advertise, no dentist shall advertise or solicit patients in any form of communication in a manner that is false or misleading in any material respect.*

5-B Name of Practice

Since the name under which a dentist conducts his practice may be a factor in the selection process of the patient, the use of a trade name or an assumed name that is false or misleading in any material respect is unethical.

Use of the name of a dentist no longer actively associated with the practice may be continued for a period not to exceed one year.*

5-C Announcement of Specialization and Limitation of Practice.

This Section and Section 5-D are designed to help the public make an informed selection between the practitioner who has completed an accredited program beyond the dental degree and a practitioner who has not completed such a program.

The special areas of dental practice approved by the American Dental Association and the designation for ethical specialty announcement and limitation of practice are: dental public health, endodontics, oral pathology, oral and maxillofacial surgery, orthodontics, pedodontics (dentistry for children), periodontics and prosthodontics.

Dentists who choose to announce specialization should use "specialist in" and shall limit their practice exclusively to the announced special area(s) of dental practice, provided at the time of the announcement such dentists have met in each approved specialty for which they announce the existing educational requirements and standards set forth by the American Dental Association.

Dentists who use their eligibility to announce as specialists to make the public believe that specialty services rendered in the dental office are being rendered by qualified specialists when such is not the case are engaged in unethical conduct. The burden of responsibility is on specialists to avoid any inference that general practitioners who are associated with specialists are qualified to announce themselves as specialists.

General Standards. The following are included within the standards of the American Dental Association for determining what dentists have the education experience and other appropriate requirements for announcing specialization and limitation of practice:

1. The special area(s) of dental practice and an appropriate certifying board must be approved by the American Dental Association.

2. Dentists who announce as specialists must have successfully completed an educational program accredited by the Commission on Dental Accreditation, two or more years in length, as specified by the Council on Dental Education or be diplomates of a nationally recognized certifying board.

3. The practice carried on by dentists who announce as specialists shall be limited exclusively to the special area(s) of dental practice announced by the dentist.

Standards for Multiple-Specialty Announcements.

Educational criteria for announcement by dentists in additional recognized specialty areas are the successful completion of an educational program accredited by the Commission on Dental Accreditation in each area for which the dentist wishes to announce.

Dentists who completed their advanced education in programs listed by the Council on Dental Education prior to the initiation of the accreditation process in 1967 and who are currently ethically announcing as specialists in a recognized area may announce in additional areas provided they are educationally qualified or are certified diplomates in each area for which they wish to announce. Documentation of successful completion of the educational program(s) must be submitted to the appropriate constituent society. The documentation must assure that the duration of the program(s) is a minimum of two years except for oral and maxillofacial surgery which must have been a minimum of three years in duration.*

5-D **General Practitioner Announcement of Services**

General dentists who wish to announce the services available in their practices are permitted to announce the availability of those services so long as they avoid any communications that express or imply specialization. General dentists shall also state that the services are being provided by general dentists. No dentist shall announce available services in any way that would be false or misleading in any material respect. The phrase "practice limited to" shall be avoided.*

*Advertising, solicitation of patients or business, or other promotional activities by dentists or dental care delivery organizations shall not be considered unethical or improper, except for those promotional activities which are false or misleading in any material respect. Notwithstanding any ADA *Principles of Ethics and Code of Professional Conduct* or other standards of dentist conduct which may be differently worded, this shall be the sole standard for determining the ethical propriety of such promotional activities. Any provision of an ADA constituent or component society's code of ethics or other standard of dentist conduct relating to dentists' or dental care delivery organizations' advertising, solicitation, or other promotional activities which is worded differently from the above standard shall be deemed to be in conflict with the ADA *Principles of Ethics and Code of Professional Conduct.*

INTERPRETATION AND APPLICATION OF "PRINCIPLES OF ETHICS AND CODE OF PROFESSIONAL CONDUCT"

The preceding statements constitute the *Principles of Ethics and Code of Professional Conduct* of the American Dental Association. The purpose of the *Principles and Code* is to uphold and strengthen dentistry as a member of the learned professions. The constituent and component societies may adopt additional provisions or interpretations not in conflict with these *Principles of Ethics and Code of Professional Conduct* which would enable them to serve more faithfully the traditions, customs and desires of the members of these societies.

Problems involving questions of ethics should be solved at the local level within the broad boundaries established in these *Principles of Ethics and Code of Professional Conduct* and within the interpretation by the component and/or constituent society of their respective codes of ethics. If a satisfactory decision cannot be reached, the question should be referred on appeal to the constituent society and the Council on Bylaws and Judicial Affairs of the American Dental Association, as provided in Chapter XI of the *Bylaws* of the American Dental Association. Members found guilty of unethical conduct as prescribed in the American Dental Association *Code of Professional Conduct* or codes of ethics of the constituent and component societies are subject to the penalties set forth in Chapter XI of the American Dental Association *Bylaws.*

*Copyright by the American Dental Association. Reprinted by permission.

Appendix B

Practice Evaluation

PHILOSOPHY AND GOALS

1. Have you set goals for a specific number of years in the future?
2. Does your staff understand and support your goals?
3. Does each staff member have individual goals that are compatible with and supportive of your practice goals?
4. Do you have a written philosophy or principles of practice?
5. Have you developed written financial objectives, both short-range (annual) and long-range?
6. Do you review and revise financial objectives annually?
7. Do you prepare an annual budget, giving consideration to previous years' experience, practice goals and objectives, and current circumstances?
8. Have you developed a long-range financial forecast? Do you revise and update it annually?

APPOINTMENT CONTROL

9. Is your appointment book (system) adequate to keep track of appointments and provide sufficient information for planning treatment procedures?
10. If you use an appointment "book," are all entries legible and in pencil?
11. Does your appointment secretary know how much time is required for each appointment—treatment, examination, and emergency?
12. Is each appointment confirmed prior to the appointment?
13. Do you record broken appointments on patient records, and do you attempt to work out scheduling problems with patients?
14. Does your appointment secretary know when you can see emergency patients?
15. Are patients informed as to the length of their appointments?
16. Does each patient making an appointment receive an appointment card with name, date, day of the week, and hour of appointment on it?
17. Does your appointment secretary use and maintain a list of patients who can and will accept an appointment on short notice?

OFFICE MANAGEMENT

18. Have you considered incorporating your practice?
19. Do you forecast your production at least twelve months in advance?
20. Do you employ a practice management consultant?
21. Do you monitor supply orders, invoices and back orders for accuracy of statements?
22. Is your patient record system adequate to provide quality care? Is the system efficient in order to maximize productivity and minimize frustration for you, your patients, and your staff?
23. Are your filing cabinets suitable for efficient filing and retrieval of patient records?
24. Are your files color coded?
25. Have you reviewed the files of those patients not on recall within the past year?
26. Are all old patient files stored securely and accessibly?
27. Does your inventory system ensure that you will always have needed items without undue capital investment?
28. Do you have enough working space?
29. Is your equipment adequate?
30. Is your equipment adequately maintained?
31. Do you know how many new patients you saw last month, last year?
32. Do you know how this compares with the previous period?

STAFF RELATIONS

33. Do you have periodic staff meetings?
34. Do your staff members rotate as chairperson for office staff meetings and have full responsibility for the agenda?
35. Do you review all staff salaries and performances at least annually?
36. Is daily attendance accurately recorded for all employees?
37. Is your on-going training program adequate?
38. Do other staff members participate when you hire new staff members?
39. Do you have an adequate procedure for reviewing employee complaints?
40. Is your procedure for termination fair to you and your employees?
41. Do you conduct an exit interview with all departing staff members?

COMMUNICATIONS

42. Do you have enough telephone lines coming into your office?

43. Do your staff members answer your phone courteously and promptly (before the third ring)?

44. Does each staff member know how to give directions to your office by telephone?

45. Do you have an adequate typewriter?

46. Do you answer all correspondence within three working days?

47. Do you employ correspondence as a means of enhancing others' understanding of your services?

48. Do you have an efficient system for communicating silently from one area of your office to another, especially between you and your receptionist?

FEES AND BILLING

49. Have you established a basic fee schedule for all routine procedures to simplify billing and treatment planning?

50. Do you have a rational method for adjusting your basic fee schedule to reflect additional effort or responsibility?

51. Are you fully aware of the effect of the rate of inflation on your practice costs?

52. Do you review and revise your basic fee schedule on a regular, periodic basis?

53. Is the patient who is not scheduled for subsequent appointments diplomatically encouraged to pay for service at the time of the visit?

54. Are pretreatment estimates given and firm financial arrangements made with the person responsible for the account prior to treatment?

55. Does your business assistant make all routine financial arrangements?

56. Does your business assistant have the knowledge and authority to handle most billing complaints?

57. Do you have a systematic and efficient billing and follow-up procedure for accounts receivable?

58. Do you include self-addressed return envelopes with your statements?

59. Is "address correction requested" printed on your outgoing envelopes?

60. Does your receptionist know the balance due for each patient coming in?

61. Do you know the average daily billings and receipts for your practice?

62. Do you have a special reminder system for patients paying over time?

63. When your accounts receivable system has run its course, does your business assistant, with your approval, turn the account over to an outside collection agency?

64. Does the total balance on ledger cards match the accounts receivable in the bookkeeping system?

INSURANCE PROCESSING

65. Do you process all insurance forms within three working days of treatment?

66. Do you use the ADA standard insurance form?

67. Can your insurance clerk easily transfer all treatment information from office forms to insurance forms?

68. Do you routinely obtain predetermination of benefits on all treatment plans?

69. Do you have a system for keeping track of insurance transactions?

70. Does your insurance clerk follow up on insurance transactions unduly delayed?

ACCOUNTING

71. Do you have confidence that your accountant is doing a good job for you?

72. Is your accountant thoroughly familiar with dental (or professional) practices in general, and with your practice in particular?

73. Does your accountant, along with your attorney, banker, insurance agent, consultant, etc., function as part of your management team?

74. Do you have at least one tax planning session per year with your tax advisor, to review the previous year and prepare for the next?

75. Do you have available to you an income and expense (profit and loss) statement each month (or at least each quarter) and a balance sheet at least annually?

76. Do you and your accountant review, evaluate and analyze your financial reports (profit and loss statement and balance sheet), compare them to the budget, cash flow projection, financial forecast and objectives, and develop appropriate courses of action as a result?

77. Does your accountant advise you when excess funds are available for investment purposes?

78. Is your record-keeping system adequate to support:
    —tax information requirements?
    —support for bank loans?
    —comprehensive, practical controls?

79. Do your practice controls include:
    —all receipts deposited to your bank daily?
    —separate checking accounts for business and personal use?
    —reconciliation of your bank statement monthly by either you or your accountant?
    —a positive record of each patient seen?

80. Is your outstanding accounts receivable no more than 1½ month's worth of gross receipts?

Appendix C

A Method for Evaluating Communities

A systematic approach to evaluating communities is to consider a list of variables, such as those on the community score sheet following,* to which you may add others that may be important to you. Before visiting the community, you (and your spouse) should establish your value (Item Value) for each variable in Column A. Your spouse may not be involved in evaluating professional variables. Any scale you choose is satisfactory, but it is suggested that you use the following:

A variable of great importance to you = 5
A variable of moderate importance = 3
A variable of limited importance = 1
A variable of no importance to you = 0

On the visit, use Column B with a similar scale to indicate the extent to which the factor is found (Presence Value). The following scale is suggested:

Variable present at or beyond your expectations = 5
Variable present at a satisfactory level = 3
Variable present to a limited degree = 1
Variable not present = 0

Important unlisted variables encountered during the visit should be added and assigned values. If you wish to change the value of variables during the visit, you may do so, cautiously. In upgrading the value of an item, be sure you are not temporarily enamored with it. Any upgraded or downgraded item should be re-examined critically at a later time to establish its value.

The site score (Column C) for each item is the product of multiplying Column A by Column B. A total site score (the sum of Column C) can be used to compare communities. Comparison of the sum of Column B with that of Column A shows how each community measures up against your criteria. Any items with which you are less than satisfied (Column B score is less than Column A score) should be examined closely against items with which you are more than satisfied (Column B score is greater than Column A score). Assessment of the off-setting of one variable by exceptional presence of another or others is an effective "trade-off" technique and can be achieved most objectively at some time after the site visit.

This rational approach should enable you to select a community that adequately meets your immediate needs and remains a satisfying area in which to live and practice.

---

*Adapted from Diseker, R. A., and Chappell, J.: Practice Location: A Rating System for Comparing Communities. Resident and Staff Physician, April 1977, pp. 161–167.

Score Sheet For Your Ratings

Date:_____

Community: _____

Items	(A) Item Value	×	(B) Presence Value	=	(C) Site Score
PERSONAL FACTORS					
1. Acceptability of location to spouse	_____	×	_____	=	_____
2. Similarity of spouse's background to the community	_____	×	_____	=	_____
3. Similarity of your background to the community	_____	×	_____	=	_____
4. Previous familiarity with the area	_____	×	_____	=	_____
5. Geography and climate	_____	×	_____	=	_____
6. Schools	_____	×	_____	=	_____
7. Adult education program	_____	×	_____	=	_____
8. Cultural activities	_____	×	_____	=	_____
9. Overall quality of life	_____	×	_____	=	_____
10. Social and cultural life	_____	×	_____	=	_____
11. Recreation	_____	×	_____	=	_____
12. Churches	_____	×	_____	=	_____
13. Size of community	_____	×	_____	=	_____
14. Kind of community	_____	×	_____	=	_____
15. Prospect of being influential in community affairs	_____	×	_____	=	_____
16. Family ties (or lack of) to the area	_____	×	_____	=	_____
17. Proximity to a metropolitan area	_____	×	_____	=	_____
PROFESSIONAL FACTORS					
18. Satisfactory practice arrangement	_____	×	_____	=	_____
19. Adequate health care	_____	×	_____	=	_____

20. Adequate population   _____ × _____ = _____

21. Age distribution of the population   _____ × _____ = _____

22. Need for dental services   _____ × _____ = _____

23. Organized effort of the community to attract a dentist   _____ × _____ = _____

24. Educational level   _____ × _____ = _____

25. Demand for dental services   _____ × _____ = _____

26. Population per dentist   _____ × _____ = _____

27. Dentist busyness   _____ × _____ = _____

28. Possibility of regular working hours   _____ × _____ = _____

29. Availability of professional colleagues   _____ × _____ = _____

30. Availability of dental specialists   _____ × _____ = _____

31. Availability of satisfactory continuing education   _____ × _____ = _____

32. Receptivity of community dentists   _____ × _____ = _____

33. Availability of qualified auxiliaries   _____ × _____ = _____

34. Available service for dental equipment   _____ × _____ = _____

35. Accessibility to dental laboratory   _____ × _____ = _____

36. Accessibility to dental supply house   _____ × _____ = _____

37. Opportunity for other professional activity   _____ × _____ = _____

ECONOMIC FACTORS

38. Per capita income   _____ × _____ = _____

39. Per capita retail sales   _____ × _____ = _____

40. Effective buying income   _____ × _____ = _____

41. Third-party funding for dental care   _____ × _____ = _____

42. Rate of employment   _____ × _____ = _____

43. Type of employment   _____ × _____ = _____

44. Growth potential   _____ × _____ = _____

45. Dental fees   _____ × _____ = _____

46. Business expenses   _____ × _____ = _____

47. Dentist income   _____ × _____ = _____

48. Availability of financing   _____ × _____ = _____

49. Cost of financing   _____ × _____ = _____

50. Tax rates   _____ × _____ = _____

51. Forgiveness of educational loans   _____ × _____ = _____

52. Investment opportunities   _____ × _____ = _____

53. Other   _____ × _____ = _____

     Sum Total   _____ × _____ = _____

Appendix D

List of Sources for Marketing and Advertising

Advertising Age
740 Rush Street
Chicago, IL 60611
    The leading weekly magazine in the advertising field.

The Advertising Dentist
P. O. Box 5175
Phoenix, AZ 85010
($48 yearly)
    A monthly newsletter providing detailed information on advertising of dental services.

Advertising and Promoting the Professional Practice (by Morton Walker)
Hawthorn Books, Inc.
260 Madison Avenue
New York, NY 10016 (1979)
    Written by a podiatrist, it's a practical guide to marketing professional services. Covers advertising and promotion techniques. Includes a useful bibliography.

The American Marketing Association
Suite 606, 222 S. Riverside Plaza
Chicago, IL 60606
(312) 648-0536
    The leading national organization of marketing professionals and academicians.

Custom Column Service
Box 488P
Lexington, MA 02173
    A service providing periodic newspaper columns on dental health to be used in your local newspaper with your photo, byline, and closing message.

Dental Dialogue, Inc.
390 West 7th Street
Columbus, OH 43201
    Provides a newspaper column on dental health, which is personalized in the name of the dentist using it.

"Dental Manpower Fact Book," March 1979 DHEW Publication No. (HRA) 79–14.

U.S. Department of HHS
Bureau of Health Manpower
3700 East-West Highway
Hyattsville, MD 20782
    A working reference guide, it includes a collection of statistical tables with supporting text on many aspects of dental manpower and utilization of dental services.

Dental Patient Report, C/O PSC, Inc.
3321 West Beltline Highway
Madison, WI 53713
    A bimonthly newsletter that can be sent to patients or prospective patients. Includes articles on dentistry, good health habits, nutrition, and so on. Also has reading list for laymen. Can be sent as is or company will customize it for individual practices. Information kit and price list available.

Do-It-Yourself Marketing Research (by George Edward Breen)
McGraw-Hill
1221 Avenue of the Americas
New York, NY 10020 (1977)
    Written for business professionals who aren't experienced in marketing, much of the information would be applicable to dentists wishing to do their own market research.

Facts About the Dental Market
American Dental Association
211 East Chicago Avenue
Chicago, IL 60611
    Written for dental manufacturers and advertisers, this brochure includes many statistics on dental manpower, distribution, and auxiliary personnel of value in market research.

How to Advertise (by Kenneth Roman and Jane Maas)
St. Martin's Press
175 Fifth Avenue
New York, NY 10010 (1976)
    This is a guide for obtaining effective advertising. Much of the material will be beyond the scope of dental practices, but the chapters on the different advertising media are useful.

Journal of Health Care Marketing
CMD-247
J. Walker College of Business
Appalachian State University
Boone, NC 28608 ($20 yearly)

Edited by B. J. Dunlap and Don C. Dodson. A quarterly journal targeted at health care professionals, it is designed as a resource for current research, ideas, and marketing practice. Regular features include articles, book and article reviews, guest editorials, a guide to meetings and conferences, letters, professional association news, a resource index, and health care marketing abstracts.

The Journal of Marketing/Management for Professions
1562 University Avenue
St. Paul, MN 55104 ($48 yearly)

A monthly magazine for professionals interested in marketing. It's edited by Dr. Richard Stallard and its emphasis is on marketing of dental services.

NEXUS
The Nexus Group, Inc.
P. O. Bin R
Cave Creek, AZ 85331

A newsletter for dentists whose aim is to build a practice based on advanced behavioral concepts with emphasis on personalized service.

Professional Communication Company
5799 Tall Oaks Road
Madison, WI 53711

Dental Care Marketing is a newsletter for dentists published under the aegis of Sycom. Intended for dentists who are purposefully and intentionally marketing their services. Provides a wide choice of marketing ideas.

Semantodontics, Inc.
Box 15668
Phoenix, AZ 85060

Provides various marketing aids such as books, audio tapes, posters, plaques. Catalog available upon request.

Appendix E

Marketing Checklist

1. Do I understand marketing?
2. Do I believe in marketing?
3. Am I applying marketing principles in my practice?

COMMUNITY

4. Do I understand the demography of my community?
5. What is the age distribution in my community?
6. What are the trends in age distribution?
7. What is the income distribution in my community?
8. What is the approximate rate of turnover of community residents?
9. What are the community attitudes toward dentists, dental services, and charges?
10. How am I dealing with these attitudes?
11. What do people in my community feel and believe about health services?
12. Do my services fit with these beliefs?

MARKETING IN THE COMMUNITY

13. Have I systematically segmented the market in my community?
14. Have I decided on what segment(s) to target?
15. Is there a sufficient number available in my target segment(s) to support me?
16. Do I understand the needs of my target segment(s)?
17. Have I designed my marketing mix to satisfy their needs?
18. Is my office location and decor appealing to them?
19. Are my hours convenient for them?
20. Am I providing clinical services they want and need?
21. Does my staff relate well to them?
22. Are my fees and billing arrangements acceptable to them?
23. Am I promoting in such a way as to get their attention and appeal to them?
24. Am I effectively communicating the uniqueness of my services and appealing to them?

25. Are other dentists aware of the uniqueness of my services?
26. Am I aware of the constituencies through whom I should market?
27. Do I market to non-dentist providers (if any)?
28. (For dentists developing a new practice) Have I called on, offered assistance to, and asked assistance from the following persons in the community: other dentists; physicians; public health nurses; pharmacists; business persons; dental laboratory technicians; lawyers, accountants, and bankers; and dental suppliers.

PLANNING

29. Have I thought through the ethics of marketing?
30. Have I established a marketing approach that conforms to the ADA Principles of Ethics and Code of Professional Conduct?
31. Does my approach conform to state laws? (unless I plan to challenge state laws)
32. Do my staff and I feel OK about my approach?
33. Does my marketing approach require change in my self-image?
34. Am I able to make the change?
35. Do I want to make the change?
36. Have I set goals (personal and practice)?
37. Are the practice goals supported by individual goals of each team member?
38. Are the goals written?
39. Do I have a plan for reviewing goals and evaluating progress?

EXPANDING SCOPE OF CARE

40. Have I considered expanding my scope of care?
41. Have I systematically assessed the strengths and weaknesses of current office procedures?
42. Have I decided to make any changes in current procedures?
43. Have I made any changes?
44. Have I assessed my strengths and weaknesses in procedures I currently refer?
45. Have I decided to offer services currently referred?

46. Have I begun performing procedures formerly referred?
47. Have I assessed the costs (financial and psychological) of offering new services?
48. Have I decided to offer any new services?
49. Am I now offering services not formerly offered?
50. Do I have a plan for strengthening areas of weakness?
51. Have I put my plan into operation?
52. Have I assessed my participation in treatment of patients referred to a specialist?
53. Could I provide more of the treatment myself?
54. Have I discussed this with specialist(s) to whom I refer?
55. Am I providing more treatment for patients referred to specialists than formerly?
56. Do I monitor the results of my expansion of care?
57. Have I investigated the possibilities of a specialist using my office part time?
58. Have I arranged for part time specialist coverage in my office?
59. Have I investigated the possibilities of co-ordination of services with other dentists?
60. Have I developed such arrangements with other dentists?

PROMOTION

61. Do I have a plan for promoting through publicity and personal contact?
62. Have I discussed publicity with a public relations specialist such as a media person?
63. Have I developed a plan for publicity?
64. Am I following through on my plan?
65. Am I a competent public speaker?
66. If I'm not, do I have plans for becoming competent?
67. Do I seek opportunities to speak to groups?
68. Do I volunteer for community activity?
69. Do I provide referral slips to persons who might refer patients to me?
70. Have I established a lay advisory panel?
71. Does the panel meet regularly?
72. Does the panel provide marketing information?
73. Do I use the information?
74. Does the information improve my marketing?

ADVERTISING

75. Have I investigated and do I understand media advertising?

76. Does it fit into my marketing program?
77. Am I aware of what appeals are effective in advertising dental services?
78.. Have I determined what unique characteristics of my practice I could feature in my advertising?
79. Do I understand the charges for advertising?
80. Have I developed a budget for advertising?
81. Do I have an advertising program?
82. Does the advertising copy appeal on the basis of needs?
83. Does it feature unique characteristics of my practice that address these needs?
84. Have I developed means for evaluating the effectiveness of my advertising?
85. Is my advertising effective?
86. Do I plan any changes, based on evaluation?

TELEPHONE

87. Do we understand how to use the telephone as a marketing tool?
88. Do we use it effectively?
89. Have we worked out telephone procedures?
90. Do we follow the procedures?
91. Has the telephone company assessed our traffic?
92. Are there sufficient telephone lines?
93. Is our telephone answered promptly? courteously?
94. Do we respond adequately to callers' problems?
95. Can each staff member give directions to the office by telephone?
96. Do we confirm appointments for those who need it?
97. Do we telephone patients about delinquent accounts?
98. Is the telephone answered around the clock?
99. Are patients provided a telephone in privacy for making calls?

CORRESPONDENCE

100. Do we market effectively through correspondence?
101. Is incoming correspondence efficiently processed?
102. Is correspondence promptly answered?
103. Is our correspondence neat?
104. Is outgoing correspondence efficiently generated?
105. Is equipment sufficient?
106. Does the stationery communicate the image I want?

107. Do we send personalized welcome letters to new patients, including children?
108. Do we send treatment confirmation letters?
109. Do we send letters upon completion of treatment?
110. Do we send checkup reminders?
111. Do we send letters to inactive patients?
112. Do we send referral letters?
113. Do we inform physicians about current developments in dentistry which are of interest to them?
114. Do we send letters to physicians about mutual patients?
115. Do we send newsletters?
116. Do we distribute brochures to patients?
117. Do we send collection letters?
118. Do I hand-write letters of appreciation to persons who refer patients?

THE HELPING PROCESS

119. Do we get to know our patients well?
120. Do we understand people's fears and anxieties about the dental office?
121. Do we help people deal with these fears and anxieties?
122. Do we give patients an opportunity to explain their problems to us?
123. Do we share information that enables them to understand their problems better?
124. Do we understand the helping process?
125. Do we try to help people?
126. Is the reception room pleasant and comfortable for our patients?
127. Are patients promptly and warmly welcomed when they enter the reception room?
128. Do we shake hands with patients?
129. Do we always introduce patients to each team member?
130. Do we use patient education pamphlets and other media *selectively*?
131. Does the interview room provide privacy and a non-threatening atmosphere?
132. In interviewing do we use open-ended questions designed to elicit information?
133. Do we follow up such questions with more specific questions?
134. During the examination do I ask the patient questions designed to heighten awareness?
135. Do we obtain a written health history *after* the interview?
136. Do we respond promptly to patients with dental emergencies?

137. Do we relate directly to small children as well as to parents?
138. Do I understand how learning occurs, as exemplified by the learning ladder?
139. Do I prepare adequately for treatment conferences?
140. Do I consider the patient's total situation as I prepare?
141. Do I conduct treatment conferences in a non-threatening, comfortable room?
142. Do I delay and modify treatment conferences according to the patient's readiness?
143. Are my patients aware of their choices and the likely consequences?
144. Is scheduling flexible according to individual patient situations?
145. Are financial arrangements flexible?
146. Do I ask questions during a treatment conference?
147. Do patients talk freely during the conference?
148. Do we come to an agreement during conference?
149. Are patients seated promptly at the appointed time?
150. Do I (and my staff) take a minute or two at each visit to get reacquainted with the patient?
151. Do I plan treatment visits with consideration for patients' total needs?
152. Am I honest with patients, and do I pay attention to their fears and anxieties?
153. Do we inform patients of what to expect at each visit?
154. Do I always obtain a patient's permission to proceed if there will be pain?
155. Do I show concern for patients' comfort by lubricating lips, providing disposable sunglasses to reduce glare, providing short rest periods, and so on?
156. Do I relate well to children in the chair?
157. Do we explain to patients what we are doing, what we have done, and what they should expect?
158. Do we give printed information sheets following surgery or major restorative procedures?
159. Do I give patients my residence telephone number after major procedures?
160. Do I call patients after major procedures?

RETAINING PATIENTS

161. Do we attempt to retain patients?
162. Do I have post-treatment conferences?

163. Do I always ascertain that patients are satisfied after treatment?
164. Do I solicit referrals from patients?
165. Are patients provided a post-treatment questionnaire?
166. Are patients aware of their untreated problems?
167. Are patients given choices about recall visits?
168. Is the recall system flexible enough to accommodate patient choices?
169. Do we audit our patient records and attempt to re-establish contact with drop-out patients?

REWARDS

170. Do I monitor my referral sources?
171. Do I reward patients and staff for referring patients?
172. Am I aware of what kinds of rewards are most appreciated?
173. Do I send flowers to ill patients?
174. Do I give special rewards to persons who refer many patients?
175. Do I give gifts for graduations and weddings?
176. Do I give a free first examination to young children?
177. Do I give rewards to staff?
178. Are the rewards based on performance?
179. Do we have occasional staff parties?

DENTAL PREPAYMENT

180. Do we market effectively through dental insurance?
181. Am I aware of the problems with dental insurance?
182. Do we help our patients to understand their insurance benefits and their financial responsibility?
183. Do we make financial arrangements with patients for their portion of the fee?
184. Do we keep a file of information on plans in effect in the community?
185. Do we process insurance paperwork within two working days?
186. Do we obtain preauthorization for all treatment plans totaling more than the maximum amount not requiring predetermination?
187. Do we have a system for keeping track of insurance authorizations and payments?
188. Do we accept assignment of benefits?
189. Do we use the superbill receipt with our pegboard bookkeeping system?
190. Do we use toll-free numbers for insurance companies?

191. Is one staff member assigned responsibility for dental insurance?
192. Do we have the name of the contact person at each insurance company?
193. Do we follow up when insurance payments and paperwork are not returned in a reasonable time?
194. Do we use the standard insurance form?
195. Do we use ADA code numbers for treatment procedures?
196. Does my insurance clerk complete paperwork ready for signature?
197. Do I justify unusual treatment in the estimate?
198. Do we know the insurance clerks (or benefits persons) in local industries with dental plans?
199. Are my insurance clerk and I familiar with the method for computing benefits of the various plans in effect in the community?
200. Doe we assist patients in obtaining maximum benefits from their dental insurance?
201. Do I actively promote new dental insurance plans and the improvement of current ones?
202. Do I participate in other third-party programs?

STAFF

203. Do I select staff members systematically?
204. Do I market through applicants not hired?
205. Do all staff members know their responsibilities?
206. Do all staff members participate in the marketing program?
207. Do all staff members treat patients with warmth and consideration?
208. Are staff members adequately trained?
209. Do I conduct periodic performance reviews?
210. Do performance reviews include marketing?
211. Do I have exit interviews with staff members who are leaving?
212. Do former staff members continue to refer patients?
213. Do I reward them for such referrals?

EVALUATION

214. Do I evaluate the effectiveness of my marketing program?
215. Do I compare productivity with that for the previous year?
216. Do we record numbers of new patients?
217. Do I compare these numbers with the previous period?
218. Do we compute the proportion of new patients who accept treatment?

219. Do I compare this with the previous period?
220. Do we survey patients about their satisfaction?
221. Are they satisfied?
222. Do I know the geographic distribution of my patients?
223. Am I achieving satisfactory penetration in various neighborhoods?
224. Do I know the number of patients referred by various referrers?
225. Have I surveyed the community regarding patient needs?
226. Does my marketing mix satisfy those needs?
227. Do we have a staff or office manual?

228. Is it complete or in the process of being completed?
229. Is the scheduling system effective?
230. Is the billing system working well?
231. Have I considered using a computer?
232. Have I determined what information I need about computers?
223. Have we analyzed our work for the purpose of simplification?
234. Do my auxiliaries know what tasks should be completed when I'm out of the office?
235. Does my office receive an annual checkup?

Index